The Digital Echo ATLAS

A Multimedia Reference

The Digital Echo ATLAS

A Multimedia Reference

Stephen David Clements Jr, MD

Emory University School of Medicine
Atlanta, Georgia

Wolters Kluwer

Philadelphia • Baltimore • New York • London
Buenos Aires • Hong Kong • Sydney • Tokyo

Senior Acquisitions Editor: Sharon Zinner
Development Editor: Ashley Fischer
Editorial Coordinator: John Larkin
Marketing Manager: Rachel Mante Leung
Production Project Manager: Bridgett Dougherty
Design Coordinator: Stephen Druding
Manufacturing Coordinator: Beth Welsh
Prepress Vendor: SPi Global

First edition

9 8 7 6 5 4 3 2 1

Printed in China

Library of Congress Cataloging-in-Publication Data
Names: Clements, Stephen David, Jr., 1940- author.
Title: The Digital Echo Atlas: A Multimedia Reference / Stephen David Clements, Jr..
Description: First edition. | Philadelphia : Wolters Kluwer, [2019] | Includes bibliographical references and index.
Identifiers: LCCN 2018015042 | ISBN 9781496356307 (hardback)
Subjects: | MESH: Echocardiography | Atlases
Classification: LCC RC683.5.U5 | NLM WG 17 | DDC 616.1/207543—dc23 LC record available at https://lccn.loc.gov/2018015042

LWW.com

To our sonographers who without their efforts we would not be able to create this work and to our cardiology fellows who put their faith in us to train them well in the specialty of cardiology.

Stephen David Clements Jr, MD
Emory University School of Medicine
Atlanta, Georgia

PREFACE

The concept of this work came from the desire to share the images that we have encountered over the years at a large university hospital system (Emory Healthcare). We felt that from viewing these images much can be learned. They illustrate the physiology and pathophysiology of underlying processes that we encounter. We discussed this idea with Dr. Itzhak Kronzon a few years back, and he suggested that we go forward with this project and that Wolters Kluwer might be interested. They were and thus work began.

One of our cardiology fellows, Dr. Jonathan Patton, initially helped extract from our logs the most important images. He selected images and converted them to appropriate formats. They were further organized and displayed. The need for legends, introductory information, normals, and guidelines became obvious, and they were incorporated into the work.

The publisher suggested a "hard copy" or printed book that would introduce a more extensive video atlas or e-book. We always worked on the principle that a "picture is worth a 1000 words" and extended that to "a video is worth a 1000 pictures." As such, you will see an throughout the print chapters to remind you that additional, expanded content (including text, figures, and video clips) is available via access to the e-book. Instructions for accessing the e-book can be found on the inside front cover of this text.

Each step of the way new ideas surfaced and the need to add more here and there arose. However, it had to stop somewhere so we could move forward. Finally, after much back and forth regarding adding additional content, the product (both print and digital) reached its goal of covering various target areas in each chapter, and it went to press and the build for the e-book.

We hope that this work is useful and adds to the basic fund of knowledge of those who read and view these images.

Stephen David Clements Jr, MD

Emory University School of Medicine
Atlanta, Georgia

ACKNOWLEDGMENTS

It took the help of many for completion of this work. Our talented sonographers at Emory University Hospital provided the wonderful images from which this work originated. They do a great job in obtaining the best images possible to answer the question at hand. They teach us and we teach them on a daily basis. The entire staff of the echo lab at Emory University Hospital offered encouragement for this project. Our fellows contributed when possible sometimes bringing images from other hospitals. Our colleagues helped when special areas of expertise was available—Dr. B. Robinson Williams III helped with the chapter on Hypertrophic Cardiomyopathy and Dr. Stamatios Lerakis and Sharon Howell with the chapter on Structural Heart imaging. Sandra Pernetz and Dr. Wendy Book helped in the production and review of the chapter on Adult Congenital Heart Disease. Other sonographers who obtained the great images in this book include Trang Truong, Tara Edwards, Randy Oum, Funmi Sanusi, Chandy Thou-Voeun, Brian Gowens, and Lamar Brown. Special thanks to them.

Special thanks to those around us who helped with the daily work. Rebekah Hills used her technical skills to move this project forward. Chris Comeou helped process the images. Patrick Strickland and Erica Okene worked on the project. Ashley Fischer was the leader from Wolters Kluwer that led us through the project.

Finally, a special thanks to my wife, Helen, who put up with my before daybreak activities on this project and tolerated my periods of silence during long drives.

Stephen David Clements Jr, MD

Emory University School of Medicine
Atlanta, Georgia

CONTENTS

For expanded versions of these chapters including additional text, figures, and video clips, please access the e-Book bundled with this text

1

The Left Atrium and the Left Atrial Appendage

SECTION 1

THE LEFT ATRIAL APPENDAGE

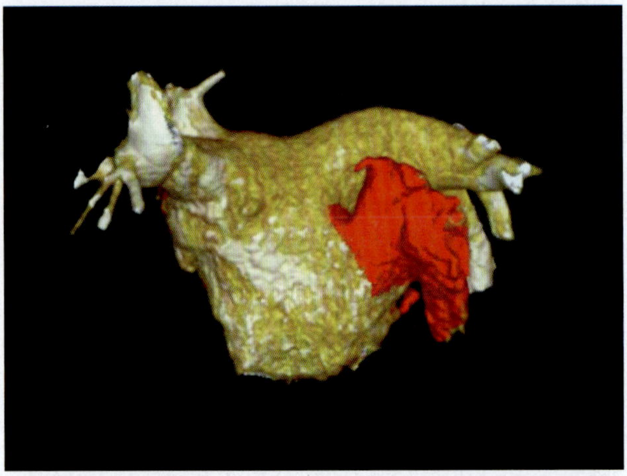

FIGURE 1.1 Three-dimensional computerized tomographic arteriogram demonstrated above. Volume rendering has been done, and the mitral annular region has been removed by cropping. The left atrial appendage is in red. The pulmonary veins and their branches appear like "horns" on the left atrium.

ANATOMY OF THE LEFT ATRIAL APPENDAGE

Interest in the left atrial appendage (LAA) has risen during recent years because of its role in thrombus formation in relationship to stroke. When thrombi are present in hearts not affected by the rheumatic process, ~90% have their origin in the LAA.[1]

The LAA is a slender fingerlike projection from the atrial body that has various shapes and sizes. The os of the LAA is narrow compared to that of the right atrial appendage and lies just above the atrioventricular groove. The atrioventricular groove itself at this point contains the circumflex coronary artery and the great cardiac vein and is also related to the left phrenic nerve in the overlying fibrous pericardium.

The LAA has a smooth lining in the area of the os and then extends to a variable cavity that contains muscle bands and pectinate muscles, which have a whorl-like configuration.

From the exterior of the heart, the LAA lies in between the pulmonary artery and the left ventricle filling in the gap between these structures. From superior to inferior in an anterior view, it is the third of the four "bumps" on the cardiac silhouette. First is the aorta, then the pulmonary artery followed by the LAA, and finally the left ventricle, all components of the left border of the heart from the anterior perspective. The fibrous pericardium over the LAA contains the phrenic nerve.

From the inside of the left atrium, the LAA is separated from the pulmonary veins by a prominent ridge termed the "Coumadin ridge" or the broad left lateral ridge.

Imaging of this structure gave rise to the descriptive sign named the "Q-tip sign."

From the exterior of the heart, the LAA usually wraps around the pulmonary artery but can have a tip that is even turned posterior. It has epicardial fat and multiple crenellations on the exterior that are associated with one or more lobes.[2-4]

Wang et al. have studied the shape of the LAA with multidetector computerized tomography (MDCT) to aid in preoperative planning for implantation of a closure device. In this group of patients, four different morphologies were defined. "Windsock," "cauliflower," "chicken wing," and "cactus" types were identified (Fig. 1.2).[5] In another study of patients with drug refractory atrial fibrillation who were about to have ablation, the "chicken wing" configuration was the most common, and in those who had a history of transient ischemic attack (TIA), the "cactus" configuration was the most common and the "chicken wing" was the least common.[5-7]

The Shape of the Left Atrial Appendage

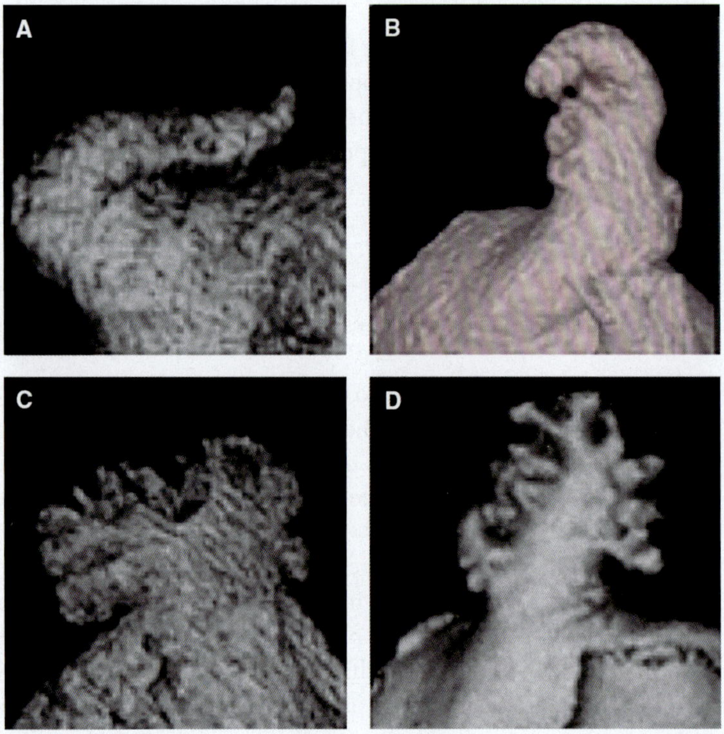

FIGURE 1.2 The left atrial appendage comes in a variety of shapes. It has been described by Wang as part of preoperative planning before device implantation to have four general shapes as viewed on computerized tomography. It is important to know the shape of the left atrial appendage, the diameter of the ostium, the orientation of the major axis of the appendage, and the depth of the appendage before a closure is performed with any device or procedure. The frequency of the anatomic types found in the individuals studied by Wang is listed below.[5] **A:** The "chicken wing" type with a short neck and a bent toward the tip (18.3%). **B:** The "windsock" type, which has a short neck (46.7%). **C:** The "cauliflower" type (29.1%). **D:** The "cactus" type (5.9%). (Source: DiBiase L, Santangeli P, Anselmino M, et al. Does the left atrial appendage morphology correlate with the risk of stroke in patients with atrial fibrillation? Results from a multicenter study. *J Am Coll Cardiol.* 2013;60:531-538.)

FUNCTION OF THE LEFT ATRIAL APPENDAGE

The LAA has similar functions to the LA. It acts as a reservoir, a conduit, an active contractile chamber, and a suction source. Experimentally, occlusion leads to increased left atrial pressure. The mechanical function of the LAA can lead to augmentation of stroke volume. Since the LAA is more distensible that the remainder of LA in can also act as a reservoir.

At a glance, the size of the LAA suggests that the left atrium may be dilated. Also, occurrences within the left atrium influence the function of the LAA. The presence of atrial fibrillation (AF) is associated with larger volumes and orifice sizes of the LAA sometimes being up to 3 times the size in those who have normal sinus rhythm. Furthermore, in individuals with AF, the endocardial surface of the dilated LAA is smoother and has more endocardial fibroelastosis than in the normal appendage.[2,4,8-10]

In addition, the LAA has endocrine function in that it contains stretch receptors that can influence heart rate and natriuretic peptides (ANP) that may account for ~30% of all ANP that in turn can influence diuresis, natriuresis, and heart rate.[8]

Analysis of the mechanical function of the LAA using echocardiography centers around the measurement of pulsed-wave Doppler flow signals into and out of the appendage using TEE. Once adequate images are obtained, the pulsed-wave Doppler sample is placed within the first one-third of the LAA with flow as parallel as possible to the cursor. A good color Doppler signal from this site has a characteristic pattern. Four distinct flow waves are usually identifiable in the presence of normal rhythm and flow. First, there is a positive wave produced by flow out of the appendage toward the transducer in atrial systole (red on color Doppler) with a velocity usually in the 60 cm/s range. This positive wave is followed by a negative or filling wave of the LAA and is of similar velocity although in the opposite direction (blue on color Doppler). In individuals with normal or high velocities of filling and emptying, a variable number of reflection waves follow before the end of systole. Early ventricular diastole is associated with a smaller positive wave and then a negative wave that follows mitral valve opening (see Fig. 1.3). Normally, the most prominent wave is the emptying wave, which is positive and ranges from 50 to 80 cm/s; the corresponding filling wave is in the 45-60 cm/s range.[4] Emptying velocities of <40 cm/s in individuals with nonvalvular atrial fibrillation have a limited chance of maintaining normal rhythm at 1 year.[11]

Spontaneous echo contrast (SEC) is associated with low flow velocities and increasing risk of thrombus formation. Sometimes, the SEC is so dense that it is difficult to discern from the jellylike thrombi that occur in the apex of the LAA. Echo contrast agents can sometimes be used to separate SEC from jellylike thrombus. In addition, when the SEC is very dense and the flow velocities are very low or absent, it sometimes assumes a tornadiclike appearance. All of these visual findings are associated with very low velocities in the LAA.

One can imagine the effects of various arrhythmias on the velocity profiles of flow into and out of the LAA. Extremely low–velocity flow leads to the formation of SEC, a precursor of thrombus. Atrial fibrillation, atrial flutter, and AV dissociation alter the velocity profile in a diagnostic manner. Other abnormalities such as diastolic dysfunction, mitral stenosis, and mitral regurgitation have significant effects on the anatomy and function of the LAA.

Normal Pulsed-Wave Doppler Velocities in the Left Atrial Appendage

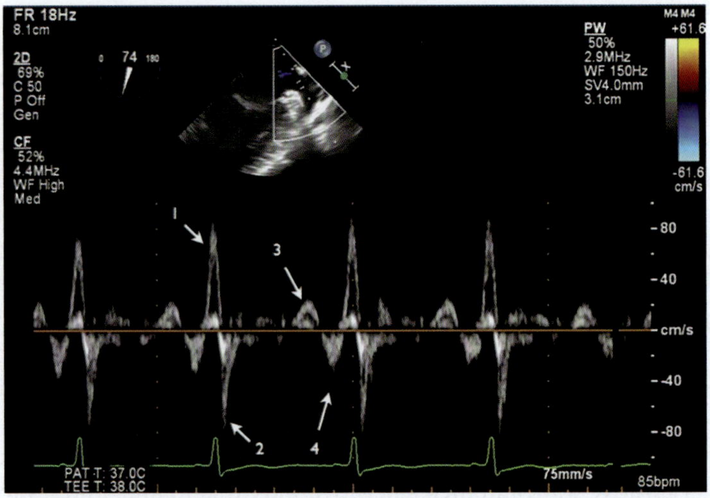

FIGURE 1.3 Pulsed-wave Doppler flow pattern in a normal individual with vigorous LAA contraction and normal relaxation. The first wave (*1*) is very prominent with a velocity of about 90 cm/s with a negative filling wave that follows of similar velocity (*2*). In diastole, there are two waves with the first being in early diastole (*3*) and second that reflects from the early diastolic filling wave (*4*). The normal emptying velocity for the appendage is >50 cm/s. In the presence of atrial fibrillation, very low velocities <20 cm/s often indicate potential for thrombus formation and decreased chances of success with cardioversion. Very low velocities also are often associated with smoke within the LAA. Good velocities suggest that the mechanical integrity of the LAA is still intact and that the duration of the rhythm may not have been so long. Additionally, the potential for thrombus formation is lessened and the chances of successful cardioversion are enhanced.[4,24]

IMAGING OF THE LEFT ATRIAL APPENDAGE

The Left Atrial Appendage on Transthoracic Echo

The LAA can be visualized from several views including the A2C view, the high cross-sectional short axis view, and less commonly the subcostal views (Fig. 1.4A and B). It is there to be visualized but often is overlooked. Although the appendage can be visualized from TTE, the views are incomplete, and the thorough investigation that is needed to exclude thrombus can only be done with TEE. When a small pericardial effusion is present, the outer borders of the LAA are often outlined. This pericardial fluid can extend around posterior to the pulmonary artery and the aorta in the space that is called the transverse sinus. Sometimes, just the tip of the appendage is visualized in this small fluid-filled space and can give the appearance of a mobile mass. The right atrial appendage also is better outlined in the setting of a small pericardial effusion.

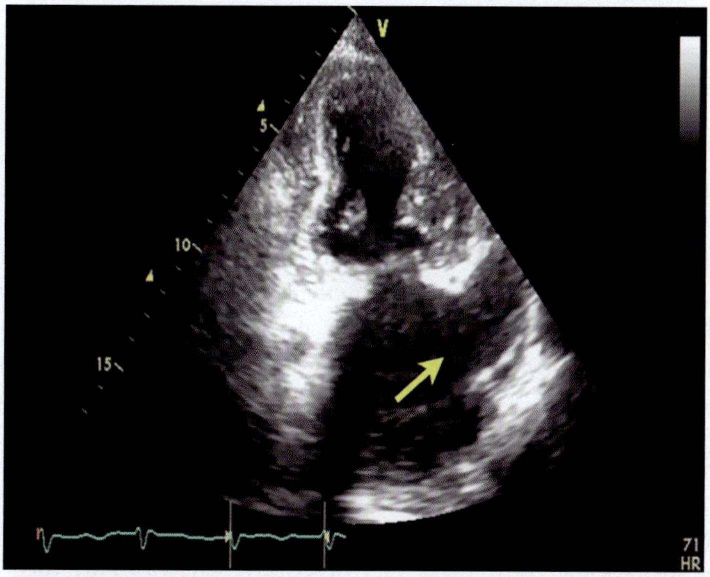

FIGURE 1.4 A very large left atrium in addition to a very large left atrial appendage shown on transthoracic echo (*yellow arrow*). The size of the left atrial appendage is related to the duration of atrial fibrillation and the left atrial pressure. TTE, A2C view.

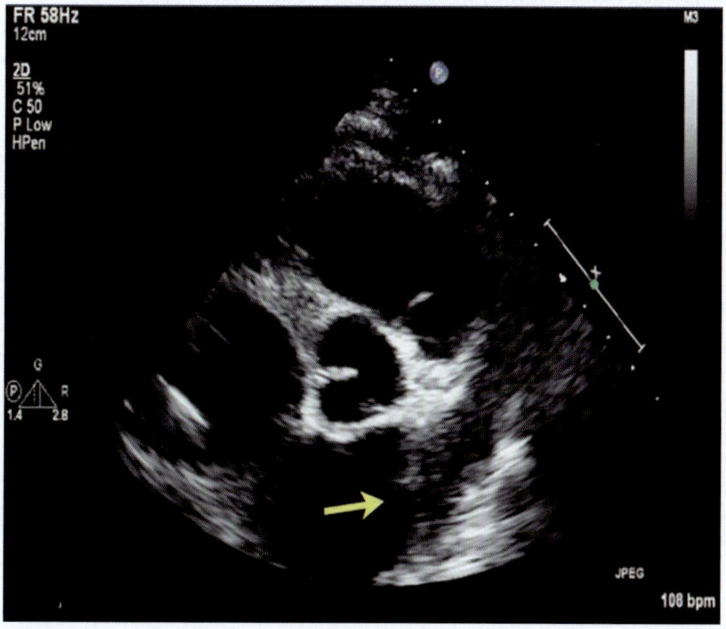

FIGURE 1.5 On the high cross-sectional views, the appendage can also be visualized; however, artifact is often prominent in this view preventing accurate determinations about the presence or absence of thrombus (*yellow arrow*). TTE, high cross-sectional view.

The Left Atrial Appendage on Transesophageal Echo

Transesophageal echo (TEE) is the primary method for analysis of the LAA. Multiplane imaging makes it possible to visualize all segments of the LAA. Three-dimensional echocardiography can also be utilized. This type of investigation is needed to evaluate for the presence of thrombus in the setting of atrial fibrillation, precardioversion, stroke, peripheral embolization, and others.[3,4]

The etiology of embolic stroke in the setting of atrial fibrillation focuses on the presence or absence of thrombus in the LAA. In individuals with nonvalvular atrial fibrillation if thrombus is present, it will be in the LAA 90% of the time and not in the body of the LA.[1] The cul-de-sac configuration of the LAA and the alterations of flow in the LAA that occur in atrial fibrillation combine to make thrombus formation more likely. Atrial fibrillation alters the normal contractility of the LAA and leads to stagnation of flow.

The anatomy of the LAA varies from one individual to another. Wang et al. using CT angiography have imaged and described the shape of the LAA in four categories (see Fig. 1.2). These very descriptive categories are the "windsock," "cauliflower," "chicken wing," and the "cactus" types in the order of their frequency. Evaluating the shape of the LAA and the size of the ostium is important as one plans for application of a LAA closure device.[5] Some of these configurations are more common in those with TIA (the cactus type).[6]

Imaging of the LAA using the multiplane TEE requires using the entire spectrum of angles. As one approaches the appendage from the midesophageal region, it is easily identified from the 60°-70° view (see Figs. 1.6 and 1.7). This is always a good starting point. It is worth noting also that the general sequence of performing TEE should be the same each time. There may be variations from operator to operator, but a repeatable sequence is important from the standpoint of not missing a view or an area of the LAA or the heart for that matter. During the procedure, when adjacent abnormalities are identified, it is tempting to move to that area, but this risks changing the sequence and leaving out something. On the other hand, when time is constrained, one has at times to go for the "money shots" first.

A thorough investigation of the lobes of the LAA is always indicated. Thrombi can be tucked away in small areas and require a search to identify. Once the "comma-shaped" LAA is identified at 60°-70°, the angle can be advanced to interrogate the appendage to higher angles at about 15° intervals and then back from about 40°-0°. At higher angles, one notes the pectinate muscles assume linear; partitioning shapes and lobes are defined. These are easily mistaken for thrombi. Usually there are two lobes, but sometimes small side lobes are present and extend superior toward the transverse sinus.

At a glance, the size of the LAA tells a story. High left ventricular filling pressures, mitral regurgitation, and stenosis all often are associated with large appendages. Similar to the left atrium, the LAA also serves as a reservoir.

As mentioned earlier, the functional analysis of LAA centers around Doppler flow patterns into and out of the appendage. Once adequate images are obtained, the pulsed-wave Doppler sample volume is placed within the first one-third of the LAA or about 1 cm within the ostium of the LAA with flow as parallel as possible to the cursor (see Fig. 1.6). A good color Doppler signal from this site has a characteristic pattern. Analysis of flow patterns should be performed from a direction that is as parallel to flow as possible. Four distinct flow waves are usually identifiable in the presence of normal rhythm and flow. First, there is a positive wave that produced positive flow toward the transducer (red in color) usually in the 60 cm/s range. This positive wave is followed by a negative or filling wave of the LAA and is of a similar velocity although in the opposite direction (blue in color Fig. 1.7). In individuals with normal or high velocities of filling and emptying, a variable number of reflections waves follow before the end of systole. Early diastole is associated with a smaller positive wave that follows mitral valve opening (see Fig. 1.3).

One can imagine the effects of various arrhythmias on the imaging of the LAA and the velocity profiles. Atrial flutter and atrial fibrillation (see Fig. 1.10) leave their mark on the profile as does AV dissociation. These flow patterns are of physiologic significance but also can be of diagnostic value. In the setting of atrial fibrillation, low flow velocities predict a lower chance of long-term maintenance of normal rhythm.[11]

Low flow velocities are associated with SEC and increasing risk of thrombus formation. Sometimes the SEC is so dense that it is difficult to discern from the jellylike thrombi that occur in the apex of the LAA. Echo contrast agents can sometimes be used to separate SEC from jellylike thrombus. In addition, when the SEC is very dense and the flow velocities are very low or absent, it can assume a tornadic appearance. All of these visual findings are associated with very low velocities in the LAA. In the setting of nonvalvular atrial fibrillation (see Figs. 1.11 and 1.12) as mentioned, thrombi when they occur are found in the LAA in contrast to rheumatic valvular disease, and atrial fibrillation thrombi are found mural and in the LAA (see Fig. 1.13).

Cursor Location for Measurement of Velocities Into and out of the LAA

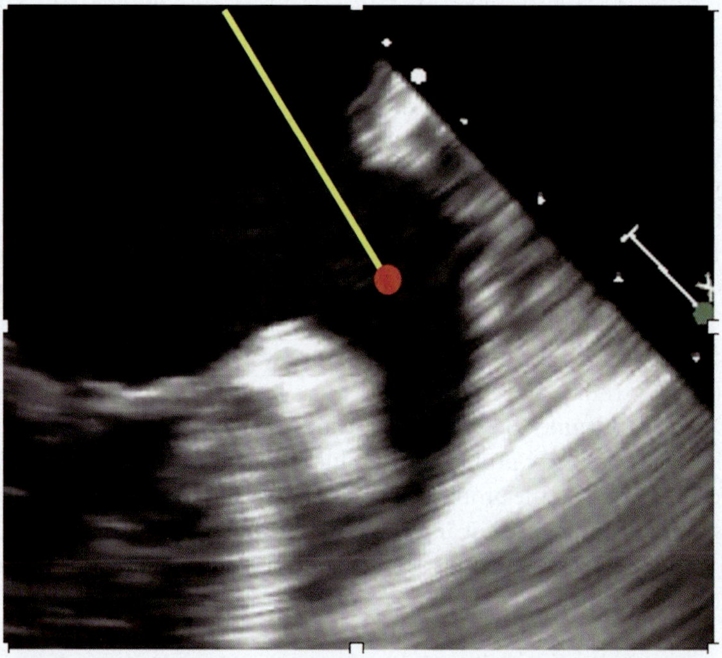

FIGURE 1.6 Measurement of the velocity of flow into and out of the left atrial appendage should be done about 1 cm from the ostium of the appendage and as parallel as possible to flow usually in the 70° view. *Yellow line* represents the pulsed-wave Doppler beam and the *red dot* the position of the sample volume.

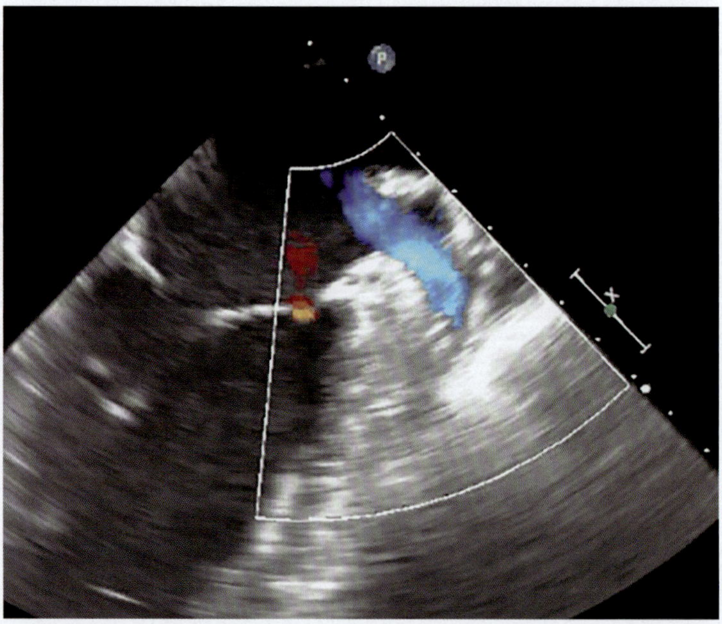

FIGURE 1.7 From the 70° view, the color Doppler image on stop frame shows a *blue color* or flow toward the transducer. This position is good for sampling of the pulsed-wave Doppler signal for analysis.

CASE PRESENTATION

The Left Arial Appendage in Arial Flutter

A 47-year-old gentleman presented to the emergency room with 5 days of palpitations and irregular heartbeat. In the ER, he was discovered to have atrial flutter with variable conduction. TEE was done, and he subsequently had ablation.

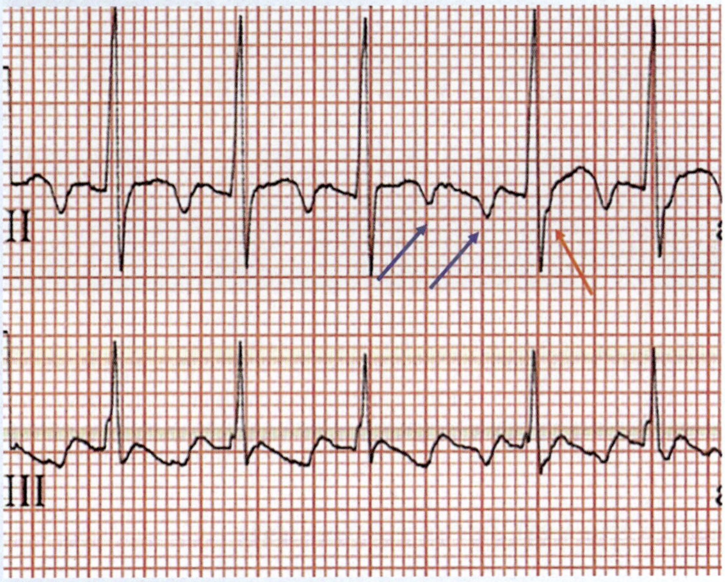

FIGURE 1.8 The EKG from the 47-year-old gentleman who presented with atrial flutter. The *blue arrows* point to flutter waves at a rate of slightly <300 BPM, and the *red arrow* points to a QRS complex that obscures the flutter wave.

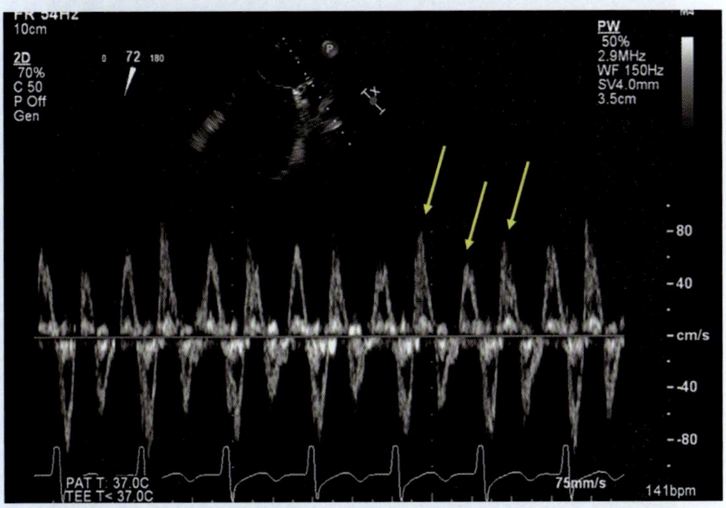

FIGURE 1.9 Pulsed-wave Doppler sampling in the first third of the atrial appendage shows rhythmic waves consistent with atrial flutter (*yellow arrows*). There is alternation of the velocities associated with the position of the mitral valve. TEE, 72° view.

The Left Atrial Appendage in Atrial Fibrillation

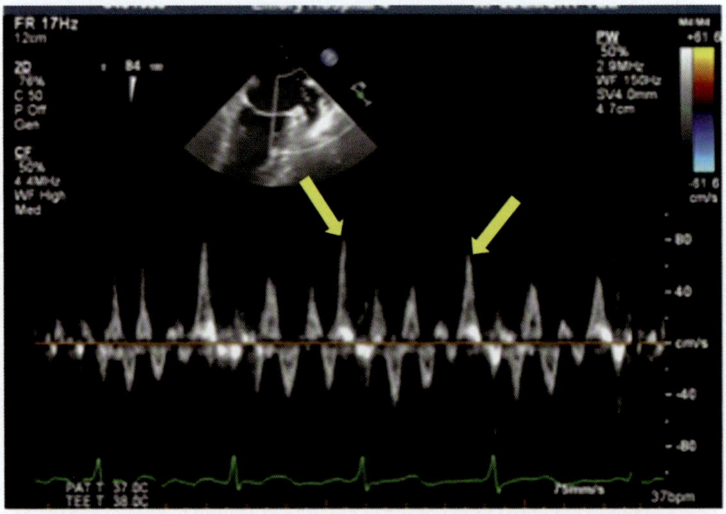

FIGURE 1.10 Sometimes the atrial rhythm is not obvious from the electrocardiogram. For example, in the setting of ventricular pacing, the atrial rhythm is often ignored. The loss of atrial kick can be a significant clinical problem. If an atrial lead is present, then interrogation of the device can make this determination; however, the TEE can make the diagnosis. In the above example, the typical atrial fibrillation Doppler velocity waves are present (*yellow arrows*) and demonstrate good velocities suggesting that the situation is favorable for long-term maintenance of sinus rhythm. The smaller velocities are related to mechanical activity, while the mitral valve is closed.

Thrombus in the Left Atrial Appendage

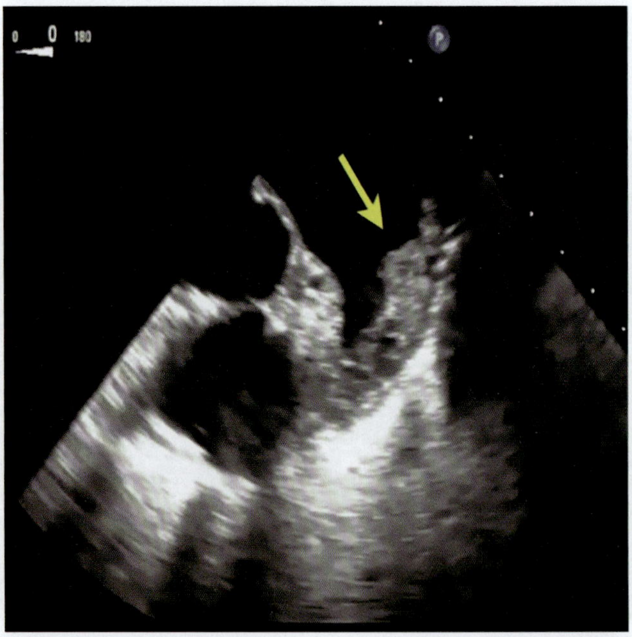

FIGURE 1.11 Transesophageal echo from 0° showing an even larger mural thrombus (*yellow arrow*) in the left atrial appendage appearing to be firmly attached to the wall. TEE, 32° view.

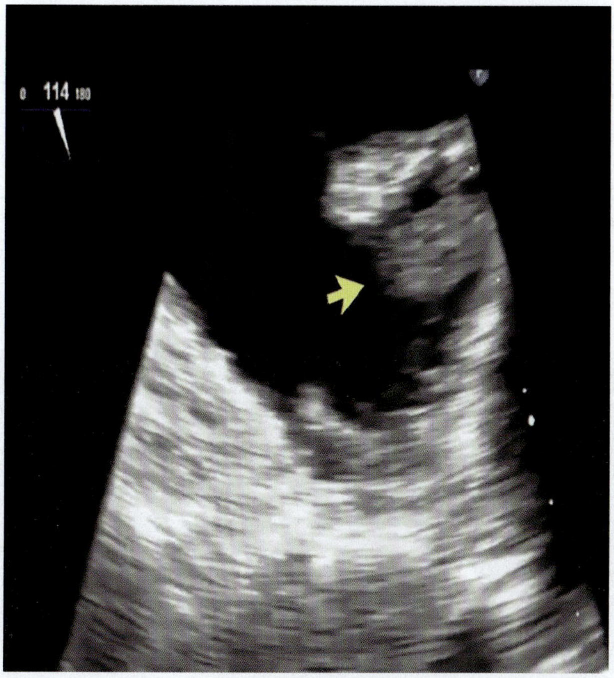

FIGURE 1.12 Small thrombus in a second lobe of the LAA (*yellow arrow*). TEE, 114° view.

Thrombus in the Left Atrial Appendage in the Presence of Mitral Stenosis

High left atrial pressures, sluggish flow, and SEC all predispose to thrombus formation in the LAA. Mitral stenosis is a setup for thrombus formation in the LAA and the body of the LA since flow is sluggish and pressures are high. SEC is often present, and atrial fibrillation and thrombus formation are common (see Fig. 1.13).

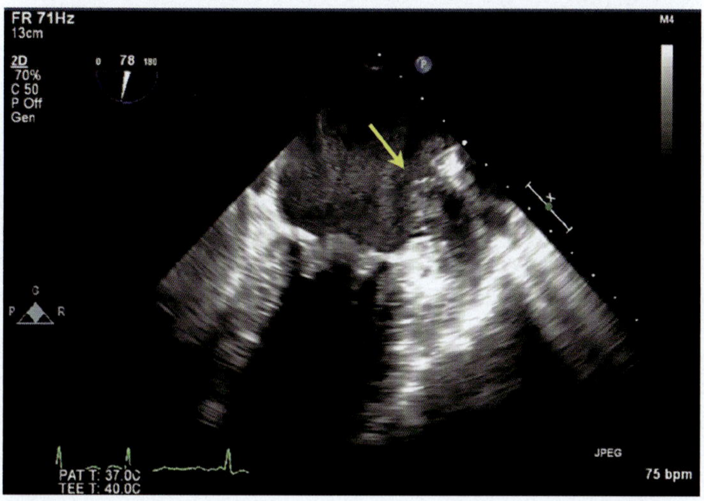

FIGURE 1.13 Individuals with mitral valve stenosis have high left atrial pressures, atrial fibrillation, and sluggish flow through the left atrium. Spontaneous echo contrast or "smoke" is common, and left atrial thrombus follows. In the example above, there is smoke within the left atrium, and the entire left atrial appendage is filled with thrombus (*yellow arrow*).

CLOSURE TECHNIQUES AND DEVICES

Closure of the LAA has been performed surgically for many years. At the time of mitral valve surgery, the ostium of the LAA is visible and can be sutured closed (see Fig. 1.10). This usually has a high rate of success; however, occasionally the appendage opens up. Other techniques have been used to include thoracoscopic ligation or clipping of the appendage. Recently, catheter-based techniques including the PLAATO device, the Watchman device, and the LARIAT device have been used.

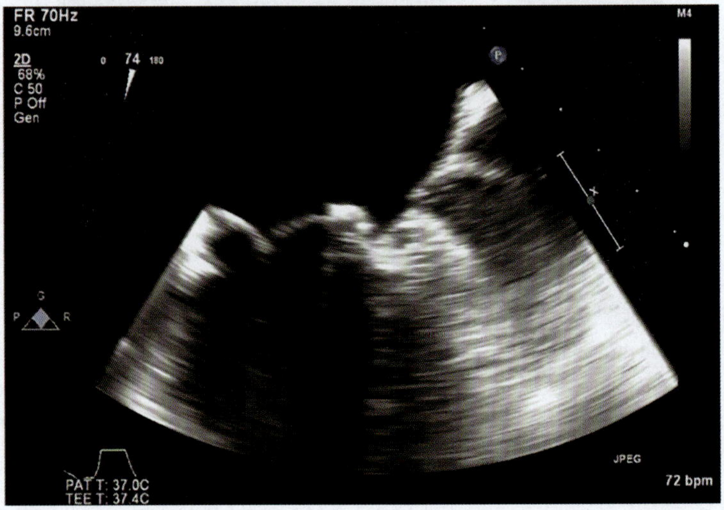

FIGURE 1.14 Surgically ligated left atrial appendage is demonstrated with thrombus within the appendage; the ostium is tightly closed and the adjacent tissue mitral prosthesis is visualized adjacent to the LAA. On color Doppler, there was no flow into or out of the LAA.

Left Atrial Appendage Occlusion Devices: The LARIAT Procedure

The LARIAT procedure uses a catheter-based delivery technique to deliver an extrudible closure device. The device is delivered by way of the transseptal approach. A second catheter system is placed in the pericardium from a percutaneous technique. The left atrial catheter and the pericardial catheter are connected by means of a magnet tip. Once appropriate positioning is obtained with fluoroscopic and transesophageal visualization, the "lasso" can be extruded from the pericardial delivery catheter and the LAA can be snared.[12]

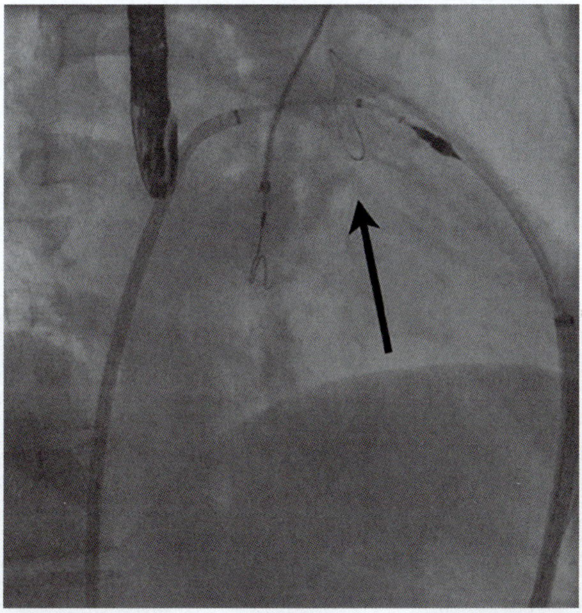

FIGURE 1.15 The LARIAT (*black arrow*) is being tightened up and monitored under fluoroscopy. The magnets have been connected, and the delivery catheter can be advanced and the device delivered.

The PLAATO Device

The PLAATO device (percutaneous left atrial transcatheter occlusion, Appriva Medical, Inc.) was a catheter-delivered expandable device that fits into and occludes the LAA. In contrast to the LARIAT, it did not use a pericardial component. The delivery catheter enters the left atrium by way of a transseptal puncture, positioned and deployed with fluoroscopic and echo guidance. This device did not get beyond clinical trials in the United States.[7]

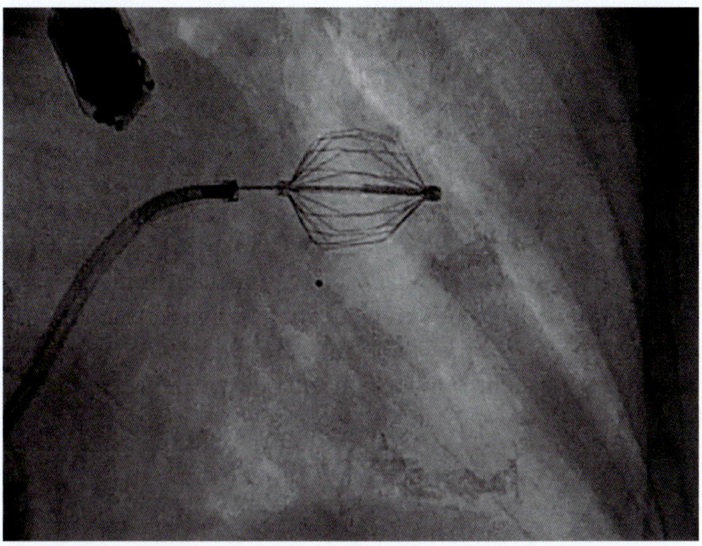

FIGURE 1.16 The PLAATO device being inserted in the cath lab under TEE and fluoro guidance. This device is no longer used; however, it did offer a flush occlusion of the left atrial appendage.

The Watchman Device

The Watchman device is currently being used in the United States and throughout the world for occlusion of the left atrium in individuals who cannot take anticoagulants for one reason or another. It is a percutaneous venous procedure using the transseptal approach to deliver an expandable parachutelike device into the ostium of the LAA. This device is inserted under fluoroscopic and TEE guidance.[13,14]

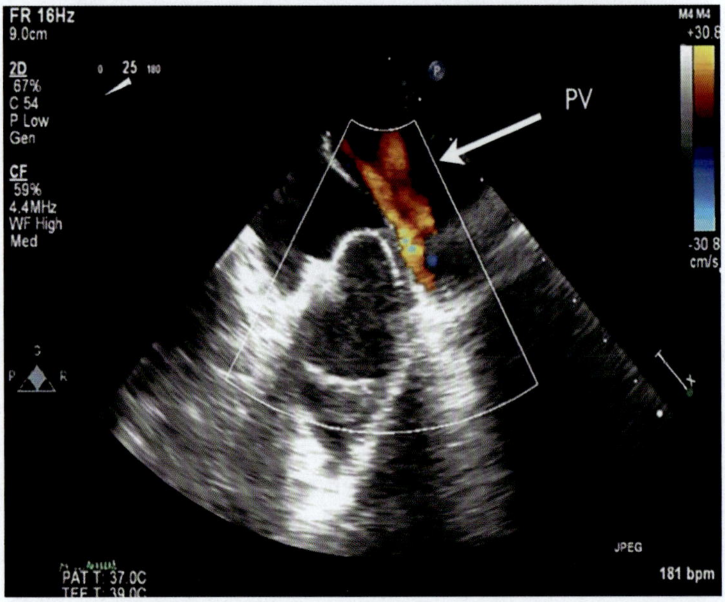

FIGURE 1.17 The device has been deployed into the left atrial appendage and color Doppler applied to check for leaks. Turning the Doppler gain down can be helpful. Flow in the adjacent pulmonary vein is noted above (PV). TEE, 25° view.

Left Atrial Appendage Thrombus Visualized on a Computerized Tomography (CT) and Cardiac Magnetic Resonance Imaging (CMRI)

Often, a thrombus within the LAA is an incidental finding during a computerized tomography (CT) scan. The scan might be ordered for pulmonary embolus, aortic aneurysm size, or left or right ventricular abnormalities. In general, iodinated contrast is needed to fully visualize the LAA unless a thrombus has been present so long that it has calcified. Filling defects of various sizes may be identified on these scans. Often, when they are being read, no knowledge has been put forth as to whether the patient is in atrial fibrillation or flutter, so these findings just appear.

Examples of CT scans that revealed LAA thrombi will be shown in the following panels. Computerized Tomography (CT) and Cardiac Magnetic Resonance Imaging (CMRI).

Both CT and MRI can very accurately define the LAA and the left atrium. Iodinated or gadolinium contrast is usually needed to define filling defects. Usually, these modalities are used for other purposes but in the presence of atrial fibrillation or low-flow states can demonstrate the presence or absence of a thrombus in the left atrium or the appendage. Thrombi are noted in the CT (see Fig. 1.18) and CMRI (see Fig. 1.19).

Thrombus as Visualized by Computerized Tomography

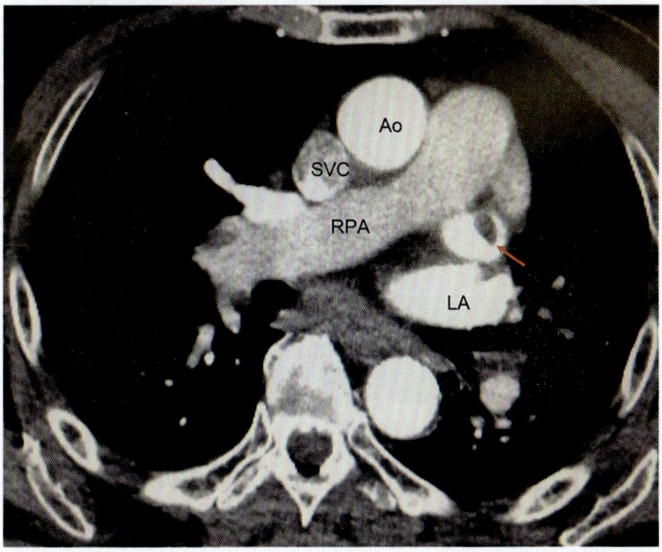

FIGURE 1.18 On occasion with the use of contrast, one can visualize a left atrial appendage thrombus (*red arrow* points to the thrombus within the left atrial appendage). Ao, aorta; LA, left atrium; RPA, right pulmonary artery; SVC, superior vena cava.

Thrombus as Visualized by Cardiac Magnetic Resonance Imaging

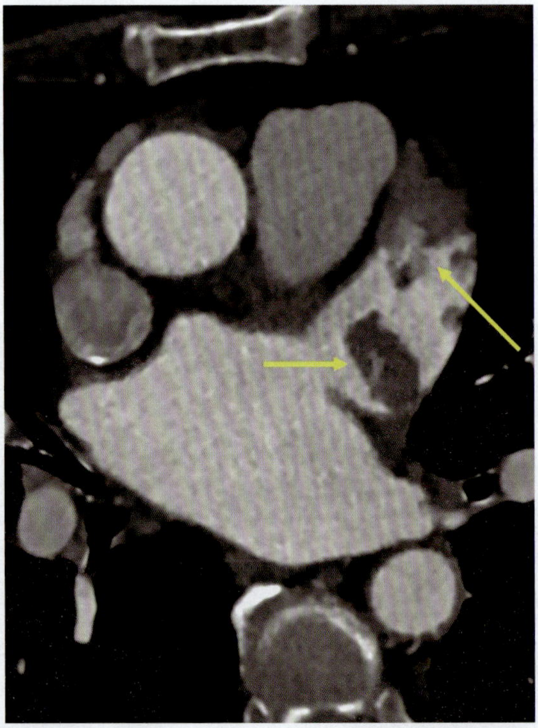

FIGURE 1.19 The MRI in an 87-year-old gentleman with chronic atrial fibrillation who was unable to take anticoagulants. The patient did not have a history of stroke and no history of stroke. *Yellow arrows* indicate multilobulated thrombus on CMRI within the left atrial appendage of such a duration that calcification has occurred.

UNUSUAL PROBLEMS WITH THE LEFT ATRIAL APPENDAGE

The LAA like other cardiac structures can be involved in unusual problems. The walls of the appendage especially between the pectinate muscles can be paper thin. This anatomical feature predisposes the appendage to being perforated by either wires or catheters or even at the time of surgery by a cannula. Figure 1.20 illustrates the consequences of perforation of the appendage and subsequent development of a large pseudoaneurysm extending into the pericardial space. Flow went in and out of this structure until the defect was closed with an Amplatzer device.

A second unusual occurrence is illustrated in Figure 1.21. A large mass was noted to have its origin in the LAA and extended out to the LA and even prolapsed into the orifice of the mitral valve. At the time of surgery, this was a sarcoma that had its origin in the floor of the LAA.

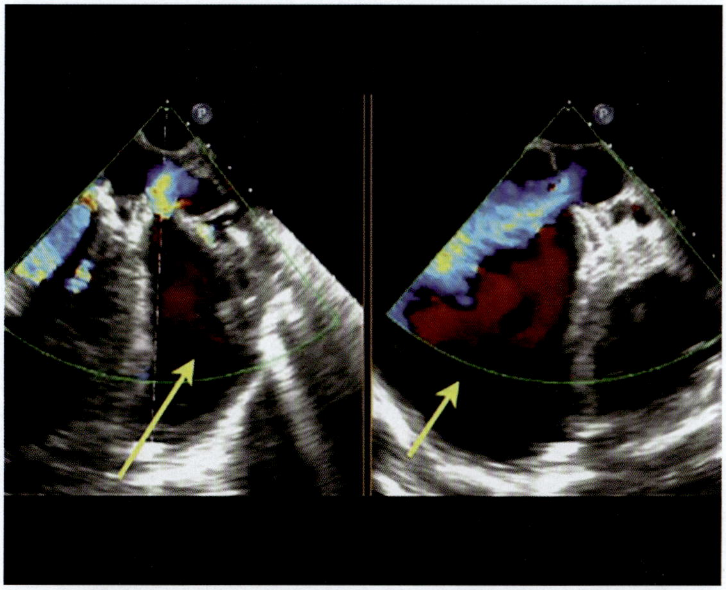

FIGURE 1.20 Color Doppler demonstrates flow into the pseudoaneurysm (*yellow arrows*). Once this was identified, plans were made to close the defect with an Amplatzer device. TEE with color Doppler.

Malignant Tumor Arising in the Left Atrial Appendage

One would not think of the LAA as a potential origin of a malignant tumor. However, it does have various types of tissue to include muscle and connective tissue with each of these have that potential. This LAA mass has a fixed component and a mobile component as demonstrated on CMRI (Fig. 1.17) and on TEE (Fig. 1.18).

The following example is that of a young woman who had a primary tumor of the LAA that was extremely malignant. The tumor fills the LAA and extends down upon the mitral leaflet. The LAA mass has a fixed component and a mobile component as demonstrated on CMRI (see Fig. 1.14) and on TEE (see Fig. 1.15). The primary tumor was removed surgically. The surgeon described having to "peel" the tumor from the floor of the LAA being careful not to disturb the coronary sinus or the circumflex coronary artery. At the time of surgery, it was known that areas of metastasis existed; however, impending obstruction of the mitral valve orifice was present. She was treated vigorously for 6 months with potent chemotherapy; however, the tumor continued to progress and she entered hospice care.

The pathological diagnosis of the atrial mass was a "myxoid sarcoma" and was further described as a "high-grade intimal sarcoma with rhabdomyoblastic differentiation." It was positive for MDM2 gene amplification.

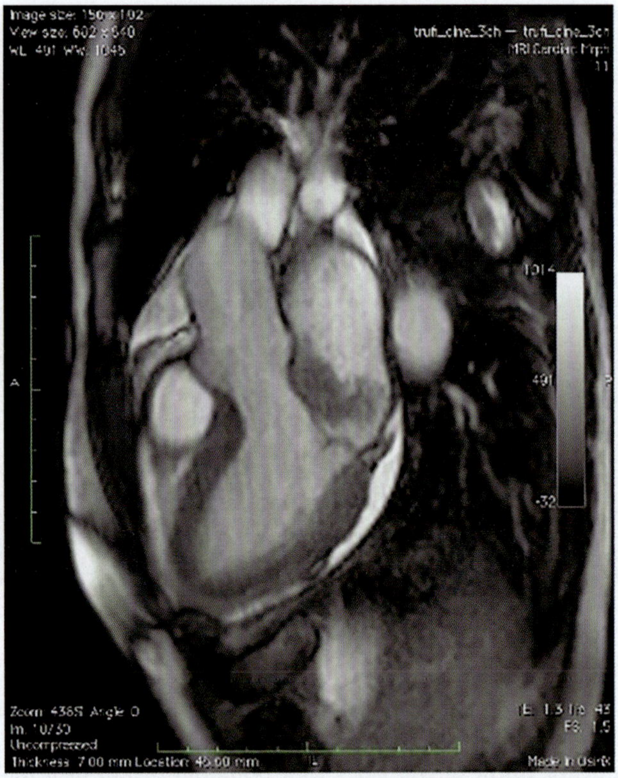

FIGURE 1.21 The CMRI demonstrates the tumor that arose in the floor of the LAA and extended down upon the AMVL. The mobile component prolapsed through the mitral orifice in diastole. From Raphael K, Martimez A, Clements S, Isiadinso I. A Rare Left Atrial Mass. "In press" likely to be published in the Journal of the Texas Heart Institute.

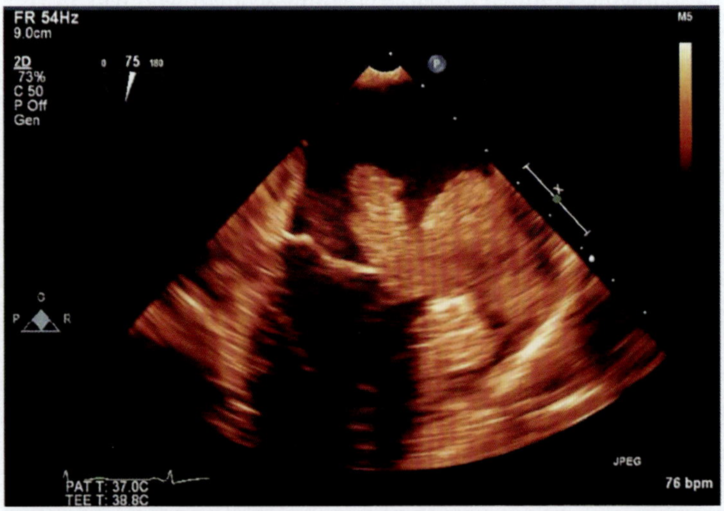

FIGURE 1.22 Visualization of the tumor with TEE demonstrating that it fills the LAA and extends down upon the mitral leaflet. This image shows the tumor being attached to the floor of the LAA near the coronary sinus and circumflex coronary suggesting that the origin was in this area. The surgeon described the tumor as having its origin in the floor of the left atrial appendage. TEE, 75°. From Raphael K, Martimez A, Clements S, Isiadinso I. A Rare Left Atrial Mass. "In press" likely to be published in the Journal of the Texas Heart Institute.

SUMMARY

The LAA probably is of more significance than was once thought. It has pump function that augments the normal pump function of the left atrium and when the heart has a normal rhythm adds to the function of the left atrium. It has in addition reservoir function, and in the presence of high pressures and volumes in the left atrium, it has been noticed to dilate. After all, it is the most compliant segment of the left atrium and in conditions such as mitral regurgitation, mitral stenosis, left ventricular diastolic dysfunction, and others, it is often very prominent in size. In the presence of atrial fibrillation, it becomes hazardous in that it acts like an isolated corner of the atrium, has very sluggish flow, and often demonstrates the most SEC, and therefore it is the most vulnerable location for thrombus formation. In the setting of embolic stroke, it is the first place in the heart to be investigated and often is the culprit if atrial fibrillation is present. Efforts to eliminate the LAA from the circulation are long-standing and are still in the development phase, and the effects of the LAA not being a participant in the circulation are still being investigated. In the cardiac catheterization laboratory, we are reminded that it has paper-thin walls that can be easily perforated resulting in various consequences. Our awareness of this structure is still gaining momentum.

SECTION 2

QUANTITATION OF THE LEFT ATRIUM

The left atrium is located more posterior than it is to the left making the name somewhat of a misnomer. It is posterior to the aorta and anterior to the esophagus. These relationships are important in that for the interventionalist, puncture of the aorta needs to be avoided, and to the electrophysiologist during ablation, disruption of the posterior wall of the left atrium can damage the esophagus. The relationship of the left atrium to the esophagus makes the heart easily visualized with TEE, offering opportunity to use higher ultrasound frequencies for better resolution and not compromising on penetration depth. From the inside of the left atrium, the impression of the adjacent aorta on the left atrium produces a "moundlike" area in the region of the mitral aortic intervalvular fibrosa. Posteriorly the left atrium is separated from the esophagus by only a few millimeters of left atrial wall and epicardial membrane.

When the heart is viewed from the anterior perspective, the only portion of the left atrium that is visible is the tip of the LAA. This structure usually wraps around the pulmonary artery and covers a portion of the atrioventricular groove and the origin of the left coronary artery.

From the inside of the left atrium, the boundaries include the superior wall, the posterior wall, the left lateral wall, the interatrial septum, and the anterior wall. The mitral valve annulus and the leaflets allow blood to exit the left atrium in an inferior and lateral direction.

The interatrial septum is a composite of septum primum (on the left) and septum secundum (on the right). These fuse, and on the right side of the septum, the incomplete septum secundum covers the defect in the septum primum. Most of the time, this is totally fused; however, when it is incomplete, a flaplike valve closes the defect from the higher-pressure left atrium. From the left side of the atrium, only a thin portion of the interatrial septum is present. On this side, the rims are indistinct. From the right side, the rims form the borders of the fossa ovalis.

The more posterior portion of the left atrium receives the pulmonary veins. The entrance point of these structures creates ridges of electrophysiologic importance. Often, each has a short main stem at the entrance into the left atrium, and within, there is a bifurcation into the main branches arising from the various pulmonary lobar segments. It is know well known that a sleeve of atrial tissue is present that extends 1-2 cm up into the veins. This anatomic finding is related to the discovery that the origin of abnormal electrical impulses that lead to atrial fibrillation is often located in this area. The only functional significance of these muscular extensions could be that they offer some resistance to reflux of the left atrial blood back into the vein during atrial contraction.

One major ridge that is present to a variable degree is that at the superior border of the entrance to the LAA. This ridge has been described as being shaped like a "Q tip" or "drumstick" and earlier was mistaken for a clot and thus has been termed the "Coumadin ridge." When viewed with the TEE, this ridge lies between the LAA and the left upper pulmonary vein. It has a variable length from a simple ridge to a membrane extending across the atrium. When very prominent, this ridge divides the atrium into two parts, the vestibule area and the posterior portion of the atrium. The posterior portion of the left atrium receives the pulmonary veins.

When the ridge extends across the atrium and assumes the shape of a membrane, a third atrium is created and thus the name "cor triatriatum sinister." Defects in this membrane create a pressure gradient within the left atrium as blood approaches the mitral valve.

The roof of the left atrium is not well visualized since it is parallel to most of our echo beams. It is important to surgeons since they sometimes identify and dissect the groove between the two atria called the "Waterston groove." The vein of Marshall or its residual extends down from the posterior roof of the left atrium and joins the coronary sinus. Bachmann bundle is located in the anterior portion of the roof and electrically connects the right and left atria. Remembering the influence and relationship of the left atrium to the left mainstem bronchus, one can see that with enlargement of the left atrium as seen in mitral stenosis that the main stem is shifted in a superior direction on the plain chest x-ray.

The size of the left atrium has become recognized as a prime index of left ventricular systolic and diastolic function. Enlargement of the left atrium is probably more related to pressure than volume. It has become one of the important factors in the diagnosis of diastolic dysfunction. Simple measurement of the diameter of the left atrium is no longer adequate. Methods of measurement have varied as technology has advanced. Recent ASE guidelines have endorsed left atrial volume index to be superior to simple diameter measurements. Methods of measurement include the ellipsoid method and the Simpson method of disks (see Fig. 1.23). 3D echo also offers a measurement of left atrial volume. Each of these has its geometric challenges but still offers more than simple diameter dimensions.[2]

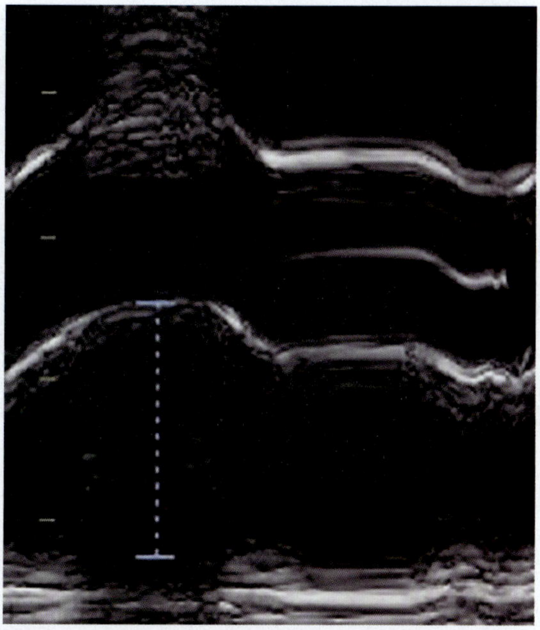

FIGURE 1.23 The standard and often used and standardized dimension of the left atrium is from the M-mode tracing measured at end systole and using the leading edge-to-leading edge convention.

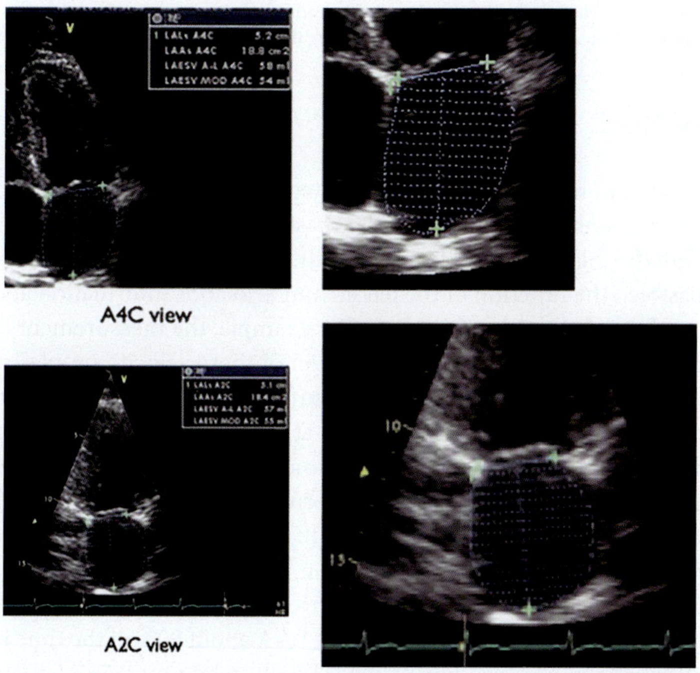

FIGURE 1.24 Measurements of the left atrial volume offer the more accurate representation of left atrial size. This can be done using the A4C view and the A2C view and the Simpson method of disks. The atrium in its largest dimension can be traced at end systole with care to excluding the pulmonary veins and the left atrial appendage. The inferior border is the plane of the mitral annulus. These two tracings are then placed into the software computer algorithm, and a left atrial area is produced. This value can be indexed and compared to current guidelines suggesting that the upper limit of normal for both genders is 34 mL/m^2. The ellipsoid model can also be used to calculate the left atrial volume, but more recently, the Simpson method of disks is recommended.[15,25,26]

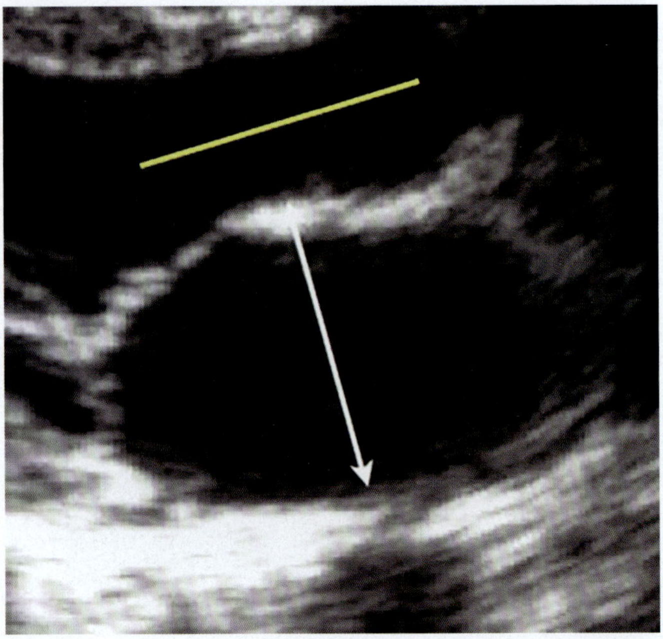

FIGURE 1.25 Measurement of the LA dimension. *Yellow line* is the center line of the LVOT and the *double-headed white arrow* is perpendicular to that line. On two-dimensional echo, the left atrial dimension is measured at end systole and at the level of the tips of the aortic valve leaflets and along a line that is perpendicular to the left ventricular outflow tract (*white double headed arrow*). The leading edge-to-leading edge method is used with the posterior dimension starting at the center of the line denoting the posterior left atrial wall.

LEFT ATRIAL FUNCTION

The left atrium has functions in three categories. The reservoir function acts as a collection chamber during ventricular diastole. Secondly, the left atrium serves as a conduit during early diastole, and thirdly, it performs as a booster pump during late diastole. The function of the left atrium also adds information about various abnormalities that might be present. For example, the measurement of velocities entering the left ventricle and the duration of these velocity profiles relate to left atrial function in addition to providing information about the left ventricle. The velocity profile of blood entering the left atrium from the pulmonary veins offers information about left ventricular systolic and diastolic function. Reversal of flow during atrial contraction also offers information about mitral regurgitation and left ventricular diastolic function. More recently, tissue Doppler techniques have allowed quantitation of left atrial function using strain parameters.

An enlarged left atrium can harbor thrombus. However, it is well known that left atrial thrombi have their origin in the LAA about 90% of the time in individuals with nonvalvular atrial fibrillation. Usually, when there is a left atrial thrombus, there is also one in the LAA. The isolated anatomy of the LAA especially in the presence of atrial fibrillation sets the stage for stasis, endothelial dysfunction, and thrombus formation. Layers of thrombus involving the left atrial wall can organize and even calcify giving rise to a hardened thick walled chamber that has been termed a "coconut left atrium."

Tumors can involve the left atrium either by direct extension from the pulmonary veins and from contiguous regions or even by primarily arising within the left atrium. The most famous of these is the left atrial myxoma that almost always arises from the region of the fossa ovalis. Lung cancers extend into the pulmonary veins and sarcomas can arise from atrial tissue.[15]

Normal Left Atrial Strain

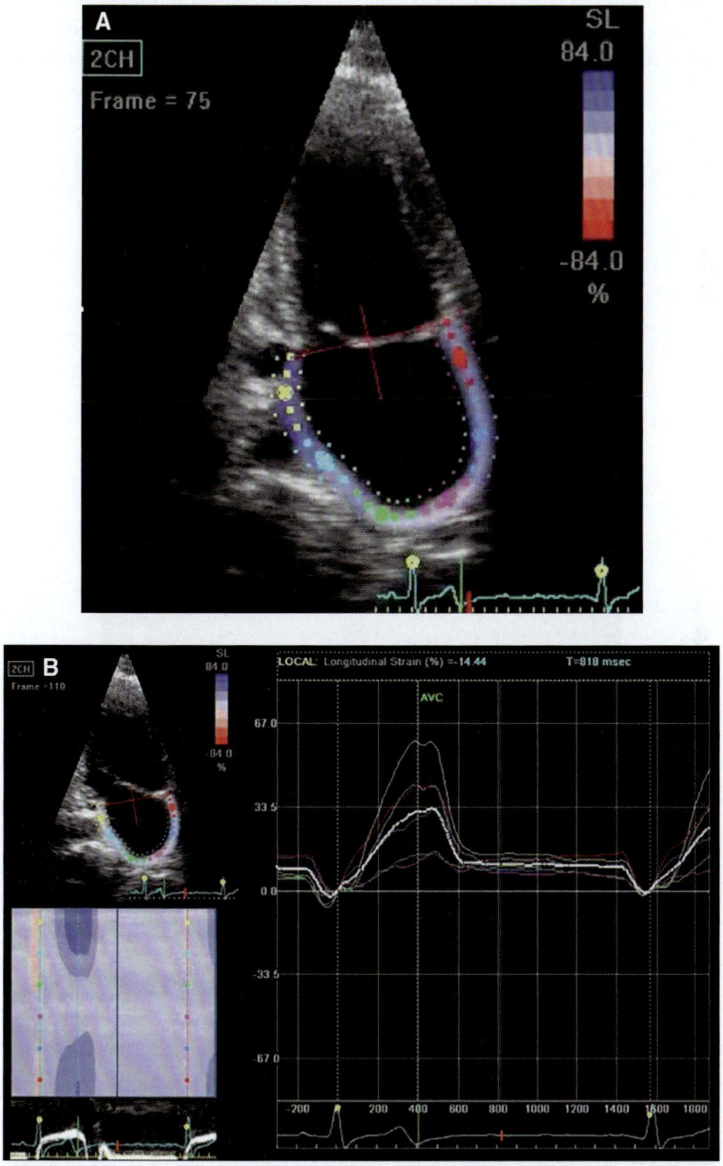

FIGURE 1.26 **A:** 2D speckle tracking or tissue Doppler echocardiography can be used for measurement of atrial strain. In the speckle tracking method, one has to choose a starting point relative to the P wave or that of the QRS complex since different displays will be obtained with each method. In this example the QRS was chosen (*yellow dots* on the QRS complexes) as a reference and the atrial borders were defined as was the mitral annulus. The machine then displayed the segments of the left atrium. **B:** The graphic display of strain in the color coded segments is displayed in a linear color display and an instantaneous display with the QRS as a reference. The *dotted white line* represents the mean peaking at +33.5% which is a normal value.

CASE PRESENTATION

Left Atrial Strain in Amyloidosis

A 54-year-old gentleman who has been treated for systemic amyloidosis. Multiple systems were involved including renal, peripheral nerves, and the heart. Atrial flutter has been present and deep vein thrombosis had also occurred.

In this individual with cardiac amyloid, the left atrial strain numbers are very low peaking out at +16 in contrast to the individual on the previous panel whose strain numbers peaked out at +33.5. Note that these numbers come out in a positive direction on the display.

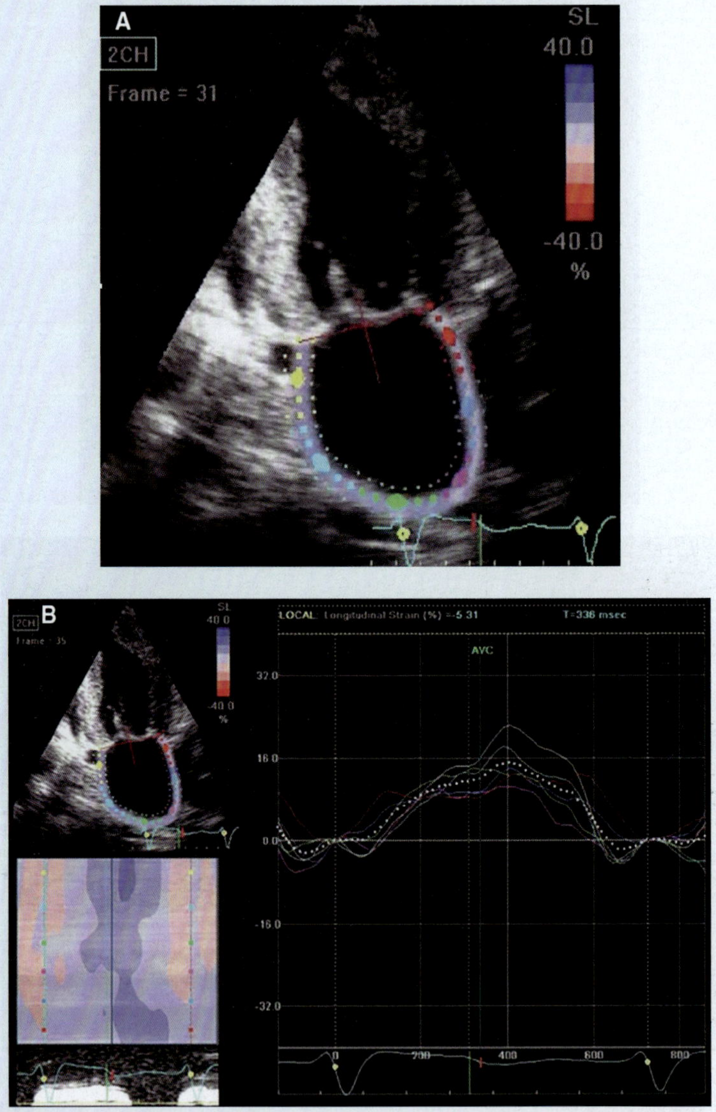

FIGURE 1.27 **A:** In this example of amyloid involving the heart the apical two chamber view has been chosen, the atrium outlined and the mitral annulus has been defined. The machine displayed the segments for analysis. **B:** The graphic display of the left atrial strain with color display and linear instantaneous display. The numbers are very abnormal with the mean peaking at only +16%. Note that these are only half of those displayed in the normal example which was +33.5%.

ABNORMALITIES OF THE LEFT ATRIUM

The left atrium is a vulnerable structure from the standpoint of becoming dilated, having electrical instability, developing thrombi, being invaded by malignancy, or having a congenital abnormality. Most commonly, the pressures and volumes within the LA cavity become high, and it becomes dilated. Happenings within the left ventricle very much influence the size of the left atrium, especially high filling pressures of the left ventricle associated with diastolic dysfunction. Problems with the mitral valve to include mitral stenosis and regurgitation result in a dilated LA. Once flow is slowed through the left atrium as a part of its reservoir function, thrombi form the appendage and sometimes on the walls of the left atrium. Mural thrombi are especially prominent when mitral stenosis is present. In the case of mitral regurgitation, the incidence of LAA thrombi and LA thrombi is not as common perhaps because of the washing effects of the regurgitant jet. The left atrium can be congenitally septated resulting in the clinical entity of cor triatriatum, and benign and malignant tumors can occur in this structure. Some illustrations will follow.

INTERATRIAL SEPTAL ANEURYSM

CASE PRESENTATION

Left Atrial Appendage Aneurysm and LVAD

A gentleman in his 20s who is waiting on heart transplant had these images made during a left ventricular assist device interrogation.

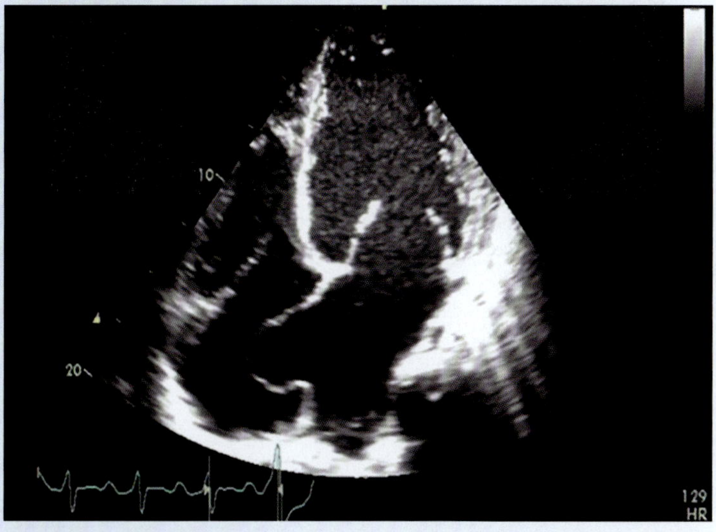

FIGURE 1.28 The very thin interatrial septum bulging toward the right. This qualifies as an interatrial septal aneurysm, and the septum is so thin that it is easily influenced by changes in relative pressures between the two atria. TTE, A4C view.

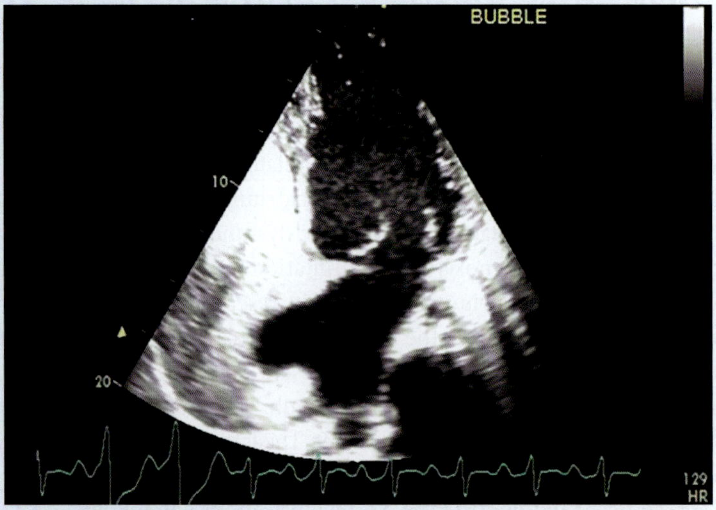

FIGURE 1.29 Bubble study outlining the shape of the bulging IAS, which at this time is under the influence of a higher left atrial pressure. TTE, A4C view.

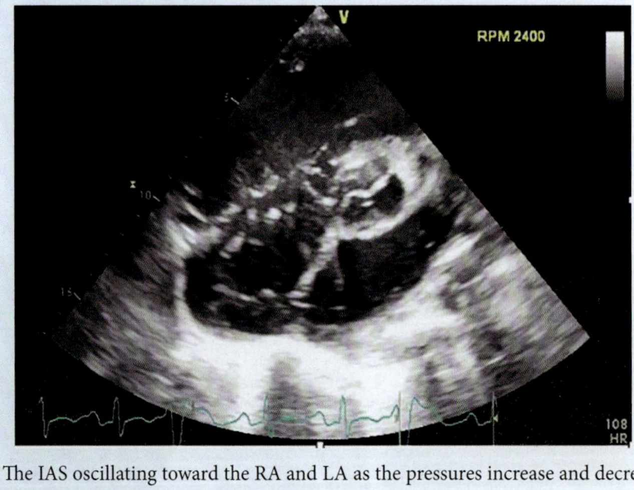

FIGURE 1.30 The IAS oscillating toward the RA and LA as the pressures increase and decrease in each chamber. At this point, the patient has received a left ventricular assist device and left atrial pressures have been lowered. TTE, RV inflow view.

CASE PRESENTATION

Interatrial Septum Aneurysm, Smoke, and History of Embolization

A 70-year-old gentleman who has chronic atrial fibrillation and a recent embolus to his left arm.

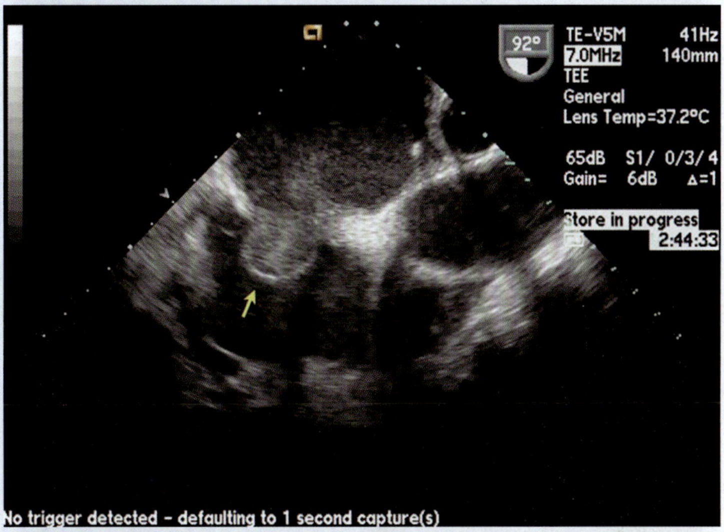

FIGURE 1.31 In this image, both atria are dilated and there is a bulging interatrial septum toward the right forming an aneurysm (*yellow arrow*). Within the aneurysm, there is dense smoke that is swirling around. Changes in right atrial pressure might evert this structure and empty the contents, or they might spontaneously empty resulting in a systemic embolus if thrombus is present. This aneurysm can even become larger and almost fill the right atrium. If a patent foramen is present, it can be stretched open resulting in a communication between the two circulations. TEE, 92° view.

COR TRIATRIATUM SINISTER

Cor triatriatum sinister is an interesting and rare condition. The left atrium can be divided into two components. One is slightly more tabulated and contains the LAAs and the more anterior portions of the left atrial chamber including the orifice of the mitral valve. The more posterior portion of the atrium has a smooth endocardium and harbors the confluence of the pulmonary veins from each side. The prominent ridge that separates the LAA from the left pulmonary veins or the "Coumadin ridge" represents the involution of the area that earlier in the evolution process separated these two sections of the left atrium. Failure of this area to fully involute results in a membrane either partial or nearly complete that offers resistance to flow in the direction of the mitral valve orifice. This results in a two-chambered atrium on the left and one on the right. In the case of the left side, "cor triatriatum sinister" results. An example of this is shown in the text and figures that follow.[16,17]

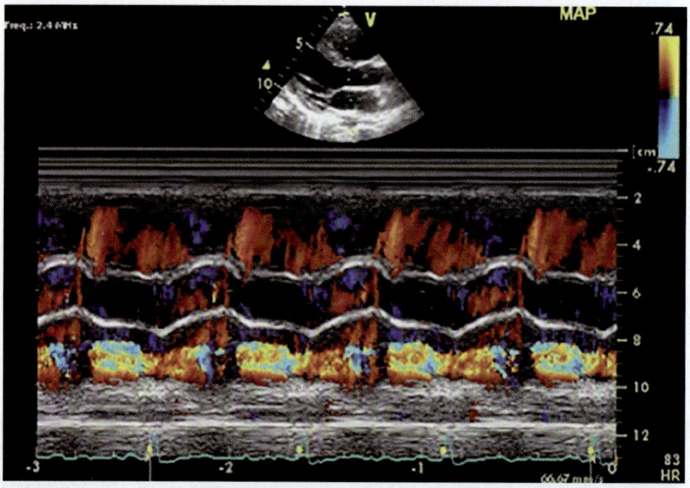

FIGURE 1.32 Color mode shows a near continuous area of turbulence in the mid left atrium. (Adapted from Strickland PT, Peretz MA, Jokhadar M, Hartlage G, Clements S. Cor triatriatum sinister: a patient, a review, and some unique findings. *Echocardiography.* 2014;31(6):792, Fig 4.)

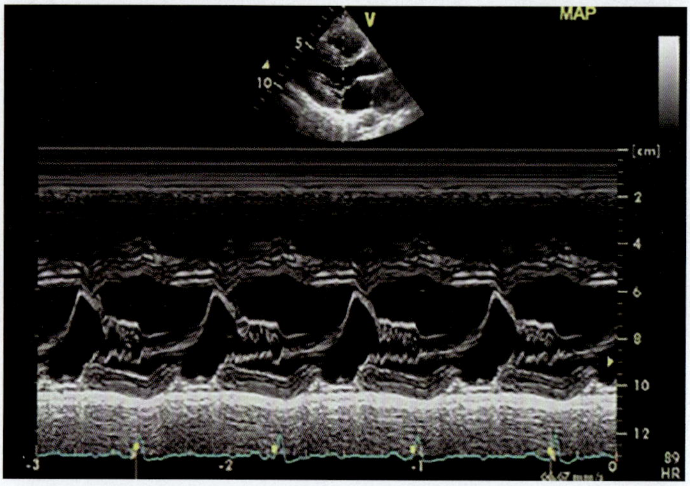

FIGURE 1.33 M-mode tracing through the mitral valve showing flutter of not only the anterior mitral leaflet but flutter on the posterior mitral leaflet. This is consistent with a jet coursing through the central portion of the mitral orifice. (Adapted from Strickland PT, Peretz MA, Jokhadar M, Hartlage G, Clements S. Cor triatriatum sinister: a patient, a review, and some unique findings. *Echocardiography.* 2014;31(6):792, Fig 4.)

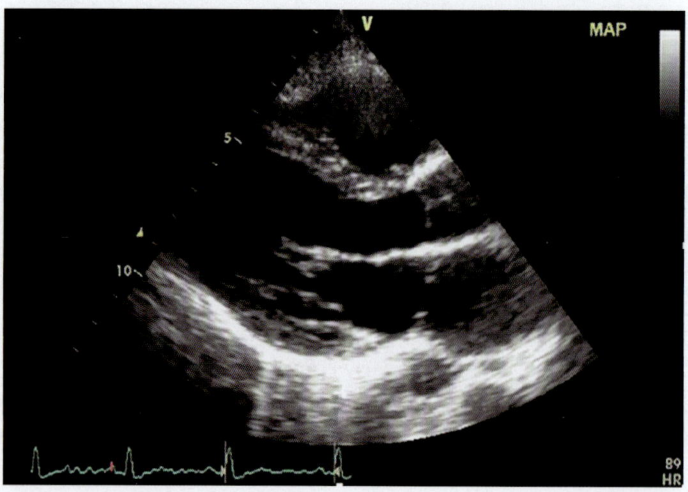

FIGURE 1.34 Two-dimensional echo showing a membrane in the midportion of the LA that gives rise to the turbulent flow illustrated to the right.

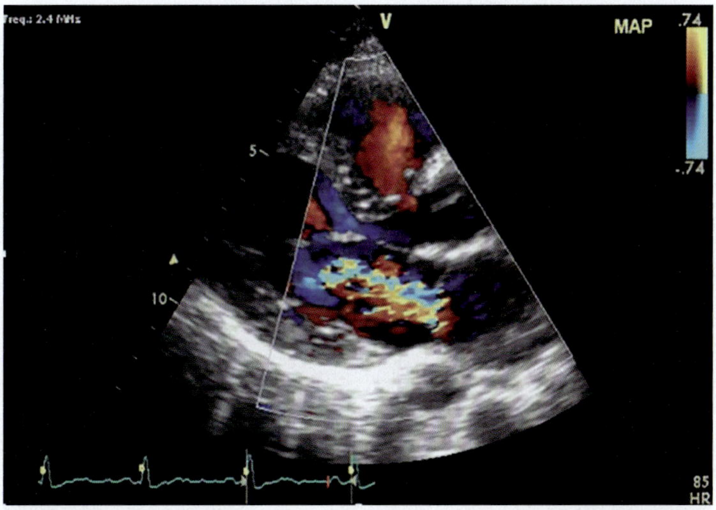

FIGURE 1.35 Turbulence coming through the hole in the cor triatriatum membrane indicating significant obstruction at that level. (Adapted from Strickland PT, Peretz MA, Jokhadar M, Hartlage G, Clements S. Cor triatriatum sinister: a patient, a review, and some unique findings. *Echocardiography.* 2014;31(6):793, Fig 5.)

Cor Triatriatum and the Associated Gradient on Continuous Wave Doppler

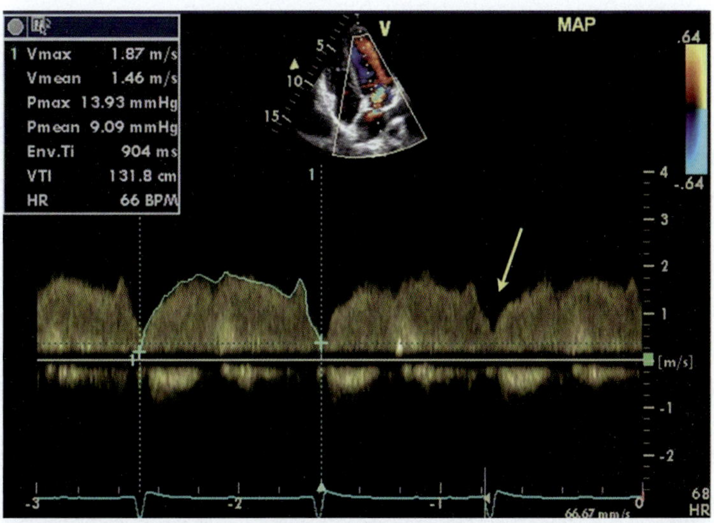

FIGURE 1.36 The gradient across the membrane in the left atrium on CW Doppler demonstrates the turbulence seen in the color Doppler displays in addition to the near constant gradient except for the phase of isovolumetric contraction, which creates a competing pressure associated with the mitral leaflets closing and shifting blood in the direction of the membrane, thus transiently decreasing velocity (*yellow arrow*). The mean gradient was 9 mm Hg. TTE, CW tracing through the turbulent jet of the cor triatriatum membrane defect.

Cor Triatriatum From Transesophageal Echo and the Associated Gradient

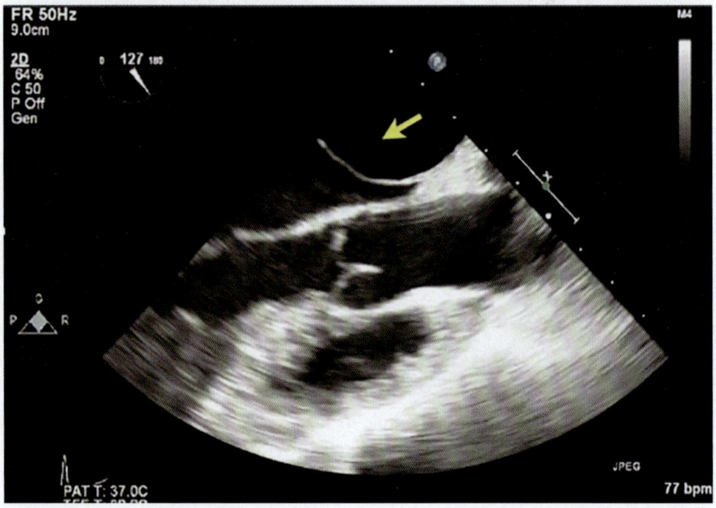

FIGURE 1.37 Long-axis view demonstrating the aortic valve and sinuses of Valsalva and an abnormal thin membrane (*yellow arrow*). This is the part of the attachment of the cor triatriatum membrane to the left atrial wall. TEE, 127° view.

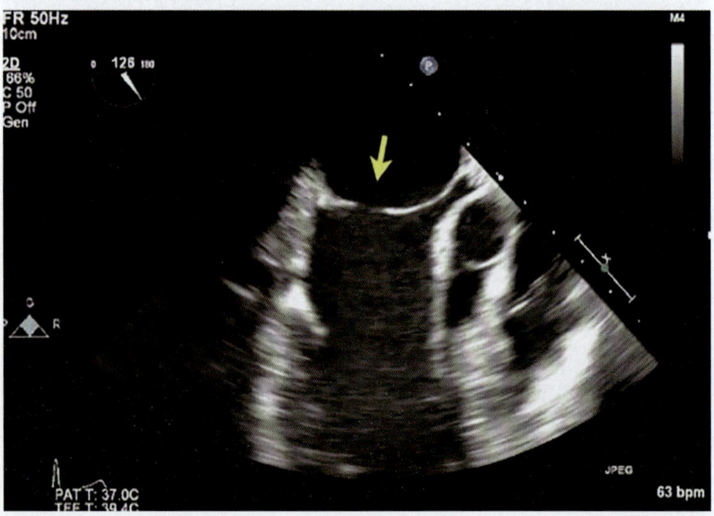

FIGURE 1.38 The long-axis view shows more of the left atrium and demonstrates the membrane and the defect (*yellow arrow*). TEE, 126° view.

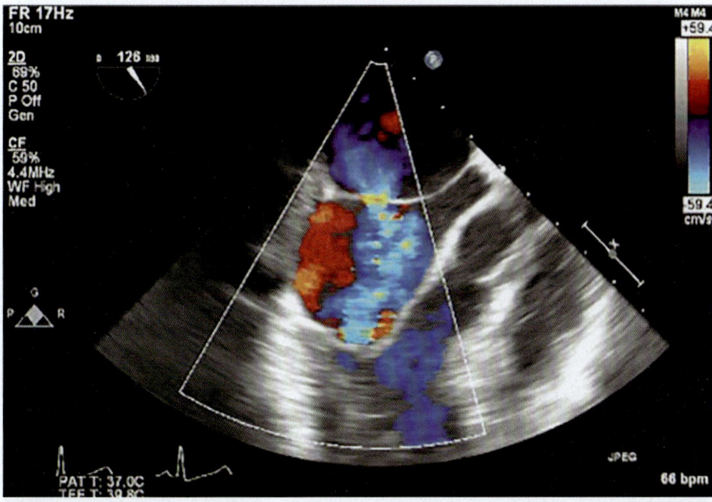

FIGURE 1.39 Color Doppler applied and the PISA of the membrane noted with the turbulence that follows. TEE, 126° view.

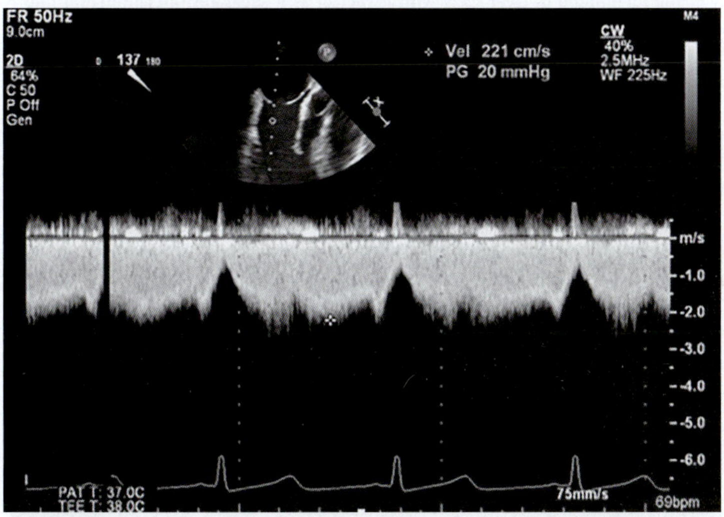

FIGURE 1.40 CW applied across the membrane and the mitral valve showing almost continuous flow. The gradient is transiently affected by early systole as the mitral valve closes. TEE, 137° view.

Cor Triatriatum on Transesophageal Echo—The Defect and the Jet

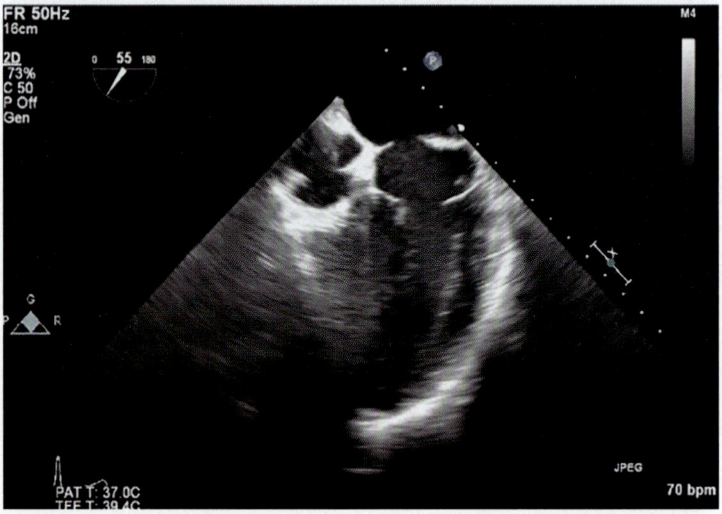

FIGURE 1.41 The membrane in clear view with its defect as it separates the left atrium into two chambers. These two chambers in addition to the right atrium result in three chambered atria—thus the name "cor triatriatum." TEE, 55° view.

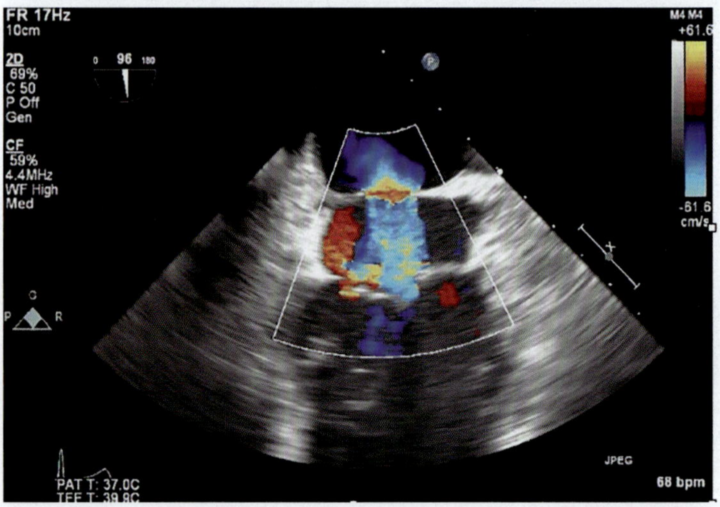

FIGURE 1.42 The color jet of turbulent flow from the upper chamber to the low chamber as it courses toward the mitral leaflets resulting in them shuttering in diastole as demonstrated in an earlier display. TEE, 96° view.

Cor Triatriatum, the Surgical Specimen, and the Postoperative Echo

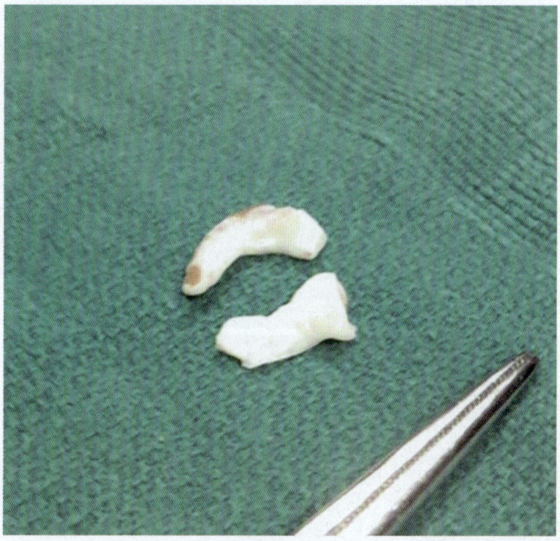

FIGURE 1.43 The surgical specimen from the patient in the previous display showing that a relatively small membrane can be associated with a higher than expected gradient.

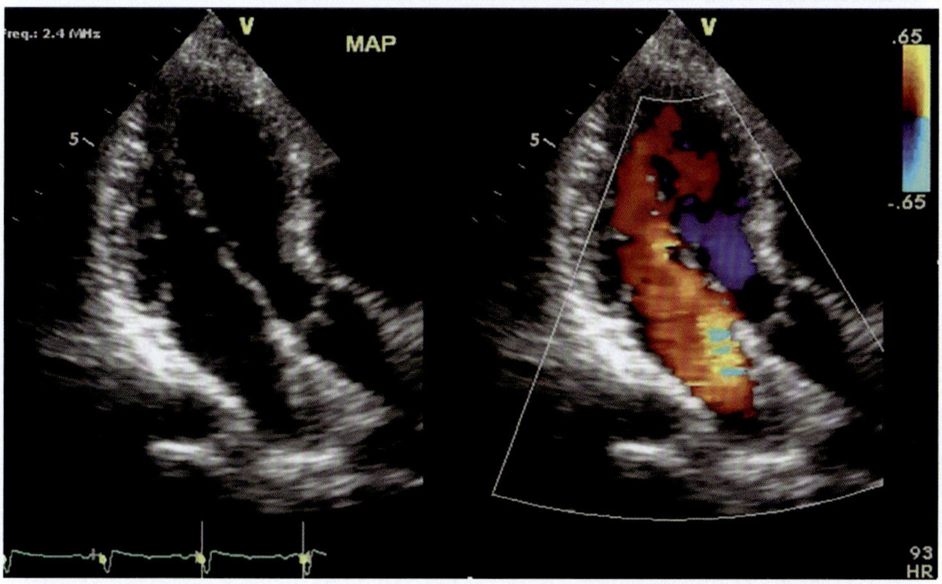

FIGURE 1.44 Postoperative echo using color compare from the apical long-axis view of the patient with cor triatriatum showing neither membrane in the left atrium nor any turbulence. TTE, PLX view.

Another Patient With Cor Triatriatum: Cor Triatriatum and 3D Echo

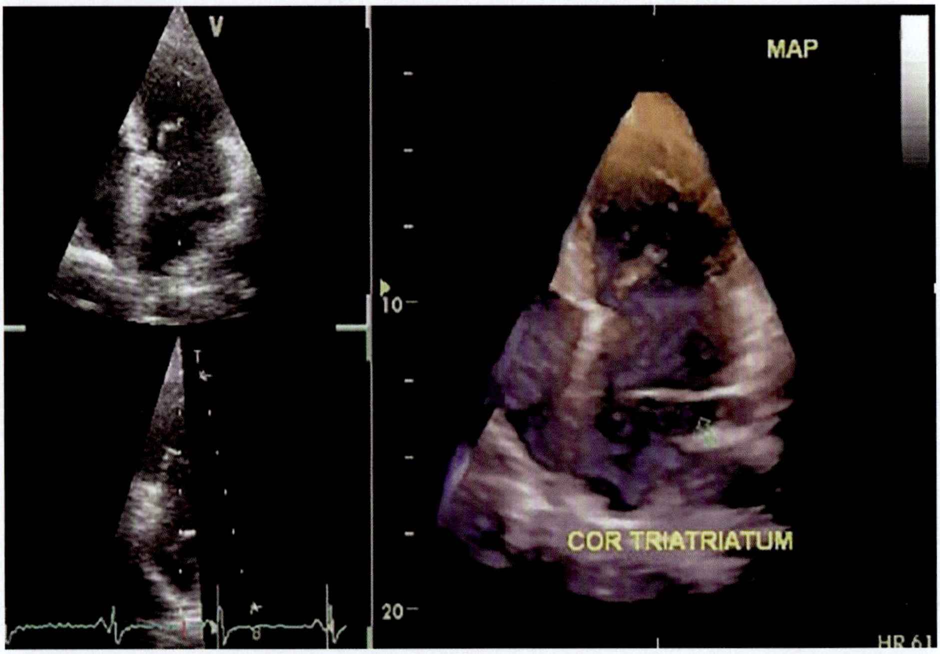

FIGURE 1.45 Another person with cor triatriatum with the membrane noted in the images on the left and illustrated in the 3D image on the right (*open green arrow*).

LEFT ATRIAL MYXOMA

Myxomas are rare cardiac tumors. They are slightly more common in males than females, may be familial, and may form one of the three components of the Carney complex (myxomas, spotty pigmentation of the skin, and endocrine overactivity).

They can be deceptive in their presentation but generally present as hemodynamic obstruction, embolization, or, with constitutional symptoms, the triad of myxomas. They are located most commonly in the left atrium, less in the right atrium, and rarely in either ventricle. In the atrium, they are usually attached to the limbus of the fossa ovalis. They are usually pedunculated but can be more sessile. They have various shapes and sizes from rounded to those with very irregular surfaces. The discovery of these has been much enhanced by the use of echocardiography.[18-22]

Left atrial myxoma is one of the most discussed abnormalities of the left atrium. These find themselves on rounds, medical conferences, textbooks, and board examinations. They have a variety of clinical manifestations, physical findings, and appearances on imaging techniques. The triad of clinical manifestations may vary from fever, anemia, and high sedimentation rate to diastolic rumbles and "tumor plops" and obstructed peripheral vessels. The common manifestations are consequences of embolization and mitral valve obstruction. A diastolic rumble and symptoms of exercise-induced shortness of breath as seen in mitral stenosis can be mimicked by a large left atrial myxoma. A diastolic rumble can be present with mitral valve obstruction as seen in rheumatic mitral stenosis, but in the case of a myxoma, the "tumor plop" is substituted for the opening snap. It is a rare opportunity nowadays to hear such a sound since these tumors are often discovered earlier in the course of their natural history. Once discovered, they should be removed as soon as possible for fear of embolic consequences.[23]

Imaging techniques are responsible for higher discovery rates of myxoma. Echocardiography has played a major role in the discovery of atrial myxoma before the dreaded consequences of embolization have occurred. CT and CMRI have also played a role in this early diagnosis. CT scans with contrast for such abnormalities as pulmonary embolus can uncover atrial myxoma. CMRI has the same potential to discover these masses. They have a special myxoid appearance on microscopic examination. Even coronary arteriography can reveal a mobile tumor blush that is characteristic of myxoma.

Atrial myxomas have characteristic findings under the microscope. They contain myxoid tissue and very few cells. They have an endocardial lining and myxoid cells that congregate about the vascular structures. Venous lakes are present that empty into the surrounding chamber. These features are illustrated in the following figures.

Large Left Atrial Myxoma on 2D and 3D Echocardiography

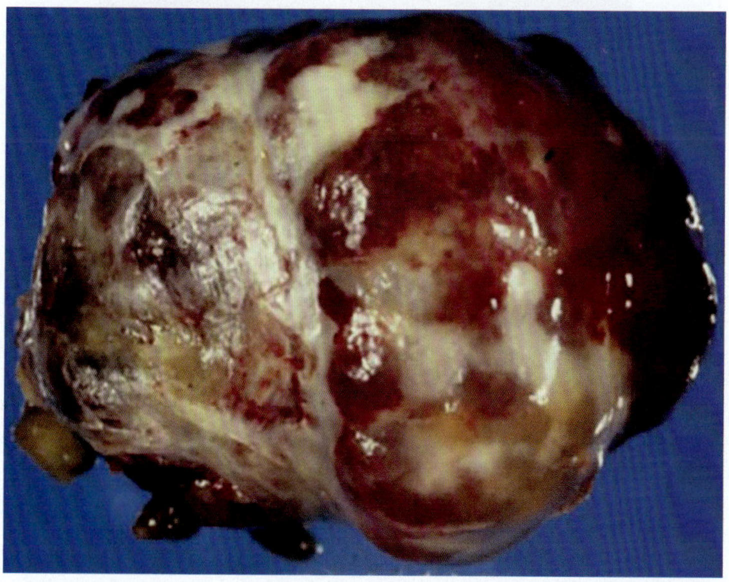

FIGURE 1.46 Image of myxoma removed at surgery. This large right atrial myxoma has multiple different components. On the left is scarring on the surface. Down the "waist" is the scarring from prolapsing through the valve orifice. On the right surface, there is hemorrhage, yellowish areas, and gelatinous areas on the far right. This tumor was actually removed from the right atrium. (Source: Clements SD, Cobbs BW, Perkins JV, Wingard T, King S, Craver JM. Echocardiographic and scintiangiographic observations in a patient with a right atrial myxoma. *J Med Assoc Ga.* 1979;68(9):827-830.)

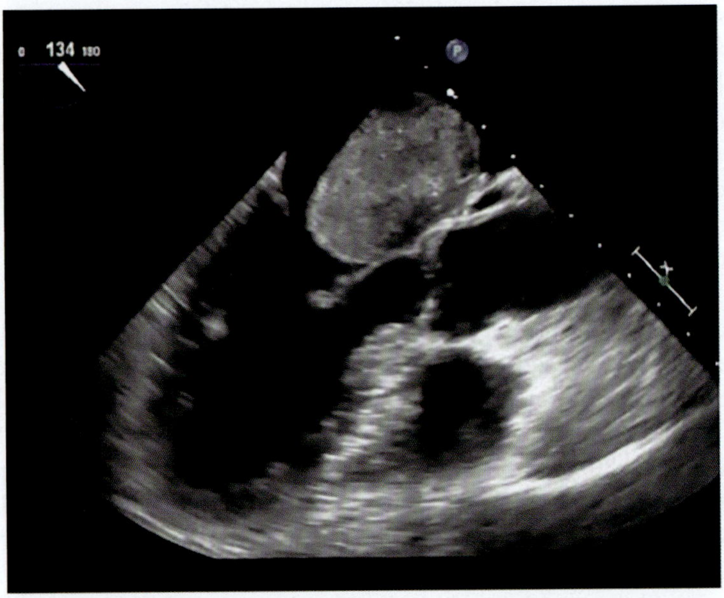

FIGURE 1.47 Still frame of a left atrial myxoma as it prolapses toward the mitral valve. The tumor is tugging on the interatrial septum adjacent to the aorta. TEE, 134° view.

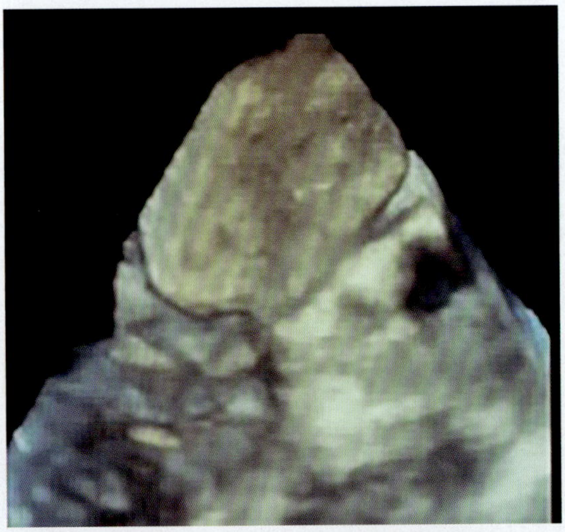

FIGURE 1.48 Live 3D still frame of the LA myxoma demonstrating its attachment to the septum and having a potatolike appearance. Visualized with its attachment to the wall of the interatrial septum. The tumor prolapses into the mitral orifice in diastole.

A Large Bilobed Left Atrial Myxoma, the "Clear Zone"

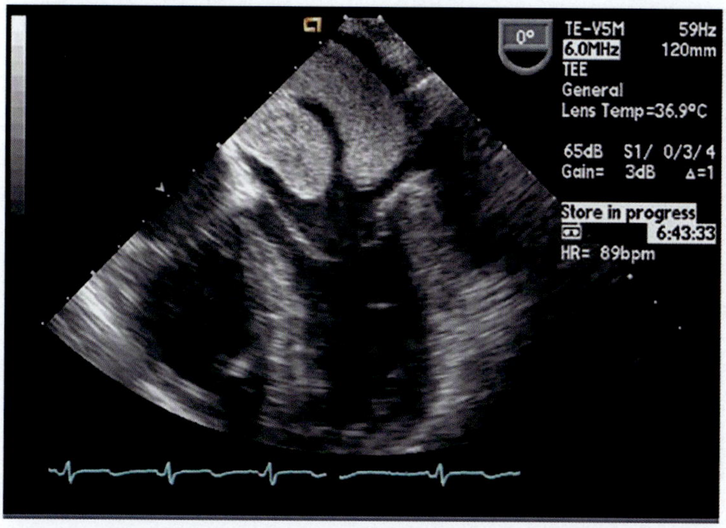

FIGURE 1.49 "Pac-man"-shaped left atrial myxoma prolapsing into the mitral orifice in diastole and rubbing against the mitral leaflets. Sometimes this repeated friction against the mitral leaflets can cause damage to them—the so-called wrecking ball effect (noted in the previous patient also). TEE, 0°.

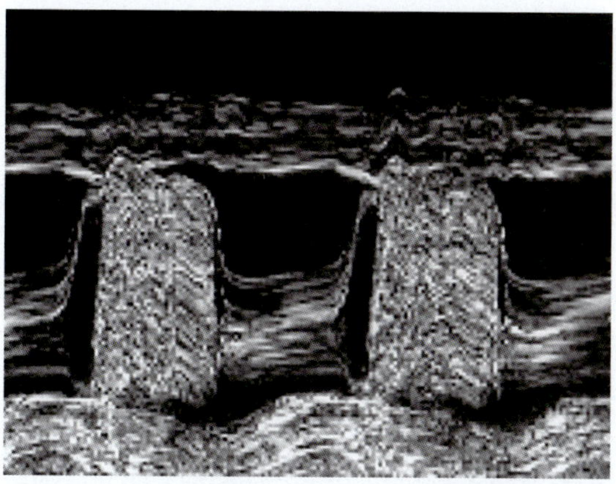

FIGURE 1.50 A zoomed view of the "clear zone"—the echo-free space that occurs in early diastole before the tumor "plops down" through the mitral orifice (*yellow arrow*). The low-pitched early diastolic sound called the "tumor plop" is caused by tensing of the stalk of the tumor, the tumor hitting the septum, or early obstruction of the mitral orifice. The myxoma abruptly stopping as it enters the mitral orifice. TTE, M-mode.

Large Left Atrial Myxoma With Very Irregular Edges

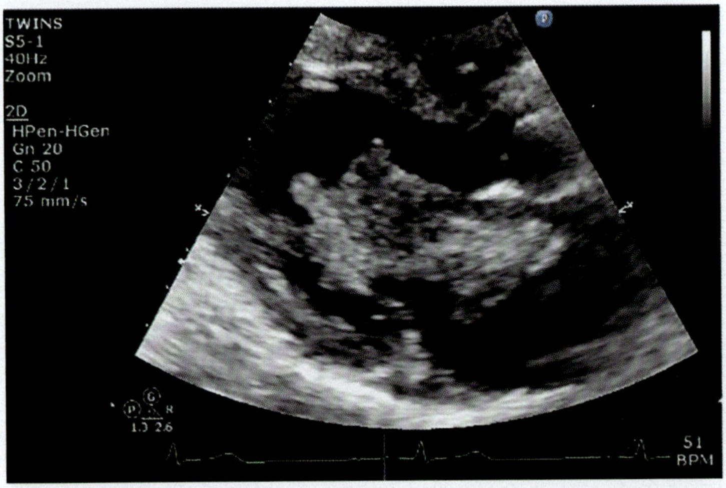

FIGURE 1.51 Still frame of a very large left atrial myxoma that has a very irregular leading edge that certainly has embolic potential. TTE, PLX view.

Microscopic Views of Atrial Myxoma

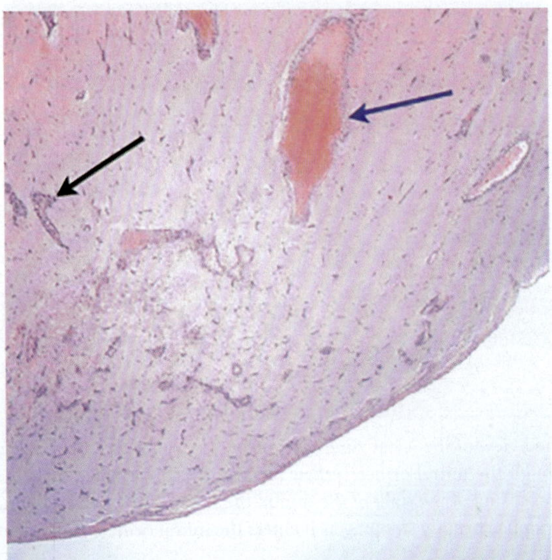

FIGURE 1.52 Microscopic view of a myxoma demonstrates an endothelial-like surface lining, venous lakes (*blue arrow*), and sparse cellular populations. Perivascular accumulation is present in some areas (*black arrow*).

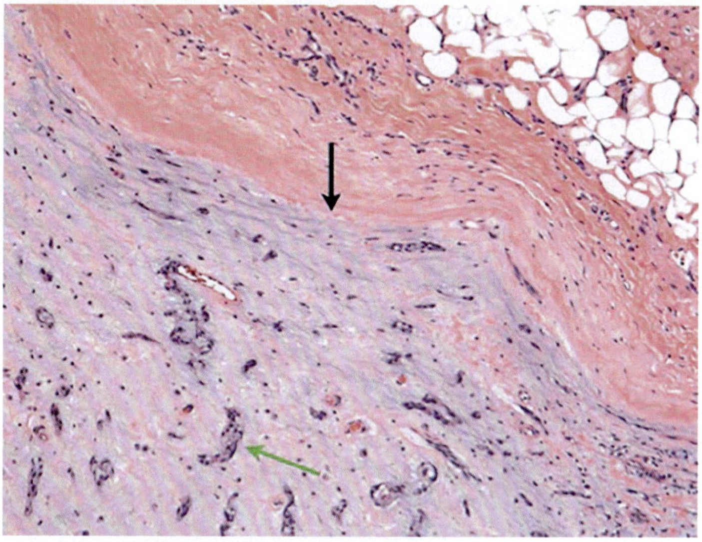

FIGURE 1.53 The junction of the myxoma and the atrial wall shows no invasion and well-defined boundaries (*black arrow*). Perivascular myxoma cells are present (*green arrow*).

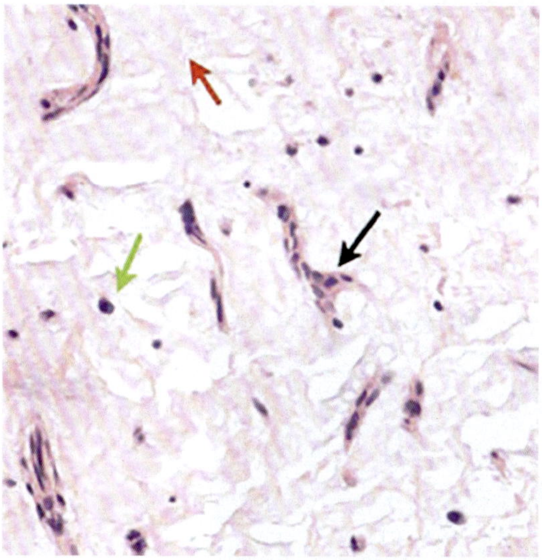

FIGURE 1.54 Multinucleated myxoma cells with a spindle shape (*black arrow*) and eosinophilic cytoplasm suspended in a myxoid matrix (*red arrow*) that is sparsely populated with smaller individual cells (*green arrow*).

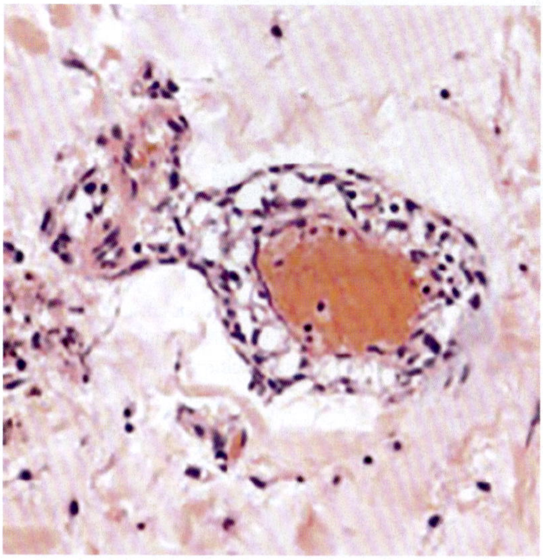

FIGURE 1.55 A halo of myxoma cells surrounding a vessel.

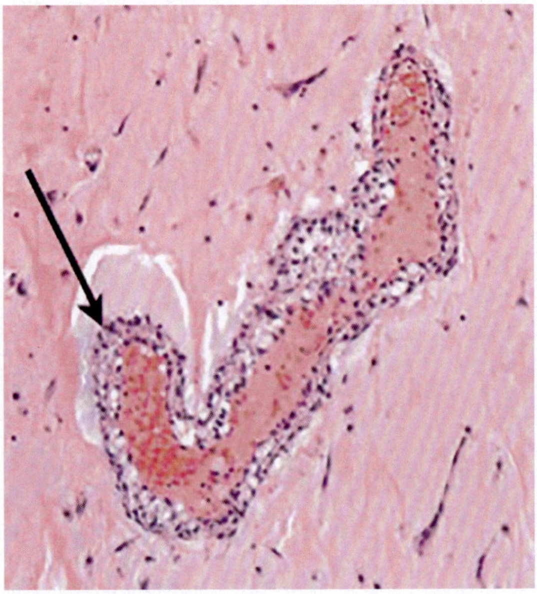

FIGURE 1.56 Perivascular arrangement of myxoma cells (*arrow*) as if they are part of the vessel itself is illustrated above. They are surrounded by an eosinophilic myxoid matrix with a sparse cellular population.

The Coronary Arteriogram in Left Atrial Myxoma: Myxoma in the Cardiac Catheterization Laboratory

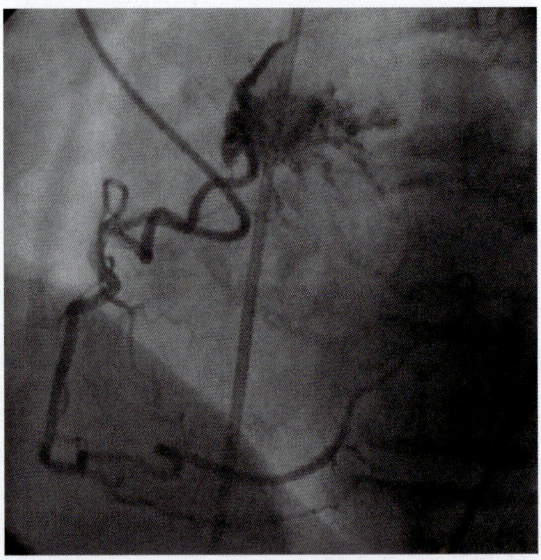

FIGURE 1.57 Coronary arteriogram in an individual with a left atrial myxoma. The venous lakes demonstrated in the previous microscopic slides show up on the arteriogram. They seem to empty directly into the left atrium from the tumor vessels. This type of angiographic appearance is characteristic of myxoma and not the fine microvascular "blush" that might be seen in a vascular malignant tumor.

REFERENCES

1. Blackshear JL, Odell JA. Appendage obliteration to reduce stroke in cardiac surgical patients with atrial fibrillation. *Ann Thorac Surg.* 1996;61:755-759.
2. Ho SY, McCarthy KP, Faletra FF. Anatomy of the left atrium for interventional echocardiography. *Eur J Echocardiogr.* 2011;12:i11-i15.
3. Agmon A, Kandheria B, Gentile F, Seward J. Echocardiographic assessment of the left atrial appendage. *J Am Coll Cardiol.* 1999;34:1868-1877.
4. Beigel R, Wunderich NC, Ho SY, Arsanjani R, Siegel RJ. The left atrial appendage: anatomy, function, and noninvasive evaluation. *JACC Cardiovasc Imaging.* 2014;7(12):1251-1265.
5. Wang Y, DiBlase L, Horton RP, et al. Left atrial appendage studied by computed tomography to help planning for appendage closure device placement. *J Cardiovasc Electrophysiol.* 2010;21:973-982
6. DiBiase L, Santangeli P, Anselmino M, et al. Does the left atrial appendage morphology correlate with the risk of stroke in patients with atrial fibrillation? Results from a multicenter study. *J Am Coll Cardiol.* 2013;60:531-538.
7. DeBacker O, Arnous S, Ihlemann N, et al. Percutaneous left atrial appendage occlusion for stroke prevention in atrial fibrillation: an update. *Open Heart.* 2014;1. doi:10.1136/openhrt-2013.000020.
8. Regazzoli D, Ancona F, Trevisi N, et al. Left atrial appendage: physiology, pathology, and role as a therapeutic target. *Biomed Res Int.* 2015;2015:205013. http://dx.doi.ort/10.1155/2015/205013
9. Ernst G, Stollberger C, Abzeiher F, et al. Morphology of the left atrial appendage. *Anat Rec.* 1995;242:553-561.
10. Shirani J, Alaeddin J. Structural remodeling of the left atrial appendage in patients with chronic non-valvular atrial fibrillation: implications for thrombus formation, systemic embolism, and assessment by transesophageal echocardiography. *Cardiovasc Pathol.* 2000;9:95-101.
11. Antonelli E, Pizzuti A, Palinkas A, et al. Clinical value of left atrial appendage flow for prediction of long-term sinus rhythm maintenance in patients with non valvular atrial fibrillation. *J Am Coll Cardiol.* 2002;39:1443-1449.
12. Bartus K, Han FT, Bednarek J, et al. Percutaneous left atrial appendage suture ligation using the lariat device in patients with atrial fibrillation. *J Am Coll Cardiol.* 2013;62(2):108-118.
13. Fountain R, Holmes DR Jr, Hodgson PK, et al. Potential applicability and utilization of left atrial appendage occlusion devices in patients with atrial fibrillation. *Am Heart J.* 2006;152(4):720-723.
14. Sick PB, Schuler G, Haumpmann KE, et al. Initial worldwide experience with the WATCHMAN left atrial appendage system for stroke prevention in atrial fibrillation. *J Am Coll Cardiol.* 2007;49(13):1490-1495.
15. Lang RM, Badano, LP, Mor-Avi V, et al. Recommendations for chamber quantification by echocardiography in adults: an update from the American Society of Echocardiography and the European Association of Cardiovascular Imaging. *J Am Soc Echocardiogr.* 2015;28:1-39.
16. Strickland PT, Peretz MA, Jokhadar M, Hartlage G, Clements S. Cor triatriatum sinister: a patient, a review, and some unique findings. *Echocardiography.* 2014;31(6):790-794.
17. Nassar PN, Hamdan RH. Cor triatriatum sinistrum: classification and imaging modalities. *Eur J Cardiovasc Med.* 2011;1(3):84-87.
18. Reymem K. Cardiac myxomas. *N Engl J Med.* 1995;333:1610-1617.
19. D'Alfonzo A, Catinia S, Pierri M, et al. Atrial Myxoma: a 25-yr single institution follow-up study. *J Cardiovasc Med.* 2008;9:178-181.
20. Pinde L, Duhaut P, Loire R. Clinical presentation of left atrial myxoma. A series of 112 consecutive cases. *Medicine.* 2001;80:159-172.
21. McCarthy P, Pilcher J, Schaff H, et al. The significance of multiple, recurrent and "complex" myxomas. *J Thorac Cardiovasc Surg.* 1986;91:389-396.

22. Carney JA, Gordon H, Carpenter PC, Shenou BV, Go VL. The complex of myxomas, spotty pigmentation and endocrine overactivity. *Medicine (Baltimore).* 1985;64:270-283.
23. Symbas PN, Hatcher CR Jr, Gravanis MB. Myxoma of the heart: clinical and experimental observations. *Ann Surg.* 1976;183:470-475.
24. Argmon Y, Khandheria BK, Gentile F, Seward JB. Echocardiographic assessment of the left atrial appendage. *J Am Coll Cardiol.* 1999;34(7):1867-1877.
25. Oh JK, Seward JB, Tajik AJ. *The Echo Manuel.* 3rd ed. Philadelphia, PA: Wolters Kluwer/ Lippincott Williams & Wilkins; 2007:23.
26. Nagueh SF, Smiseth OA, Appleton CP, et al. Recommendations for the evaluation of left ventricular diastolic function by Echocardiography: an update from the American Society of Echocardiography and the European Association of Cardiovascular Imaging. *J Am Soc Echocardiogr.* 2016;29:277-314.
27. Holt BD. Left atrial size and function: role in prognosis. *J Am Coll Cardiol.* 2014;63(6):493-505.

2

The Left Ventricle

SECTION 1

ANATOMY OF THE LEFT VENTRICLE[1]

The normal left ventricle has been described by various geometric shapes with the most common being an ellipsoid. An elongated sphere (prolated) creates an ellipsoid, the three-dimensional equivalent of an ellipse. An ellipsoid is formed when an ellipse is rotated about a long axis. A football is an ellipsoid; however, in the case of the left ventricle, it has short axes of different dimensions. Efforts to fit the real shape of the left ventricle into one of these geometric shapes have been extensive. The asymmetry of the short axes of this ellipsoid poses difficulties in using standard formulas that apply to classic geometric shapes. The biplane method of disks (modified Simpson rule) overcomes some of this asymmetry when calculating the ventricular volumes. This method analyzes orthogonal planes of the left ventricle (apical 4C view and apical 2C view) and uses software that allows the left ventricle to be divided into small disks (~20 in number) that can be integrated for full volumes for systole and diastole and calculation of the ejection fraction. Three-dimensional echo takes this a step further and puts together even smaller parts of this uneven geometric shape to give systolic and diastolic volumes. Three-dimensional methods either use a tomographic approach or a surface rendering technique and offer even more accurate display of information allowing analysis of regional left ventricular function and calculation of ejection fraction.

In the normal heart, the anterior leaflet of the mitral valve directs blood to the left ventricular outflow tract during systole. The axis of the left ventricular outflow tract is about 45° anterior to the central long axis of the left ventricle. The papillary muscles are part of the left ventricle but also are components of the mitral valve apparatus. They lie in a posteromedial and anterolateral position. From the left ventricular outflow tract, which has no trabeculations, to the apex of the ventricle, there is an increasing prominence of trabeculations. The degree of the trabeculations are not near that found in the right ventricle. The interventricular septum is shared with the right ventricle. The membranous portion of the interventricular septum on the left supports the right coronary cusp and on the right gives rise to a portion of the origin of the septal leaflet of the tricuspid valve.

The muscle fibers are arranged in a double helix formation, which has important functional significance. This is described in the section on the function of the left ventricle.

SECTION 2

CHAMBER QUANTIFICATION OF THE LEFT VENTRICLE

Recently, the guidelines for chamber quantifications have been published in the Journal of the American Society of Echocardiography by Lang et al.[2] This document represents the latest recommendations for chamber quantification and is an extensive and complete document offering the latest information regarding this issue. These recommendations are not absolute but represent a framework from which to work. It should be recognized that in time, these may change as they have done in the past.

THE NORMAL DIMENSIONS OF THE LEFT VENTRICLE

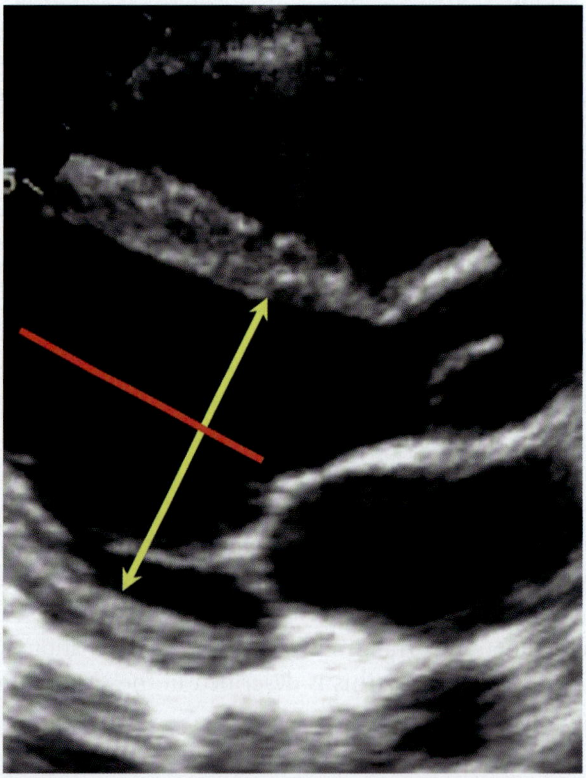

FIGURE 2.1 A diastolic frame taken at the onset of the QRS complex and extending from the blood to tissue border at or immediately below the mitral valve leaflet tips (*yellow double-headed arrow*) and perpendicular to the long axis (*red line*) of the left ventricular chamber at the interface of the LV cavity wall both anterior and posterior. In this individual, the dimension was 4.9 cm.

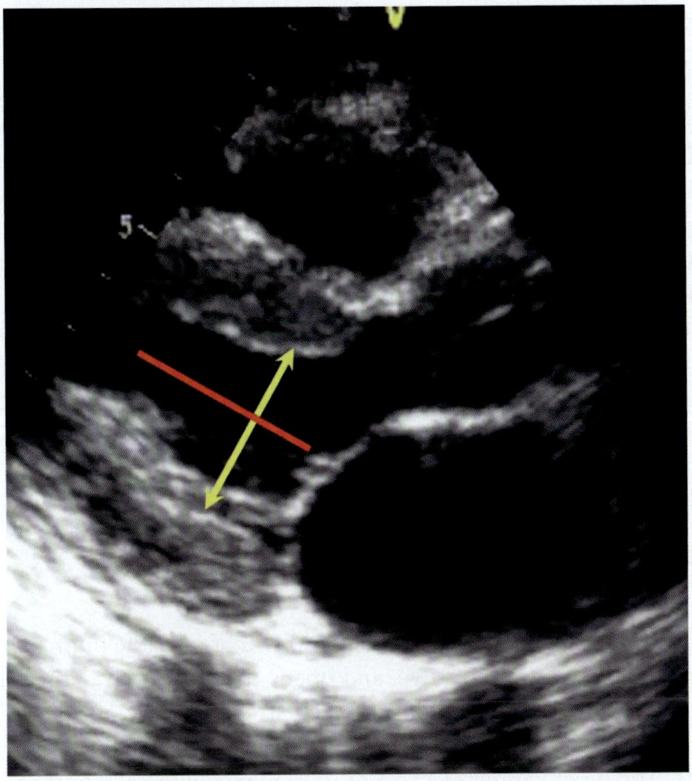

FIGURE 2.2 Measurement of the systolic dimension of the left ventricle is done by taking a point of the maximal excursion of the interventricular septum and an opposing point on the posterior wall at the level of the papillary muscle tips (*yellow double-headed arrow*) and perpendicular to the long axis of the left ventricular chamber (*red line*). In this individual, the dimension was 3.0 cm.

NORMAL VALUES FOR 2D ECHOCARDIOGRAPHIC PARAMETERS OF LV SIZE ACCORDING TO GENDER[2]

	Male		Female	
Parameter	Mean ± SD	2-SD range	Mean ± SD	2-SD range
LV internal dimension				
Diastolic dimension (mm)	50.2 ± 4.1	42.0-58.4	45.0 ± 3.6	37.8-52.2
Systolic dimension (mm)	32.4 ± 3.7	25.0-39.8	28.2 ± 3.3	21.6-34.8

FIGURE 2.3 Source: Lang RM, Badano LP, Bor-Avi V, et al. Recommendations for cardiac chamber quantification by echocardiography in adults. *J Am Soc Echocardiogr.* 2015;28:1-39.

These numbers and their ranges are taken from a normal group of individuals. One has to always remember that body size at times has to be taken into consideration. For example, in the very large person or the very small person, one has to consider the proportional size of a vessel or chamber and indexed to body surface area as is done in children. In other situations, such as the athletic individual, the "normal" may be outside of the standard limits. Therefore, these values are relative and must be individualized for each clinical situation.

LEFT VENTRICULAR MASS[3]

In addition to left ventricular dimensions, left ventricular mass can be calculated by several methods. Using M-mode and assuming that the left ventricle is prolate ellipse, one can calculate the LV mass, and using 2D, the mass can also be calculated. The 2D calculations are based on either the formula for a truncated ellipse or the area length method. Once the volume is calculated, the myocardial density is factored as 1.05 g/mL. The most validated measurements are from the M-mode method, and normal values are 95 g/m^2 for women and 115 g/m^2 for men. 2D measurements are slightly different with 88 g/m^2 for women and 102 g/m^2 for men. 3D may show the most promise but is a work in progress at this point in time. These parameters offer information about the prognosis and longitudinal follow-up of conditions such as left ventricular hypertrophy. Three-dimensional methods may be more accurate but at this point need more validation.

FUNCTION OF THE LEFT VENTRICLE

The function of the left ventricle has to do with a pulsatile pump. Once filled, it squeezes, closes the mitral valve, and opens the aortic valve. The output of the pump is measured by the volume of each stroke and the pulse rate. The stroke volume results from filling of the left ventricle and ejection of a fraction of this volume. The heart cannot eject all of its contents with each beat. At rest, about 55% or 60% of the contents of the left ventricle are ejected with each beat, and with exercise, this number can increase to the 80% range. If the myocardium becomes weakened by a disease process, it becomes dilated, and a new position on the Frank-Starling curve becomes operative to maintain stroke volume. Larger volumes of blood that are present at the end of diastole along with larger dimensions of the chamber tend to compensate for the weakened myocardium and maintain cardiac output and cardiac reserve. Volume increases do not come without the price of increased pressures within the left ventricle, the left atrium, and secondarily the pulmonary circuit.[4]

The shape of the left ventricle allows for efficient squeezing and twisting to take place. The normal left ventricle consists of three layers, an epicardial layer (arranged in a left-handed helix), a midlayer (with a circumferential arrangement), and an endocardial layer (arranged in a right-handed helix), which allow for the twisting motion of the left ventricle. The longer left-handed helical epicardial fibers pull the apex in a counterclockwise in the short axis and the base clockwise when both are viewed from the apex. Once this rotation has occurred, energy is stored and later used in the untwisting process that allows blood to be sucked into the left ventricle in diastole. Untwisting is also an energy-using process. The combination of the action of each of these layers allows the twisting motion of the left ventricle to have efficient squeezing effect and ejection of blood yet takes advantage of the limited capability of sarcomeres to contract in their narrow range of efficiency (optimally in the 13% range).[1]

Each of these layers has its own specific function both mechanically and electrically. The thickest region of the left ventricle is the basal portion with the thinnest region being the apex. The smaller radius and the thinner will of the ventricle at the apex allow maintenance of wall stress as described by the law of Laplace. The myocardial wall may hypertrophy in response to afterload or may thin in response to injury and dilatation. The walls may be compliant and respond to volume at a low pressure or be "stiff" and respond to volume at high pressure. This can be a global or a regional effect.

The rotation and the twisting effect in addition to longitudinal shortening cause the annular areas to descend toward the apex in systole.

Methods to assess the systolic function of the left ventricle center around the ejection fraction as calculated by various methods, analysis of segmental myocardial mechanics, indirect methods of analysis of Doppler profiles of flow, and time intervals between events.

The other half of the cardiac cycle, diastole, is evaluated by analysis of mitral Doppler inflow parameters, tissue Doppler velocities, and measurement of left atrial size.

In addition, the myocardium can be infiltrated by substances such as amyloid resulting in stiffening of the myocardium and dysfunction in systole and diastole. In rare instances, tumors can originate or metastasize to the myocardium. The myocardium can be constricted by a scarred pericardium or compressed by tense fluid present within the surrounding pericardial space. The left ventricle can also be affected by adjacent structures such as tumors of various origins. This section illustrates some of these abnormalities.

THE CARDIAC CYCLE[5]

A lot takes place from P wave to P wave and also from the onset of the QRS complex and the end of the T wave. Not only is there systole and diastole but periods of isovolumic contraction and relaxation occur that have their boundaries as pressure curves intersect. It is an oversimplification to consider systole the period between aortic valve opening and closing and diastole the remainder of the time. Myocardial relaxation begins after ventricular ejection reaches its peak pressure and extends well into the period after aortic closure but not throughout the period from aortic closure and opening. Echocardiography offers a unique look at these events that occur during mitral and aortic opening and closing and their temporal relationships. Analysis of these intervals offers information about the contraction and reaction of the left ventricle.

The combination of Doppler parameters with imaging information allows for more analysis of cardiac function.

SECTION 3

SYSTOLE

Evaluation of systolic function of the left ventricle by echocardiography is possible from several methods. The left ventricle can be analyzed simply by the eyeball method and systematically looking at all segments in the orthogonal parasternal and apical views. The ejection fraction can be calculated using the Simpson method of disks or using three-dimensional echo. Many other parameters are available on M-mode and 2D and 3D images for analysis of systolic function. In addition, Doppler profiles offer information about ventricular systole, and tissue Doppler and speckle tracking techniques also have added new dimensions to the understanding of systole. Tissue Doppler techniques have given information from the longitudinal view but also from the circumferential view. Systolic time intervals also offer information about the mechanical function of the left ventricle.

Illustrations of these methods are in the following panels and are listed in the following table.

ECHOCARDIOGRAPHIC EVALUATION OF GLOBAL LEFT VENTRICULAR SYSTOLIC FUNCTION[6]

- M-mode echocardiography
  - E wave height, MV excursion/LV size ~ ejection fraction.
  - E wave septal separation (normal <6 mm).
  - Rounded closure of the aortic valve suggests low stroke volume.
- Two-dimensional echocardiography
  - "Eyeballing" ejection fraction
  - Ejection fraction by the biplane method of disks (Simpson rule)
- Three-dimensional echocardiography
  - Tomographic and surface rendering techniques for volumes and ejection fraction
- Doppler echocardiography
  - Stroke volume as calculated from velocity time integral of the left ventricular outflow track (LVOT) and the LVOT diameter
  - dP/dT of the upstroke of the mitral regurgitation velocity profile
- Tissue Doppler imaging
  - Systolic velocity of the mitral annulus
  - Strain and strain rate* as determined by tissue Doppler
  - Tei index as determined by tissue Doppler[7]
- Speckle tracking echocardiography
  - Global longitudinal strain and strain rate
  - Radial and circumferential strain, strain rate, and torsion

*Evaluates systolic and diastolic function.

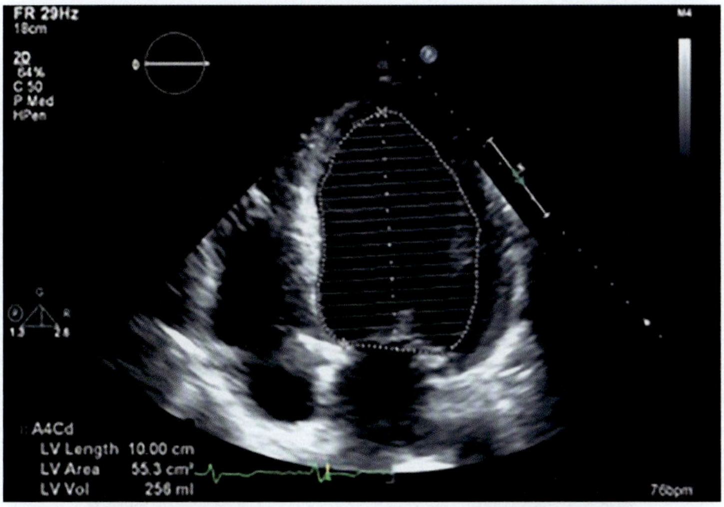

FIGURE 2.4

EJECTION FRACTION BY THE SIMPSON METHOD OF DISKS, THE 3D VOLUME RENDERING METHOD, AND THE 3D SURFACE RENDERING METHOD

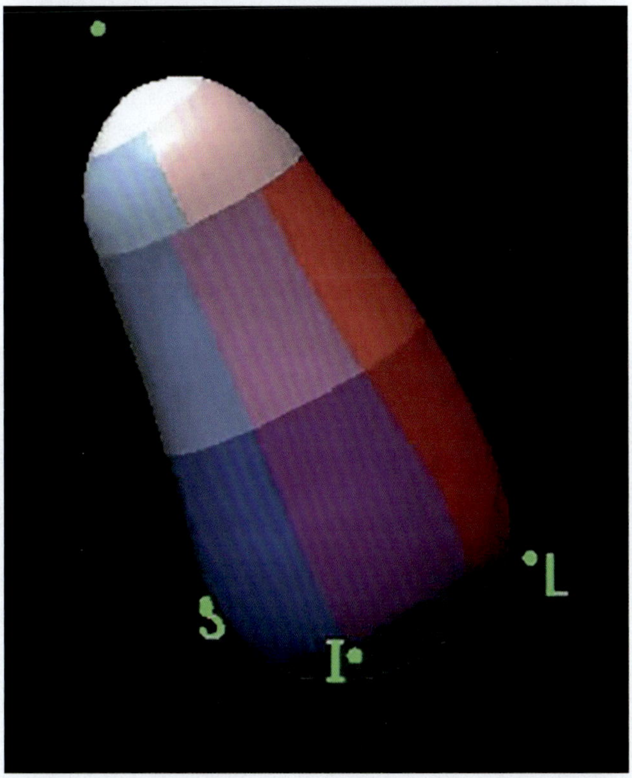

FIGURE 2.5 The apical four-chamber view in diastole with endocardial borders traced and the mitral annulus line drawn to form one of the two views needed to obtain a diastolic volume by the Simpson method of disks. This volume combined with the systolic volume allows for calculation of ejection fraction. S = septum, I = inferior and L = lateral.

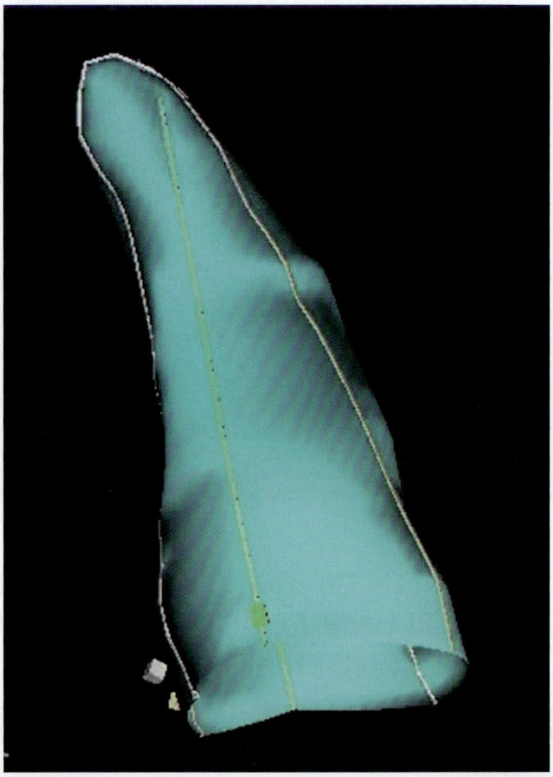

FIGURE 2.6 The composite three-dimensional display from three views, the A4C, the A2C, and the ALAX views. This display uses either the tomographic technique based on the Simpson method of disks or the surface rendering method. This compares to the 2D composite ejection fraction calculated from two orthogonal views and offers more information.

THE MITRAL REGURGITATION JET PROFILE AND LEFT VENTRICULAR SYSTOLIC FUNCTION

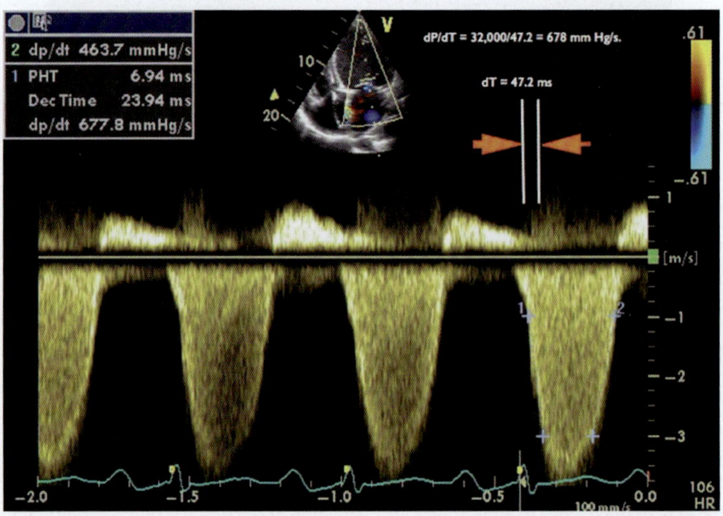

FIGURE 2.7

During the isovolumetric contraction period, the left atrial pressure remains relatively constant, so the gradient between the left ventricle and atrium remains relatively constant. The rate of rise (d*P*/d*T*) of the velocity curve reflects systolic function. If the velocity is calculated at 1 and 3 seconds, then the change in velocity in mm Hg can be calculated if the time interval is known. According to the Bernoulli equation, the pressure differential is $(4 \times 3^2) - (4 \times 1^2) = 32$ mm Hg for the time interval between 1 and 3 m/s. In this individual, the time interval was 47.2 ms. Therefore, the d*P*/d*T* for 1 second is 32 mm Hg/0.0472 = 678 mm Hg/s. The normal is >1000 mm Hg/s.[8]

STRAIN

Speckle tracking echocardiography allows identification of points or speckles in the myocardium and tracking of these speckles in time. The change in the length between two speckles from diastole to systole offers information about regional myocardial function. If one designates the initial length of a segment of the myocardium identified by speckles as L_0 and a final length as L, then this difference can be expressed as a percentage. This linear description of lengthening and shortening or deformation is referred to as Lagrangian strain.

$$\frac{L - L_0}{L_0} = \text{Strain}$$

Strain is a negative number for the left ventricle, and global strain is −20% or a more negative number such as −24%.

Since the initial length (L_0) is longer than the final length (L), the numerator will be a negative number and strain will be a negative number or percentage (normal for the left ventricle −20% or higher). In the case of circumferential strain, the same is true in that the strain is expressed as a negative number for normal segments. For radial strain that represents thickening, the initial numbers are smaller than the final numbers, so a positive percentage is obtained. Rotation of the base of the heart in a clockwise direction and the apex in a counterclockwise direction results in a twisting motion. When these angles of rotation are quantified and added together, they give a sum that is called twist. Strain rate is an expression of the rate of change of length between two points normalized to the distance between them and calculated by $(V_a - V_b)/D$ where $(V_a - V_b)$ is the velocity difference between two points and D is the distance between them. It is expressed in 1/seconds.[9-11]

GLOBAL STRAIN IMAGING AND POLAR MAP DISPLAY

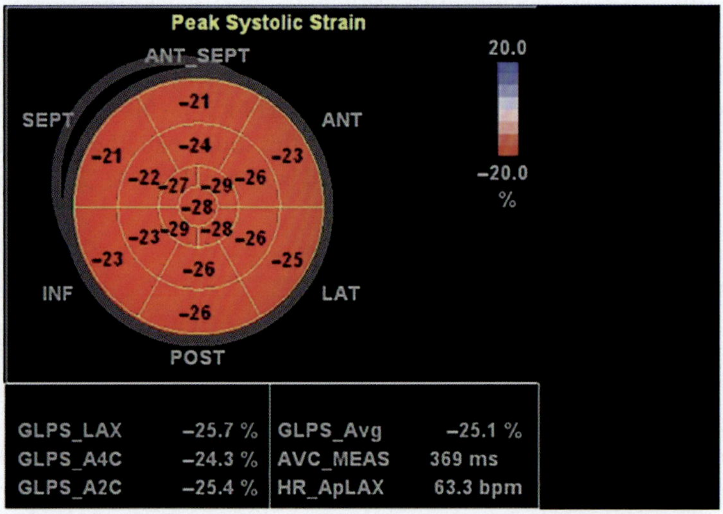

FIGURE 2.8

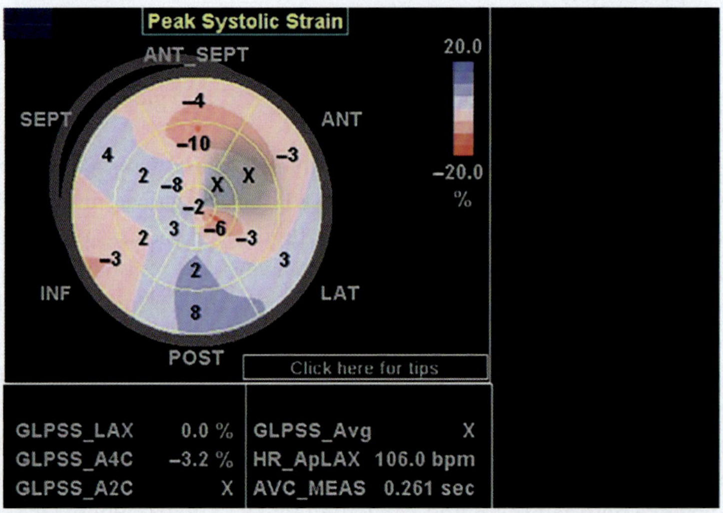

FIGURE 2.9

Longitudinal strain is measured using the speckle tracking method. These polar displays are constructed from three apical views that are combined to produce these maps. Normally, these are in the −25.1% range as is seen in Fig 2.8. In Fig 2.9, which is taken from an individual with severe dilated cardiomyopathy, the number for global strain is not calculated because some segments were not measurable and designated as "x."

ANALYSIS OF THE LEFT VENTRICLE FROM THE SHORT-AXIS VIEWS AND USING SPECKLE TRACKING ECHOCARDIOGRAPH

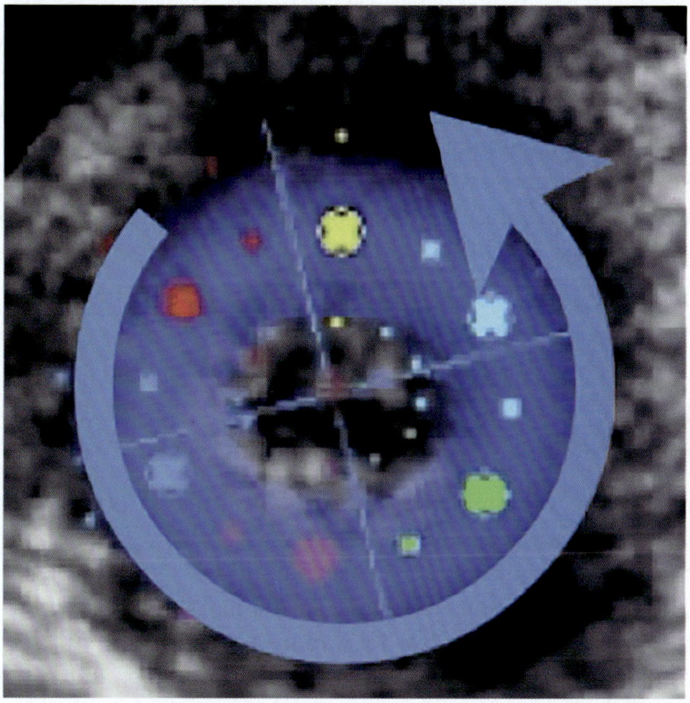

FIGURE 2.10 Stop frame at peak systolic rotational motion at the apex showing all blue or 18° of rotation in the counterclockwise direction.

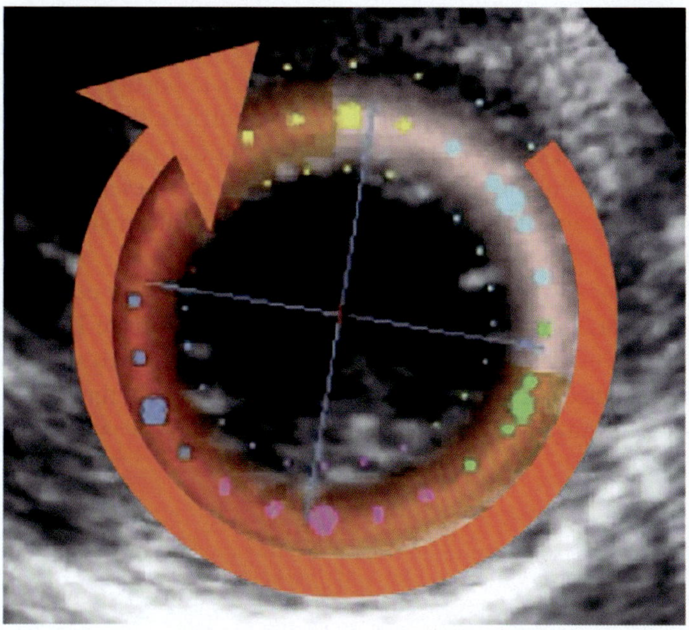

FIGURE 2.11 Stop frame at peak systolic rotation at the base showing mostly red, the clockwise designation, and peaking in the −16° range.

Rotation refers to the movement of the myocardium around the long axis of the ventricle and in the above example is +18° in a counterclockwise manner as designated and viewed from the apex. The systolic rotation in this example is −16° in a clockwise manner as viewed from the apex. Twist refers to the difference of these two angles or the net twist angle of 18 + 16 = 34°. Torsion refers to the difference in these angles as they relate from the apex to base dimension expressed in degrees per centimeter.[12]

This process evolves from infancy where apical rotation remains constant and subsequently the basal rotation transitions from counterclockwise to clockwise, the usual adult pattern. With aging, twist increases primarily due to less basal clockwise rotation and thus less opposition to apical counterclockwise rotation all due to decrease in subendocardial function.[13]

SECTION 4

DIASTOLE

During the interval from aortic closure to mitral closure, many events take place. Relaxation begins after the peak of the LV pressure curve and therefore has already begun before the isovolumic relaxation phase of the cardiac cycle. Relaxation continues after this isovolumetric phase for a variable period of time. In extreme examples, relaxation may not be completed at the end of diastole.[14] Pressure curves cross, gradients develop, and the mitral valve opens, and the early diastolic portion of left ventricular filling occurs giving rise to the E wave on the echocardiogram. Diastasis follows and on the occasion of high left ventricular filling pressures sometimes writes an L wave on the mitral Doppler inflow tracing (creating the "batman sign").[15] After diastasis, the atrium contracts associated with the P wave on the electrocardiogram and mechanically fills the left ventricle in the late portion of diastole. The left atrial pressure curve crosses that of the left ventricle, the left ventricular pressure exceeds that of the left atrium, and the mitral valve closes at the end of diastole and isovolumic systole begins. Each of these events and their respective velocities and flow volumes have important information about the state of diastole.

Short of invasive measurement of diastolic pressures, echocardiography offers our best effort to grade diastolic dysfunction and estimate LVEDP. Guidelines offer analysis of various factors used to categorize diastolic dysfunction remain to be fully validated but are the best available at this point in time.

The following panels illustrate the principles of analysis of diastolic function.[16-18]

MEASUREMENT OF PARAMETERS OF DIASTOLIC FUNCTION: THE E WAVE AND THE A WAVE

The E wave is the manifestation of early diastolic filling of the left ventricle. It is generated by the suction effect within the left ventricle by factors such as elastic recoil and the active untwisting process. This is an energy-requiring process that is produced by the undoing of the squeezing and twisting that occurs in systole. It has three components to include active relaxation, restoration of forces, and lengthening of load.[19] In young individuals, these processes are very prominent and result in a dominant E wave associated with the very vigorous suction effect associated with elastic recoil and untwisting of the left ventricle. Filling is so vigorous in early diastole that there is little left for the atrium to do and thus a small A wave is often present. In younger individuals, the E wave is dominant; however, by the sixth or seventh decade of life, the E and A waves are equal. When pressures of the left ventricle increase, filling volumes of the left ventricle in early diastole decrease, and the role of atrial systole becomes more important producing a prominent A wave that is higher than the E wave. In older individuals, the E wave decreases because of prolonged relaxation.[20] When left atrial pressure increases to compensate for the higher filling pressures, the E wave becomes prominent again and is taller than the A wave, and the pseudonormal pattern develops. High gradients between the left atrium and left ventricle allow for a high-velocity E wave of brief duration and a rapid deceleration time after reaching maximum velocity. The A wave decreases with higher grades of diastolic dysfunction, and its duration has an important relationship to the pulmonary Ar as the difference between these two parameters relates to left ventricular end-diastolic pressure. These advanced grades of diastolic dysfunction can be altered by altering left atrial pressure with Valsalva maneuver producing a longer deceleration time and thus assuming a lesser degree of diastolic dysfunction. This phenomenon is described as the reversible pattern of diastolic dysfunction and has a more favorable prognosis. Otherwise, if this reversible phenomenon does not occur, the restrictive filling pattern is irreversible and has prognostic importance.

Other parameters such as mitral annular tissue Doppler velocities, left atrial volume, tricuspid regurgitation jet velocity along with mitral inflow flow propagation, and pulmonary vein flow velocity profiles all have characteristic alterations as left ventricular diastolic dysfunction progresses from abnormal relaxation to irreversible left ventricular filling.[21]

PRESSURE CURVES AND MITRAL DOPPLER VELOCITY CURVES

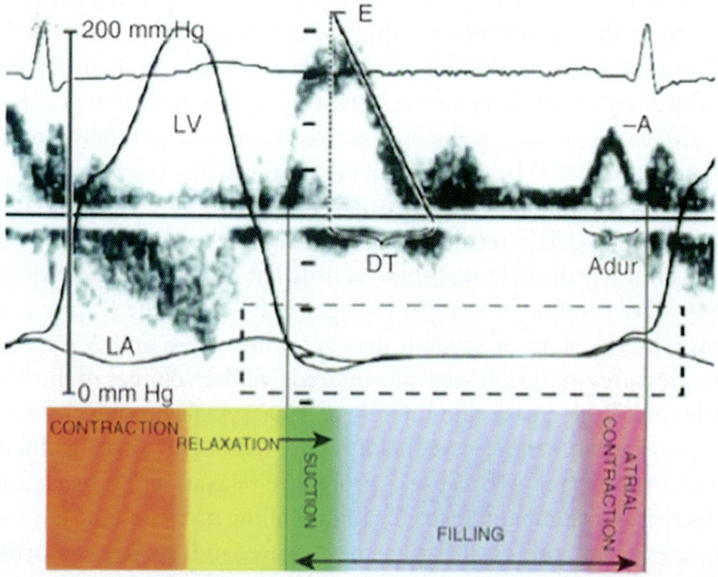

FIGURE 2.12 Mitral inflow represents pressure difference between the LV and LA; simultaneous invasive pressure curves and Doppler echocardiography during the phases of left ventricular filling (relaxation, suction, filing, and atrial contraction). A, mitral filling at atrial contraction; Adur, duration of mitral A wave; DT, mitral deceleration time; E, mitral early filling wave; LA, left atrial pressure curve; LV, left ventricular pressure curve. (Adapted from Lang RM, Goldstein SA, Kronzon I, Khandheria BK, Mor-Avi V. *ASE's Comprehensive Echocardiography*. 2nd ed. Philadelphia, PA: Elsevier (Saunders); 2016:180-184.)

In this simultaneous tracing of the left ventricular and left atrial pressure curves and mitral Doppler inflow, several points are illustrated. We must remember that gradients give rise to velocities and understanding of pressure relationships makes for understanding of velocities. Upon pressure falling within the left ventricle, relaxation occurs beginning after the peak LV pressure and extends to the point near peak diastolic flow velocity across the mitral valve. Note that relaxation begins after the peak of the LV pressure and extends into diastole to a variable degree. When the left ventricular pressure falls below that of the left atrium, the mitral valve opens and flow begins into the left ventricle. The velocity across the mitral valve is related to the maximum pressure gradient as illustrated by the difference between the two curves. Diastasis occurs after these events, and the atrium contracts later.[21]

THE APICAL FOUR-CHAMBER VIEW AT A GLANCE AND IMPORTANT POINTS FOR SAMPLING VELOCITIES

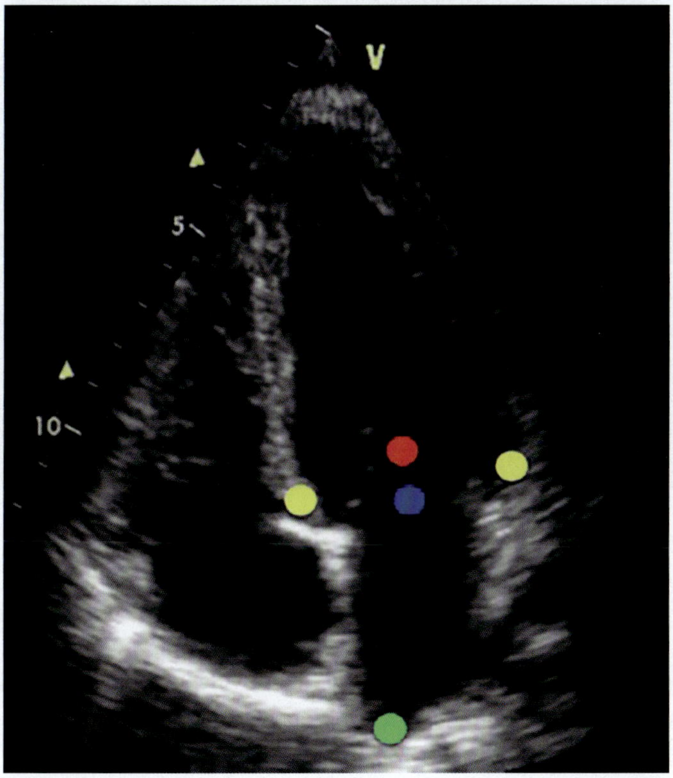

FIGURE 2.13

A stop frame in early diastole at a time when the mitral leaflets are open and early diastolic flow is taking place writes the E wave on the pulsed Doppler tracing. Sampling this phenomenon is done in the region of the red dot within the left ventricle at the tip of the mitral leaflets. The yellow dots are located at the myocardial segment within 1 cm of the mitral annulus and are the location for sampling of tissue Doppler velocities. The pulsed-wave Doppler sampling of the pulmonary vein flow velocities is done 1-2 cm within the superior pulmonary vein with the sample box adjusted to 3-4 mm. Acquisition of pulsed-wave Doppler images for measurement of mitral A wave duration is done at the level of the mitral annulus illustrated by the blue dot.

NORMAL MITRAL DOPPLER INFLOW VELOCITY PATTERN IN A 17-YEAR-OLD WOMAN

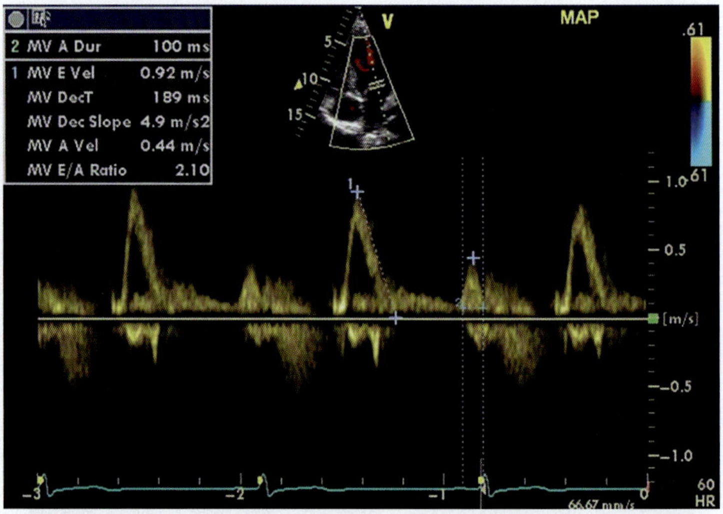

FIGURE 2.14

The normal velocity filling pattern of the left ventricle is measured at the tips of the mitral leaflets with pulsed-wave Doppler. The E wave is usually the most prominent wave and is related to active early diastolic filling. In young individuals, the initial filling is vigorous and is due to elastic recoil and the active energy-requiring untwisting process. Sometimes, early diastolic filling is so vigorous that there is little left for the atrium to do. Therefore, in young individuals, the E wave is very large and the A wave is small. A period of diastasis occurs and is followed by the velocity curve caused by atrial contraction, the A wave. Normally, the E/A ratio is between 1 and 2, and the mitral deceleration time is between 150 and 240 ms. Normally, the A wave duration is in the 79-153 ms range, and the A velocity is typically 19-35 cm/s in normal individuals 40 years or less.*[16,22]

The duration of the mitral A wave should be measured at the level of the mitral annulus and not at the tips of the leaflets. In normal individuals, these intervals are similar; however, as left ventricular filling pressures rise, the pulmonary "A" wave reversal duration begins to increase, and the difference between these two values quantitatively relates to left ventricular filling pressures. Values vary according to age and the state of atrial and ventricular function.

TISSUE DOPPLER IMAGING

Tissue Doppler imaging can be used to measure the velocities of the septal and lateral annular velocities. During systole, the apex is relatively stable and the mitral annulus descends along the long axis of the left ventricle. The rate and magnitude of this decent (manifest by the s′ wave) is related to systolic function of the ventricle. During diastole, the motion of the mitral annulus (manifest by the e′ and a′ waves) is related to the diastolic function of the left ventricle as it relaxes and fills. The magnitude of these velocities (of myocardial tissue) is about one-tenth of those of erythrocytes. That is, if the left ventricular outflow velocity (erythrocytes targeted) is 1 m/s per second, the mitral annular tissue velocities in systole and diastole are in the range of 0.1 m/s. These velocities are measured by placing sample volumes within 1 cm ventricular to the mitral annulus with sweep speed increased to the 50-100 mm/s range. Instrumentation allows recording of low velocities and filtering out of high velocities, and high frame rates are required. Values are obtained from the septal and lateral annular areas. Velocity scale should be set to about 20 cm/s above and below the baseline. There is a slight difference in the values obtained for the septal and lateral locations with the septal being slightly lower than the lateral. This is due to differences in rotational effects and the influence of the right ventricle. In healthy young individuals, the septal e′ velocities are usually >7 cm/s, and the lateral e′ velocities are >10 cm/s. Exceptions to this are in individuals with regional wall motion abnormalities such as lateral myocardial infarction, right ventricular enlargement, constrictive pericarditis, and others.[16,17,23] Constrictive pericarditis results in tethering of the lateral annular area and causes the phenomena of "annulus reversus" with the septal velocities being higher than the lateral. In the setting of constrictive pericarditis, the e′ is typically increased, and therefore, there is an inverse relationship between E/e′ and LV filling pressures, a phenomenon called "annulus paradoxus".[24,25]

In normal individuals, the E wave increases with preload and with exercise and the e′ follows. In those individuals with abnormal relaxation, the e′ is reduced and does not increase as much as preload changes. In the setting of diastolic dysfunction as preload increases and filling pressures increase, the E wave increases and the e′ wave decreases. Therefore, the ratio of these two (E/e′) is related to left ventricular filling pressures and pulmonary capillary wedge pressures. Using the guideline-recommended values for assessing diastolic dysfunction, for E/e′ average, a ratio of >14 is abnormal, and for the E/e′, a septal ratio of >15 and E/e′ lateral ratio of >13 are abnormal. These ratios along with the mitral tissue Doppler velocities, the tricuspid regurgitant jet velocity, and the left atrial volume index and other parameters are used in the assessment of diastolic function.[16,17,23]

Special situations in which E/e′ and other parameters of diastolic dysfunction may not accurately predict left ventricular filling pressures are noted in Tables 2.1 and 2.2.

TABLE 2.1 E/e′ SPECIAL SITIUATIONS PARAMETERS OF DIASTOLIC FUNCTION MAY NOT ACCURATELY PREDICT LEFT VENTRICULAR FILLING PRESSURE

1. In normal young individuals where e′ is load dependent variable
2. Constrictive pericarditis
3. Mitral valve disease
    a. Mitral regurgitation more than moderate
    b. Mitral stenosis more than moderate
    c. Calcified mitral annulus more than moderate
    d. Post-surgery, mitral annuloplasty and mitral valve replacement
4. Atrial fibrillation
5. Left bundle branch block or a paced ventricular rhythm
6. Left ventricular assist devices (LVAD, ECMO and Impella)

TABLE 2.2 OTHER SITUATIONS PARAMETERS OF DIASTOLIC FUNCTION MAY NOT ACCURATELY PREDICT LEFT VENTRICULAR FILLING PRESSURE

1. Hypertrophic cardiomyopathy with symptoms
2. Acutely decompensated heart advanced heart failure with dilated LV and impaired cardiac output
3. Cardiac resynchronization therapy

RECORDING THE TISSUE DOPPLER ANNULAR VELOCITY

The mitral annulus descends toward the apex in systole and ascends back to the baseline position in diastole. The apex remains relatively stable. The velocities of this motion can be measured with pulsed-wave Doppler using a sample volume of 2-5 mm in size and placed at the mitral annulus at or just below the leaflet attachments. The velocity scale should be set at ~20 cm/s above and below the zero-velocity baseline with minimal angulation between the ultrasound beam and the plane of cardiac motion, and sweep speed should be set at 50-100 mm/s with recordings done at end-expiration.

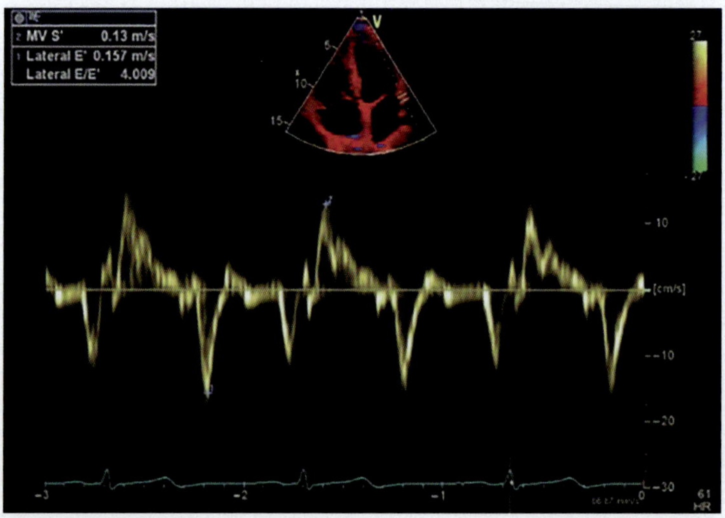

FIGURE 2.15 Sampling of the septal annular velocity 0.10 m/s.

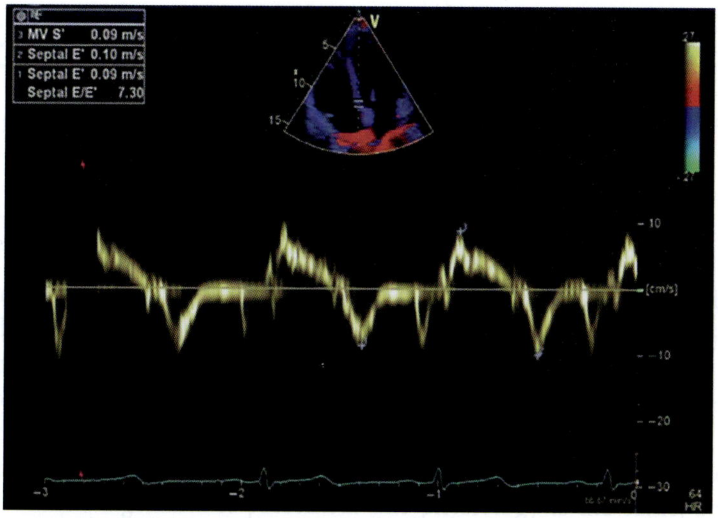

FIGURE 2.16 Sampling of the lateral annular velocity 0.157 m/s.

LEFT ATRIAL END-SYSTOLIC VOLUME INDEX (LVESV INDEX)

The left atrium is the entrance way to the left ventricle, and its size gives immediate information as to the systolic and diastolic function of the heart.

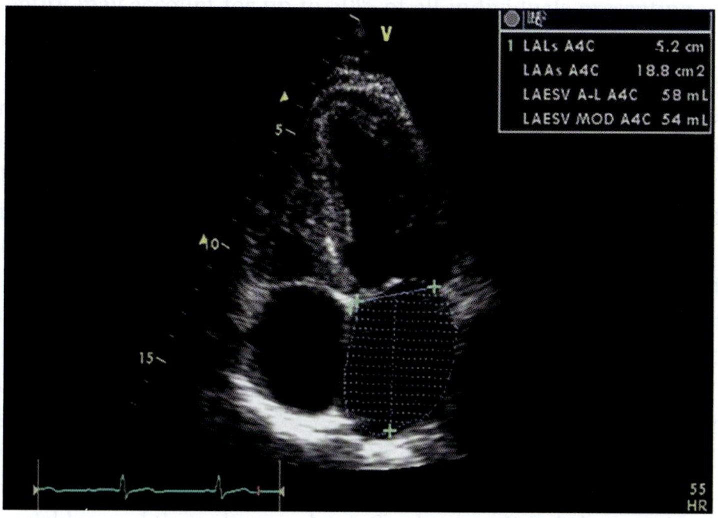

FIGURE 2.17 From the A4C view, the four chambers and their relative sizes can be assessed. One can get an idea about the size of the left atrium relative to the right. A large left atrium is a clue to diastolic dysfunction. Measurements are necessary to allow volume calculations and for indexing purposes. The atria are traced starting at the medial mitral annulus and extending around posterior and laterally making sure to exclude the pulmonary veins and left atrial appendage. Usually, the volume calculated on the basis of this view alone is a couple of mL^2 smaller than that calculated from the A2C view; the combination of these two views offer the best estimate of LAESV index.

TABLE 2.3 FACTORS IN THE ALGORITHM FOR ECHOCARDIOGRAPHIC ASSESSMENT OF DIASTOLIC FUNCTION IN INDIVIDUALS WITH NORMAL LVEF (ASE AND EACI GUIDELINES)

1. E/e′ ratio
    a. E/e′ average >14
    b. E/e′ lateral >15
    c. E/e′ septal >13
2. Mitral annular e′ velocity
    a. Septal e′ <7 cm/s, lateral e′ <10 cm/s
3. Peak tricuspid regurgitation jet velocity
    a. TR peak jet velocity >2.8 m/s
4. Left Atrial volume index
    a. >34 mL/m^2

Nagueh SF, Smiseth OA, Appleton CP, et al. Recommendations for evaluation of left ventricular diastolic function by echocardiography. An update from the American Society of Echocardiography and the European Association of Cardiovascular Imaging. *J Am Soc Echocardiogr.* 2016;29:277-314.

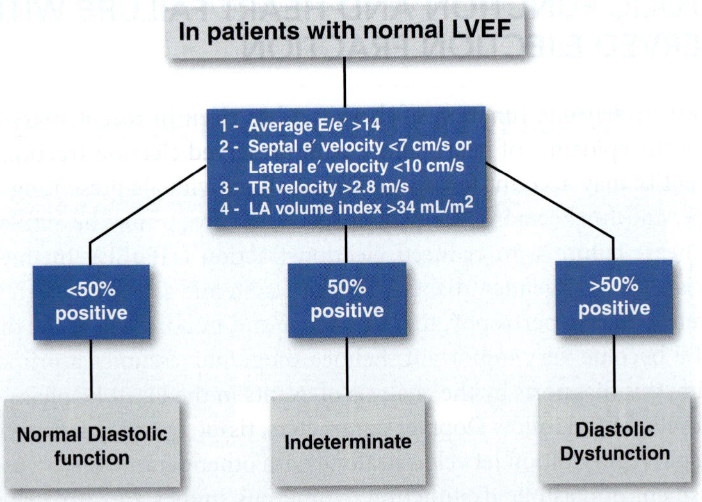

FIGURE 2.20 Algorithm for diagnosis of LV dysfunction in subjects with normal LVEF. (From Nagueh SF, Smiseth OA, Appleton CP, et al. Recommendations for the evaluation of left ventricular diastolic function by echocardiography: an update from the American Society of Echocardiography and the European Association of Cardiovascular Imaging. *J Am Soc Echcardiogr.* 2016;29:277-314.)

ECHOCARDIOGRAPHIC ASSESSMENT OF DIASTOLIC FUNCTION IN INDIVIDUALS WITH REDUCED LVEF AND GRADING OF DIASTOLIC FUNCTION

The key variables recommended by the 2016 guidelines for echocardiographic evaluation of LV filling pressures and diastolic dysfunction grade in individuals with reduced LVEF are

- Mitral flow velocities
- Mitral annular e′ velocities

- E/e′ ratio
- Peak velocity of TR jet
- LA maximum volume index†

Supplementary methods

- Pulmonary vein velocities
- LV GLS by Speckle tracking

PATIENTS WITH DEPRESSED EJECTION FRACTION

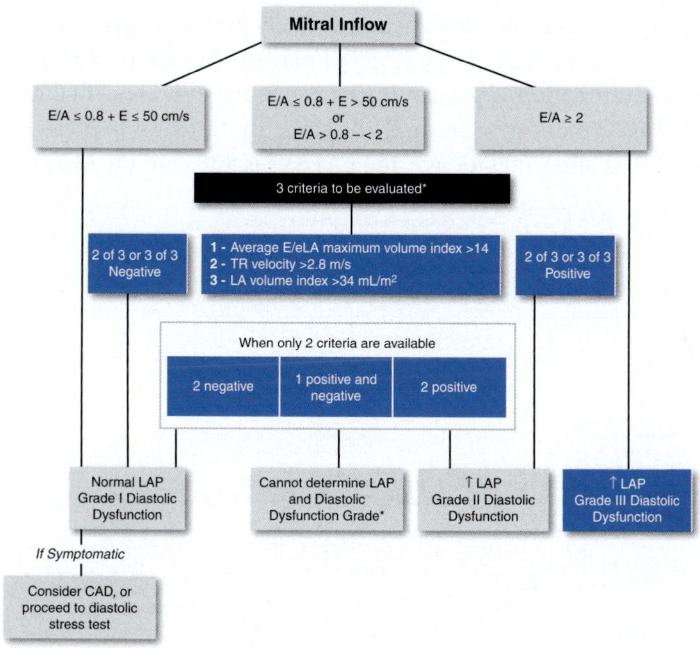

(*: LAP indeterminate if only 1 of 3 parameters available. Pulmonary vein S/D ratio <1 applicable to conclude elevated LAP in patients with depressed LVEF)

FIGURE 2.21 Algorithm for estimation of LV filling pressures and grading of LV diastolic dysfunction in patients with depressed LVEFs and patients with myocardial disease and normal EF after consideration of clinical and other 2D data. (From Nagueh SF, Smiseth OA, Appleton CP, et al. Recommendations for the evaluation of left ventricular diastolic function by echocardiography: an update from the American Society of Echocardiography and the European Association of Cardiovascular Imaging. *J Am Soc Echcardiogr.* 2016;29:277-314.)

ALGORITHM

Recently, another algorithm has been published as an alternative to the 2016 guidelines published in the Journal of the American Society of Echocardiography. Mitter et al. published their algorithm as an alternative to the ASE guidelines. This assessment of diastolic dysfunction emphasizes the effect of age and the natural and expected increase in stiffness of the left ventricle as aging occurs. In addition, the incorporation of the tricuspid regurgitant jet is not in this algorithm especially since it can be a manifestation of problems in the pre- or postcapillary abnormalities in the pulmonary circulation. In addition, the mitral valve

†See Figure 2.21.

deceleration time (MVDT) is part of the algorithm especially being important as a factor in more advanced degrees of diastolic dysfunction.[18]

Note that the lateral e′ is recommended and that this value does decrease with age. In individuals <55 years old, the normal lateral e′ is >10 cm/s; in those between 55 and 65 years, e′ lateral should be >9 cm/s. Individuals >65 years normally have e′ of >8 cm/s. Also, note that the LAESVI that is proposed is >28 mL/m^2, a number that was present in the older guidelines.

Initially, abnormalities such as tachycardia, bradycardia, AV block, mitral annular calcification, prosthetic mitral valves, mitral stenosis, or mitral regurgitation >3+ should be eliminated, and the analysis for diastolic dysfunction can begin. Grade I diastolic dysfunction is likely present if the E/A is <0.8, and the e′ is abnormal for age and the LAESVI may or may not be >28 mL/m^2. Grade II diastolic dysfunction is present if E/A is 0.8, the e′ is abnormal for age, and the LAESVI is >28 mL/m^2. Grade III diastolic dysfunction is present if the E/A is >1.5, the e′ is abnormal for age, the LAESVI is >28, and the MVDT is <140 ms.

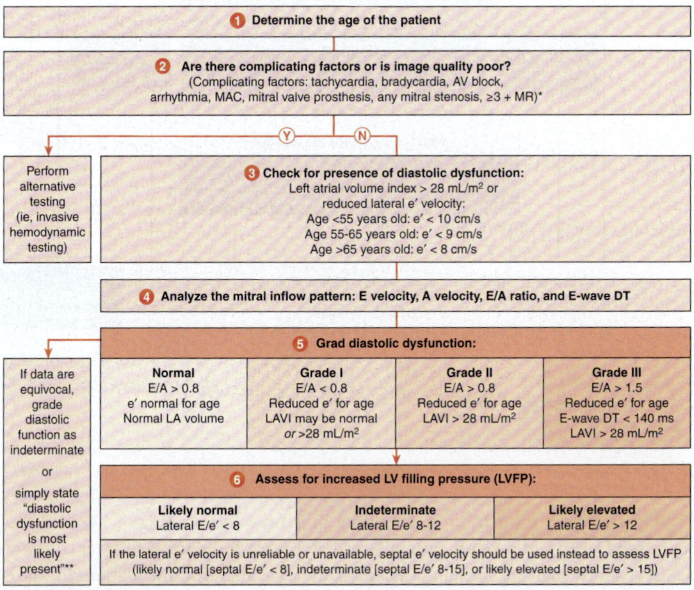

FIGURE 2.22 Algorithm for diagnosing diastolic dysfunction with Doppler echocardiography. A stepwise approach using E/A and E/e′ to diagnose diastolic dysfunction. Proper assessment is dependent on an accurate acquisition of transmitral flow and tissue Doppler imaging. A LAVI of >28 mL/m^2 (as opposed to a cutoff of >34 mL/m^2) is used in the algorithm presented to indicate an increased LA size, because obesity is a risk factor for diastolic dysfunction; thus, LAVI can underestimate LA enlargement in these individuals (due to indexing body size). *Although grading of diastolic dysfunction is not possible in these cases, the LVFP can still be estimated using surrogate markers, such as the estimated pulmonary artery systolic pressure or the end-diastolic pulmonary regurgitation gradient (as long as pulmonary arterial hypertension is not present). In older patients with normal sinus rhythm, systolic blunting of the pulmonary vein flow can be a sign of increased LA pressure. **It is not always possible to assign a diastolic dysfunction grade. In cases where equivocal data exist (eg, an E/A ratio >0.8, reduced e′ velocity, indeterminate range E/e′, and normal LAVI), one can simply state that "diastolic dysfunction is most likely present," without assigning a specific grade of diastolic dysfunction. In other cases, the e′ velocity may be normal, but LA volume may be increased and an E/A ratio of >1, which can be seen in cases of increased cardiac output or athlete's heart. In these cases, one can simply state, "diastolic function is most likely normal." A, late (atrial) transmitral flow velocity; AV, atrioventricular; DE, deceleration time; E, early diastolic transmitral flow velocity; e′, early diastolic mitral annular velocity; LA, left atrial; LAVI, left atrial volume index; LVFP, left ventricular filling pressure; LVEF, left ventricular ejection fraction; MAC, mitral annual calcification; MR, mitral regurgitation; NYHA, New York Heart Association. (From Mitter SS, Sanjiv SJ, Thomas JD. A test in contest: E/A and E/e′ to assess diastolic dysfunction and LV filling pressure. *J Am Coll Cardiol.* 2017;69(11):1451-1464.)

Further, an assessment of LV filling pressures can be made if E/e′ is analyzed. E/e′ lateral <8 suggests that LV filling pressures (LVEDP) are normal; in E/e′ lateral 8-12, the filling pressures are indeterminate, and E/e′ lateral >12 is suggestive of elevated LV filling pressures. Note that the lateral e′ is used for analysis since it is most reliably measured and is not influenced by the right ventricle and the MVDT is used especially in grade III diastolic dysfunction.

MITRAL VALVE DECELERATION TIME

Mitral valve deceleration time (MVDT) is the time interval measured from the peak of the E wave extrapolated to the baseline. It is measured by placing the sample volume at the tips of the mitral leaflets and measuring from the peak of the E wave. In normal young individuals, it is <240 ms and ranges in the normal adult from 150 to 240 ms. In grade I diastolic dysfunction, the E wave and the A wave are low and the deceleration time is prolonged >240 ms. In grade II diastolic dysfunction, the E wave has increased in height, and the mitral deceleration time is back in the normal range, 150-200 ms. In both grades I and II, the isovolumetric relaxation time (IVRT) is >90 ms; however, in the case of grade III diastolic dysfunction in which there is restrictive filling, the IVRT decreases to the 70 ms range. In grade III diastolic dysfunction, the E/A is increased, the MVDT is appreciated to <150, and if it does not reverse with Valsalva, it qualifies for grade IV or irreversible restrictive filling. These criteria have changed incorporating tissue Doppler, LAESV index, and TR jet velocity; however, a glance at the MVDT is helpful in sorting out the grades of diastolic dysfunction and estimation of LV filling pressures or mean LA pressure or mean pulmonary capillary wedge pressure. Depicted in Figure 2.23, the mitral valve deceleration slopes (red) from normal (A) to grade I diastolic dysfunction (B) and grade II diastolic dysfunction (C) and grade III diastolic dysfunction (D). The deceleration time from A to B increases as relaxation is prolonged requiring longer for LA and LV pressures to equilibrate, and as the left atrial pressure rises, the deceleration time shortens again as in C, and with marked diastolic dysfunction, it becomes very brief as depicted in D.

There is some redundancy in the use of MVDT in assessing diastolic dysfunction. In young healthy individuals with vigorous relaxation, the MVDT can be shortened due to vigorous suction effect, and the same abbreviated time can be seen with advanced diastolic dysfunction. The 2016 guidelines do not incorporate MVDT into the grading algorithm and offer a more simplified approach.[17,28]

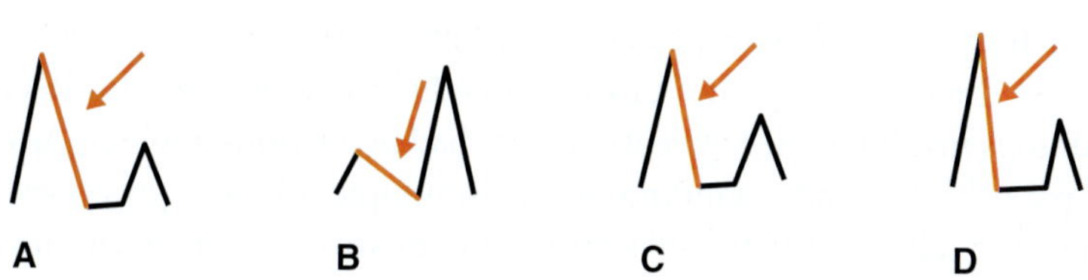

FIGURE 2.23

DIAGNOSING AND GRADING OF DIASTOLIC DYSFUNCTION

The identification and grading of diastolic dysfunction are useful in the individual presenting with the symptom of dyspnea. Left ventricular filling pressures are always elevated in individuals with dyspnea of cardiac origin. These pressures are reflected back into the pulmonary circulation and in extreme examples result in pulmonary edema and secondary hypertension.

In the day-to-day treatment of individuals with complaints of dyspnea, the echocardiogram can be helpful in assessing the clinical situation. The echocardiogram can be helpful in individuals with normal and abnormal systolic function of the left ventricle. For evaluation of diastolic function, echocardiographic parameters of diastolic function can identify the difficulty and offer some estimation of left ventricular filling pressure. Echocardiographic parameters as outlined in the guidelines include E/A ratio, mitral annular tissue Doppler velocities, tricuspid valve regurgitation velocity, and maximum left atrium volume index.[17]

Recently, an alternative classification has offered another approach to the classification of diastolic dysfunction and estimation of mean left atrial pressures or mean pulmonary capillary wedge pressure. The alternative classification focuses on the clinical setting, the age of the individual, the E/A ratio, the corresponding normal range for e′ for that age range, the LAESVI, and the MVDT.[29]

It is noteworthy that individuals do not always fit into distinct categories despite what algorithm is used, and in these situations, additional parameters can be used if needed such as analysis of pulmonary vein velocity profiles and pulmonary vein Ar velocity duration relative to mitral valve A wave velocity duration (Ar-A).

Examples of grading of diastolic dysfunction and assessment of filling pressures are in the digital version of this book.

SECTION 5

THE CARDIOMYOPATHIES

Despite extensive efforts in the past on behalf of many organizations, the classification of cardiomyopathies remains a difficult task. Interestingly, the term cardiomyopathy was first used in 1957 and was used to apply to those conditions in which the heart muscle, primarily the left ventricle, was involved in a disease process. The term idiopathic cardiomyopathy was often used to describe those conditions involving the left ventricle that had no obvious etiology. As more time has passed, the understanding of the multiple disease processes that can involve the left and right ventricles has broadened the classification categories.

In 1995, the World Health Organization proposed a classification to include dilated cardiomyopathy, hypertrophic cardiomyopathy (HCM), restrictive cardiomyopathy, and arrhythmogenic right ventricular cardiomyopathy.[30] This classification focused on structure and function. In 2006, the AHA task force proposed a new classification. The era of molecular genetics and the definition of ion channelopathies offer new categories, and classifications have expanded. This classification has major groupings of primary cardiomyopathies to include genetic, mixed, and acquired and then a grouping of secondary or acquired cardiomyopathies to include abnormalities such as amyloid.[31] Additional classifications have been proposed by the European group that are slightly different but includes those abnormalities that have molecular genetic links.[32]

These classifications tend to leave out the issues that are clinically common to include left ventricular dysfunction associated with coronary atherosclerosis ("ischemic cardiomyopathy"), the vague category of hypertensive heart disease, and left ventricular dysfunction associated with valve disease and that associated with congenital heart disease. For the clinician in daily practice, these categories are still termed cardiomyopathies associated with the underlying clinical entry.

These efforts to categorize diseases of the heart muscle or cardiomyopathies are manifestations of the expansion of understanding of the heart from the standpoints of structure, function, and molecular genetics—and are likely to further evolve in time.

The role of echocardiography has been major in our understanding of the structure and function of the myocardium not only in late stages but also in earlier stages of disease processes as they are acquired or genetic. Long-term trends in disease processes and the effects of specific treatment are definable by echocardiography.

In the following sections, various cardiomyopathies are displayed using echocardiography and other imaging techniques.

CLASSIFICATION OF CARDIOMYOPATHIES

- Dilated cardiomyopathy
  - Idiopathic dilated cardiomyopathy
  - Noncompaction
  - Tachycardia-induced cardiomyopathy
  - Takotsubo cardiomyopathy
- Restrictive cardiomyopathy
  - Amyloidosis
  - Other infiltrative processes
  - Loeffler endocarditis
- Hypertrophic cardiomyopathy

Dilated Cardiomyopathy

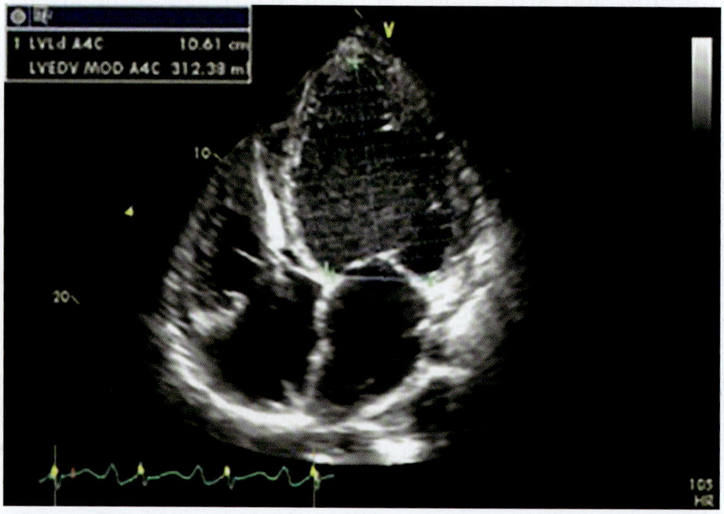

FIGURE 2.24

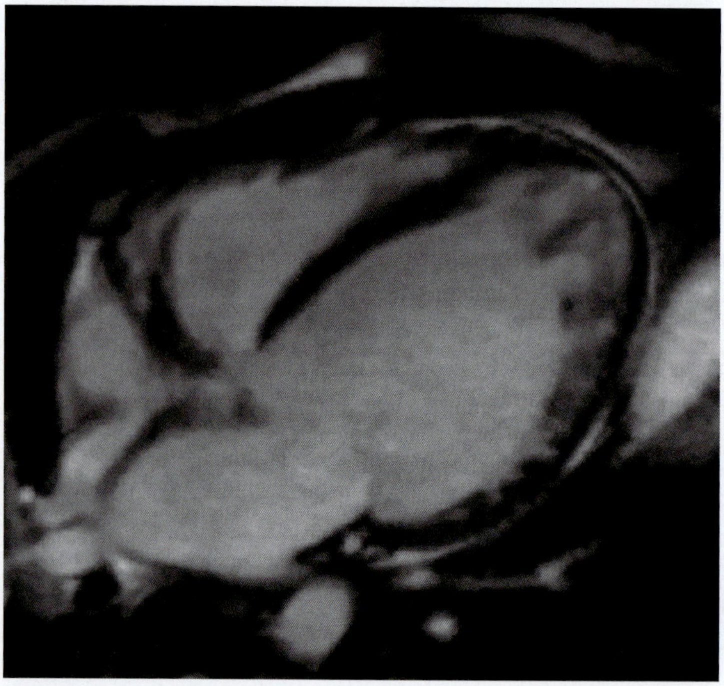

FIGURE 2.25

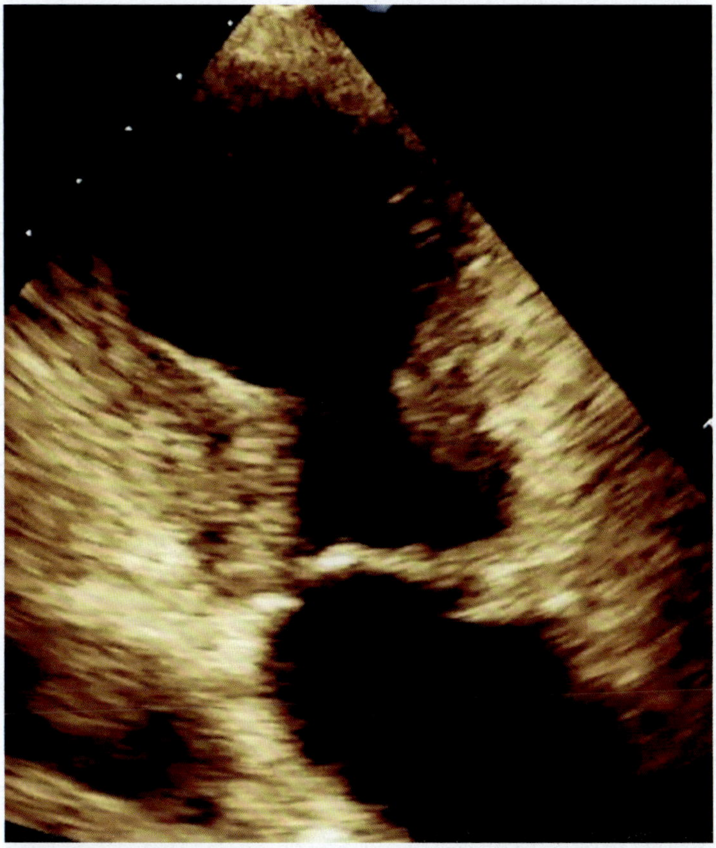

FIGURE 2.26

The three examples above are illustrations of dilated cardiomyopathy of various etiologies. The most common being idiopathic dilated cardiomyopathy. As one notes this entity at the bedside or with any imaging technique, then an etiology must be considered. Identification of an ischemic etiology, for example, could reveal a left main lesion or triple vessel disease that might require special treatment. The entity of noncompaction suggests the need to add special therapy such as defibrillator and anticoagulation. Takotsubo cardiomyopathy has precipitating factors that are often notable and implies a good prognosis on many occasions. Each encounter with this type of images requires a differential diagnosis that allows a special treatment plan for each entity. Imaging techniques and especially echocardiography offer opportunity to define etiologies and allow treatment to go forward.

Left Ventricular Thrombus in Dilated Cardiomyopathy

Left ventricular thrombus occurs in the setting of endothelial injury, a hypercoagulable state, and blood stagnation. These three conditions combined with a mural thrombus are known as Virchow triad.[33] Although Virchow in his day worked in the setting of venous thromboembolism, these principles also apply to the arterial system including the heart. In the case of coronary atherosclerotic heart disease and myocardial infarction with areas of hypokinesis or dyskinesis, the stage is set for mural thrombus formation.[34] Mural thrombi also occur in the setting of dilated cardiomyopathy and very low ejection fraction where at times very large mural thrombi form.[35] The role of antiplatelet therapy and anticoagulation with warfarin is still under investigation.[36]

The embolic potential of left ventricular thrombi is related to the characteristics of the thrombus itself. Physical characteristics that influence the embolic potential of a mural thrombus include mobility, protrusion into the left ventricular cavity, and central echo lucency.[33] The presence of a mural thrombus in the left ventricle and any of these characteristics increases the liability of embolization. In addition to echocardiography, mural thrombi can be demonstrated clearly on MRI along with the underlying wall motion abnormality. When gadolinium is used, mural thrombi do not enhance nor do they take up fluorodeoxyglucose (FDG) if positron emission testing is used. Despite of having some or all of these characteristics, some of the larger thrombi can sometimes resolve with anticoagulation without incident. In the following sections, these points are illustrated.

SECTION 6

LEFT VENTRICULAR THROMBUS

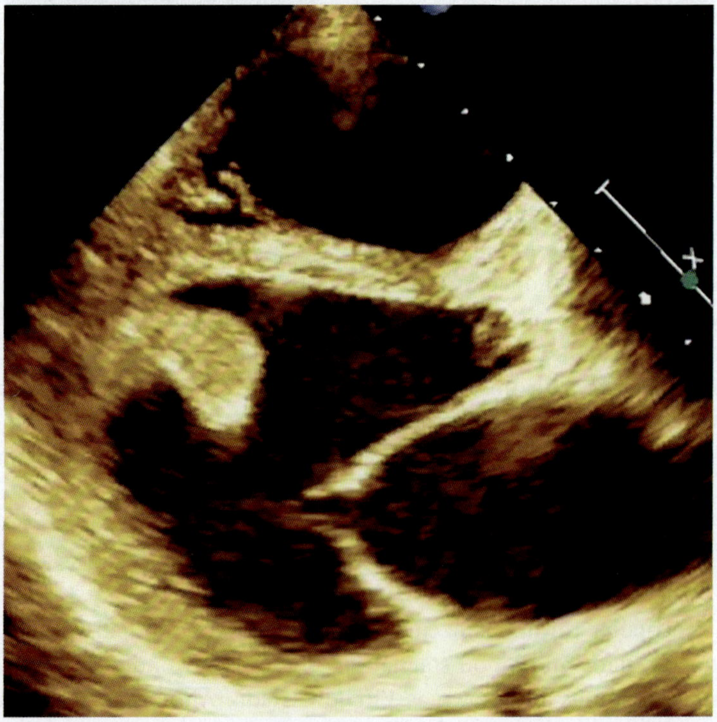

FIGURE 2.27 Apical mural thrombus with a mobile component pointing toward the LVOT is shown above. Sometimes, the "Chroma map" settings make mural thrombi more visible. TTE, PLX view with "Chroma map 2."

MRI WITH DELAYED ENHANCEMENT IMAGE

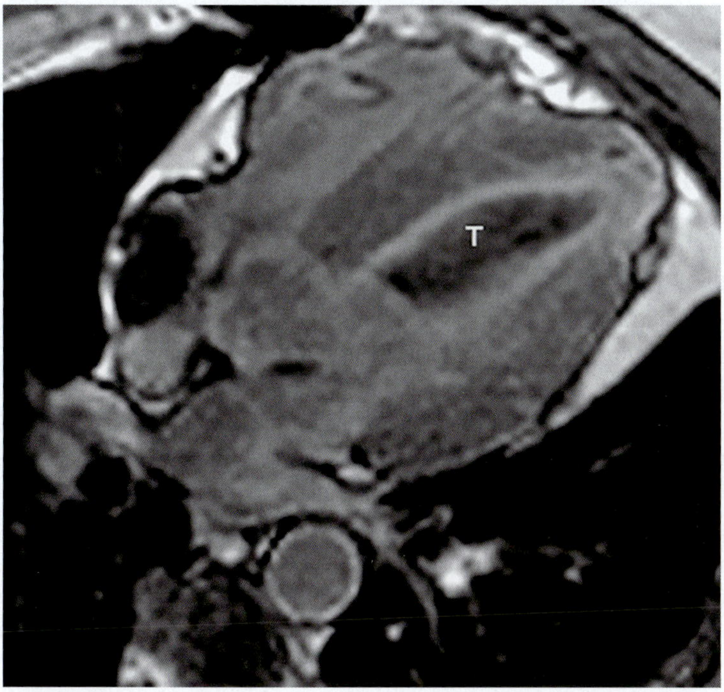

FIGURE 2.28 Delayed enhancement demonstrating that the thrombus (*T*) does not take up the gadolinium and that the heart muscle in general does. Apical four-chamber view.

SECTION 7

RESTRICTIVE CARDIOMYOPATHY[37]

The index disease process for this type of physiology is amyloidosis. This is classified as an infiltrative disorder and consists of deposition of abnormal proteins that are deposited in the endocardium, the interstitial spaces of the atrial and ventricular myocardium, and nearly every other part of the heart. There are other infiltrative cardiomyopathies to include sarcoidosis and mucopolysaccharidosis. Whereas in amyloid the proteins are deposited within the interstitial of the myocardium, another condition that produces similar physiology is associated simply with fibrotic changes in the interstitial spaces. This is termed "idiopathic fibrosis." In contrast to deposits in the interstitial spaces, the myocardial cells can be involved in a storage process as is seen in Fabry disease, hemochromatosis, and glycogen storage disease. There are a number of other conditions and disease processes that can cause restrictive cardiomyopathy and its associated physiology. These entities include the fibrotic phase of Loeffler endocarditis, endocardial fibroelastosis, carcinoid, postradiation, postchemotherapy, lymphoma, scleroderma, Churg-Strauss syndrome, and pseudoxanthoma elasticum.

CARDIAC AMYLOIDOSIS

The German pathologist Rudolph Virchow termed the condition of amyloidosis for the Greek term amylon or starch. This implies that the amyloid material is carbohydrate and not protein. This arose from the fact that amyloid proteins have an affinity for staining dyes with starch. As it turns out, the amyloid materials are proteins and not carbohydrates.[38]

Cardiac amyloidosis is an elusive diagnosis for many reasons. Earlier in our ability to recognize this condition, the focus was on searching for an etiology of heart failure, and attention was directed to the electrocardiogram and the echocardiogram. The dichotomy of low voltage on the electrocardiogram and thick walls on echo suggests the presence of infiltrative cardiomyopathy rather than left ventricular hypertrophy. Initially, systolic function was the focus, and later with techniques for evaluation of diastole, additional clues were noted. Cardiac transplantation and the subsequent development of expertise in cardiac biopsy allowed for tissue diagnosis of this condition. Special stains with Congo red and sulfonate Alcian blue offer diagnostic findings. Electron microscopy demonstrates nonbranching fibrillar architecture of the amyloid proteins.[39]

Multiple types of amyloidosis are known to be present; however, the most common is the light-chain (kappa and lambda) amyloidosis (AL). These abnormal light-chain proteins can be detected by immunofixation techniques. More recently, circulating levels of kappa and lambda light chains can be measured with quantitative techniques, and their ratio is important especially in the setting of renal impairment. Most frequently, in amyloid AL, excessive production of free lambda light chains are present and less commonly kappa light chains. A very low ratio of kappa to lambda (0.26) suggest a clone of cells producing excessive lambda light chains, whereas a ratio of kappa to lambda light chains (>1.65) suggests abnormal production of kappa light chains. Multiple myeloma should be searched for and is present in only a minority of the cases.[40] Another type of amyloidosis is that of familial amyloidosis in which the liver produces an unstable variant of the serum protein transthyretin (ATTR amyloidosis). A more common variety of this is seen in the black population in which the substitution of isoleucine for valine in position 122 is found in older individuals. Liver transplant as the treatment of this abnormality has been considered. Senile systemic amyloidosis is another type of amyloid that involves the wild type of transthyretin with heart involvement. Subtyping of amyloid is important to move to available and future treatment modalities.

The proteinaceous material is wrapped around the myocardial cells encasing them and producing a stiff muscle with abnormal diastolic and systolic properties. Diastolic dysfunction may precede systolic dysfunction and gives initial clues to the diagnosis.

More recently, abnormal patterns of strain have been demonstrated by speckle tracking techniques that show relative preservation of longitudinal strain toward the apex with a bull's-eye pattern on the map of global strain and have allowed for further recognition and understanding of this disease process. Magnetic resonance imaging has added to this diagnosis with abnormal gadolinium patterns being demonstrated.

Despite all of these modalities, we still often make this diagnosis very late in the course of illness, and therapy is limited and prognosis is poor.

CARDIAC AMYLOIDOSIS, 2D ECHO, HEART BIOPSY, AND GLOBAL PEAK SYSTOLIC STRAIN MAP

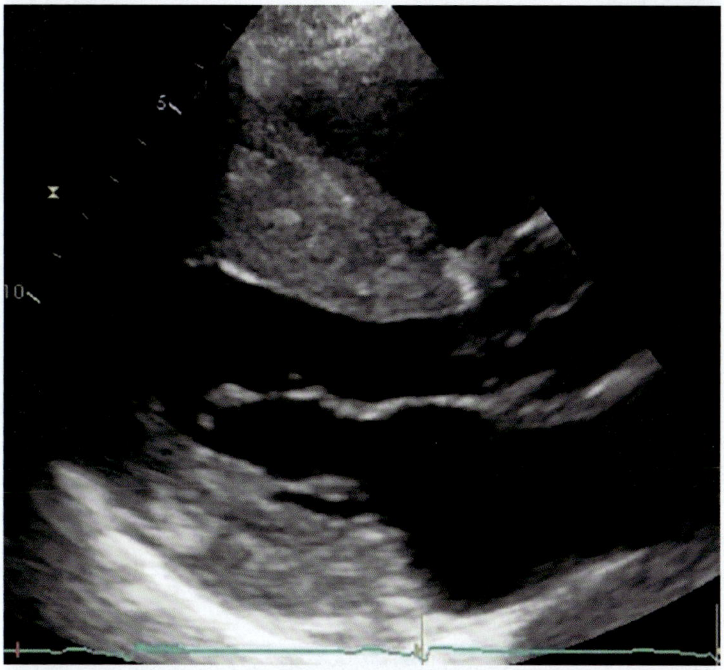

FIGURE 2.29 Illustrated above are thick walls of the left ventricle and bright sparkling echos from the myocardium all consistent with infiltrative cardiomyopathy. TTE, PLX view.

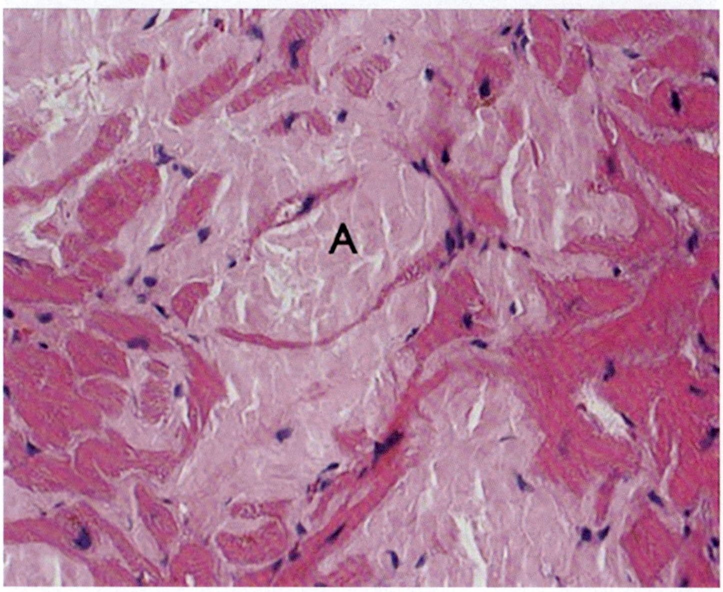

FIGURE 2.30 Hematoxylin and eosin stain showing amyloid material (*A*) in the interstitial space and surrounding the myocardial cells.

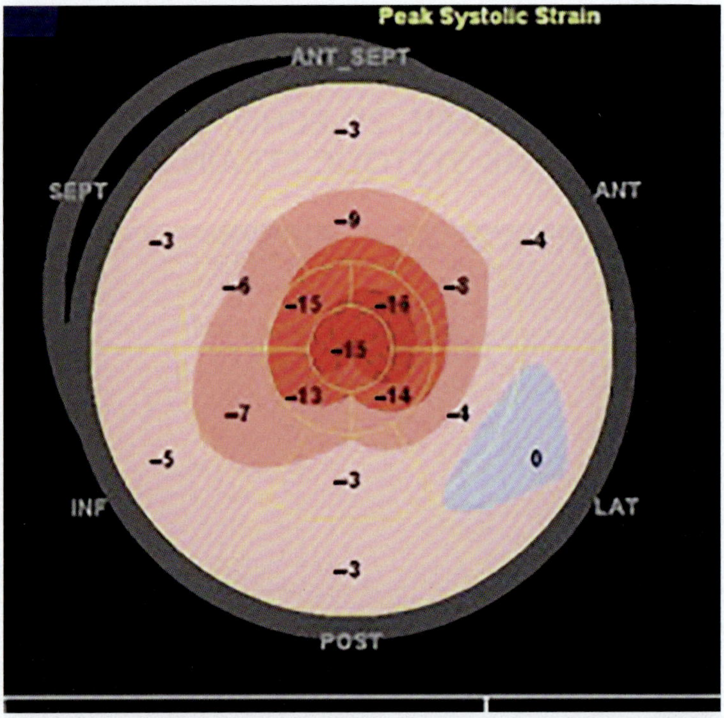

FIGURE 2.31 Peak systolic strain showing a "bull's-eye"–type pattern of global peak systolic strain using the speckle tracking technique demonstrates preservation of strain (to a degree) at the apex, a pattern known to be present when amyloid involves the left ventricle.

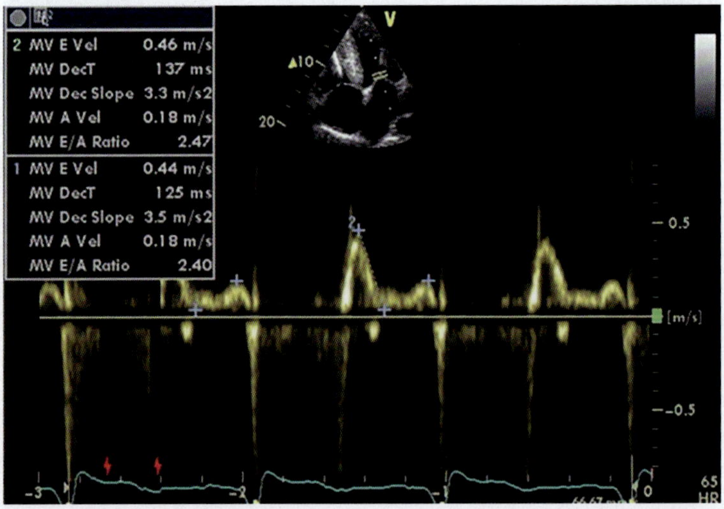

FIGURE 2.32

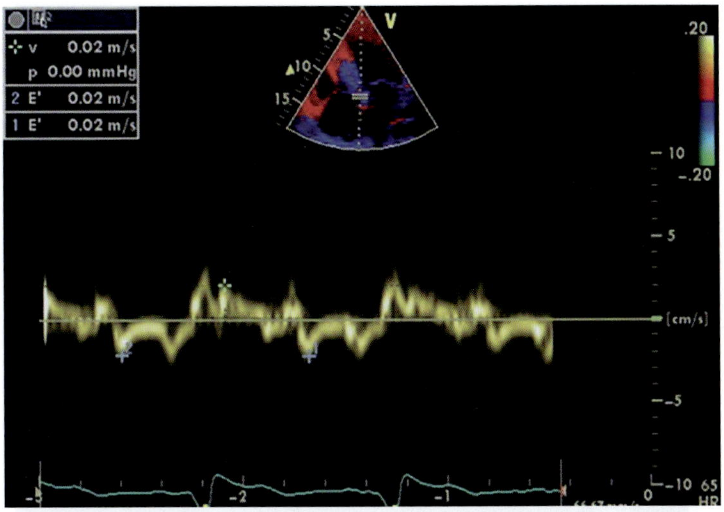

FIGURE 2.33

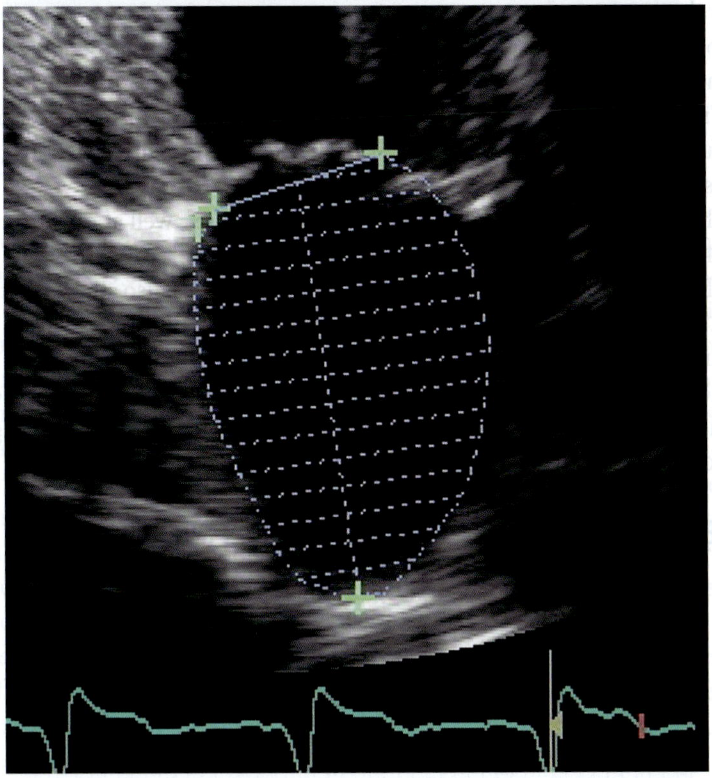

FIGURE 2.34

There are signs and symptoms that are clues to the diagnosis. They may be symptoms of shortness of breath on exertion from restrictive changes in the myocardium or a dynamic murmur of left ventricular tract obstruction noted on physical exam. Arrhythmias such as atrial fibrillation bring out the underlying left ventricular dysfunction or left ventricular hypertrophy, or even ventricular preexcitation is noted on the electrocardiogram. Unusual electrocardiograms with infarction patterns and the dramatic ST and T changes in the apical variety of this disease all give clues to the diagnosis. In the catheterization laboratory, characteristic pressure tracings that display quick upstroke and the "spike and dome" pattern in addition to a recordable intraventricular gradient may be present. The echocardiogram has been the "go-to" modality that has "nailed" the diagnosis after clinical clues point in that direction. The thickened interventricular septum, the systolic anterior motion of the aortic valve, and the systolic fluttering of the aortic valve are the "big three" for the diagnosis. Additional information from Doppler allows measurement of left ventricular outflow gradients, identification of turbulence in the left ventricular outflow tract and strain maps despite what appears to be a dynamic left ventricle reveal very abnormal measurements. CMRI demonstrates the anatomy and physiologic features of this entity with detailed displays of images from multiple views. Despite our classifications, the CMRI can detect unclassified regions of hypertrophy that help with the clinical diagnosis. The presence of myocardial scarring using this modality is key to the indications for insertion of a cardiac defibrillator.[50-54]

Certain physiologic situations offer opportunities at the bedside, the echocardiography laboratory, and the cardiac catheterization laboratory to make or confirm the diagnosis of HCM with obstruction. The postextrasystolic beat with enhanced contractility results in the appearance or accentuation of the left ventricular outflow gradient. Standing with the decreased venous return to the chest causes the heart to have less filling and accentuates the left ventricular outflow gradient as does the breath-holding phase of the Valsalva maneuver. Pharmacologic intervention with sublingual nitroglycerin causes venous pooling and some drop in arterial pressure and also accentuates the murmur. Other physiologic states such as hypovolemia and the use of adrenergic agents can accentuate the murmur and the left ventricular outflow tract gradient. In individuals with nonobstructive HCM, there may not be a murmur, and the electrocardiogram, echocardiogram, and CMRI may be needed to make a diagnosis.[55]

The mitral regurgitation that accompanies HCM has been studied in detail. The systolic anterior motion of the anterior mitral leaflet pulls apart the coaptation zones of the mitral leaflets and results in a variable degree of regurgitation. One factor in this mechanism is the length of the posterior mitral leaflet. The longer the posterior leaflet, the more of a chance it has of maintaining coaptation as the anterior leaflet is pulled away by systolic anterior motion.[56]

Therapy for HCM consists of medical therapy and septal reduction therapy. The three medications that are used include beta blockers, verapamil, and disopyramide. Each of these has negative inotropic qualities as well as some antiarrhythmic qualities. Septal reduction techniques include surgical myectomy and alcohol septal ablation (ASA).

Surgical treatment modalities for obstructive HCM have evolved over the years. Septal myectomy was developed by Andrew Morrow MD at the National Institutes of Health in the early 1960s. The operation involves the resection of a small amount of muscle (2-5 g) from the basal interventricular septum. Over the years, the procedure has been modified to include a more extensive resection (wider and deeper into the ventricle), modification of papillary muscles, removal of muscle bands, and, at times, modification of the anterior mitral leaflet. The goal is to widen the LVOT and thereby reduce systolic anterior motion of the mitral valve. The resulting reduction in LVOT obstruction and mitral regurgitation generally translates into improved symptoms.[57]

Septal reduction therapy (surgical myectomy or the catheter-based ASA) is generally reserved for patients with obstructive HCM (peak resting or provoked LVOT gradient >50 mm Hg) with significant symptoms despite adequate medical therapy. Surgical myectomy is the gold standard treatment for patients with obstructive HCM, suitable septal thickness (>15 mm), and acceptable surgical risk. In addition, ASA is a viable and effective treatment option for those with symptomatic obstructive HCM deemed not to be suitable surgical candidates.[58,59]

Treatment modalities are several and the use of echocardiography is key to guidance of these applications.

THE THREE ABNORMALITIES ON 2D AND M-MODE OF HOCM

1. Asymmetric septal hypertrophy
2. Systolic anterior motion of the aortic valve
3. Early closure and fluttering of the aortic valve

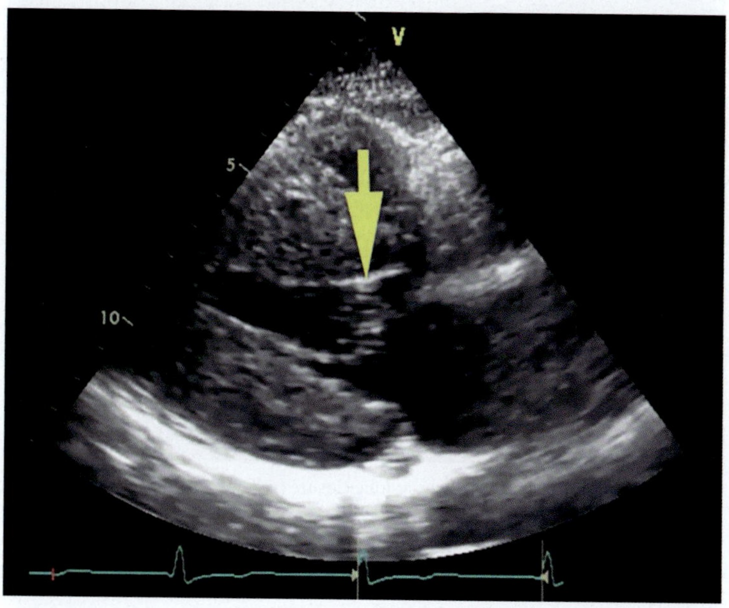

FIGURE 2.41 Hypertrophic cardiomyopathy with asymmetric hypertrophy and systolic anterior motion of the mitral valve producing subaortic obstruction. The tips of the AMVL come in contact with the interventricular septum (*yellow arrow*) and create obstruction and turbulence. TTE, PLX view.

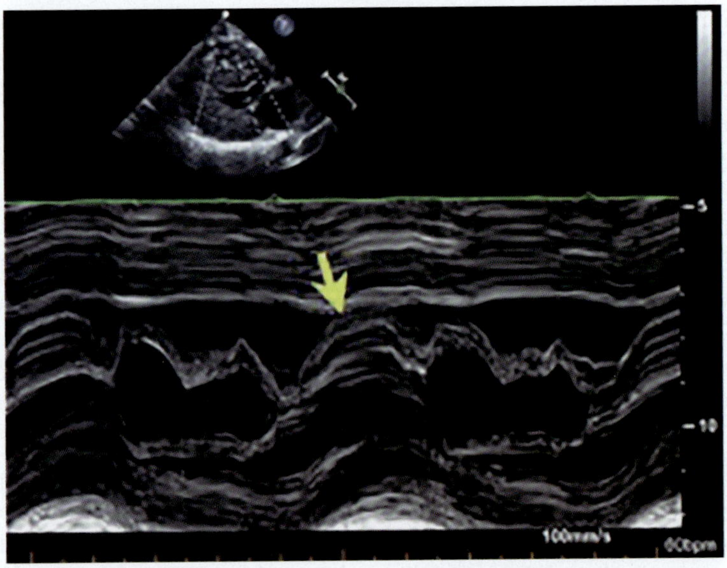

FIGURE 2.42 Systolic anterior motion of the mitral valve (*yellow arrow*) creating septal contact and obstruction to outflow. The degree of contact is related to the severity of obstruction. PLX view, M-mode tracing.

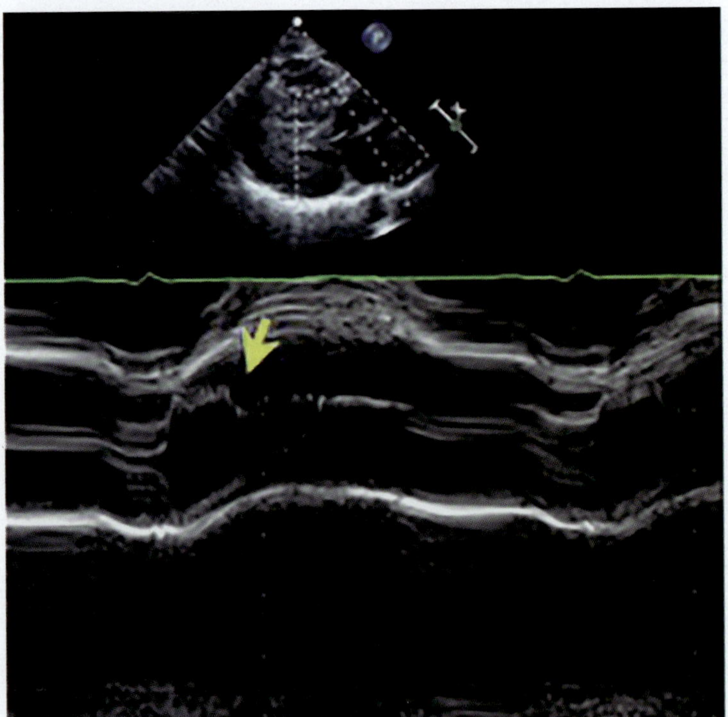

FIGURE 2.43 The aortic valve that shows early systolic closure (*yellow arrow*). PLX view, M-mode tracing.

ANATOMIC VARIANTS OF HYPERTROPHIC CARDIOMYOPATHY

- Hypertrophic obstructive cardiomyopathy (HOCM)
  - Left ventricular outflow obstruction
  - Mid ventricular obstruction
- Hypertrophic cardiomyopathy, concentric
- Apical hypertrophic cardiomyopathy

THE ELECTROCARDIOGRAM

Electrocardiographic Changes

- Left ventricular hypertrophy
- Unusual patterns of infarction
- Ventricular preexcitation
- Bazaar ST and T waves with giant negative T waves in the precordium

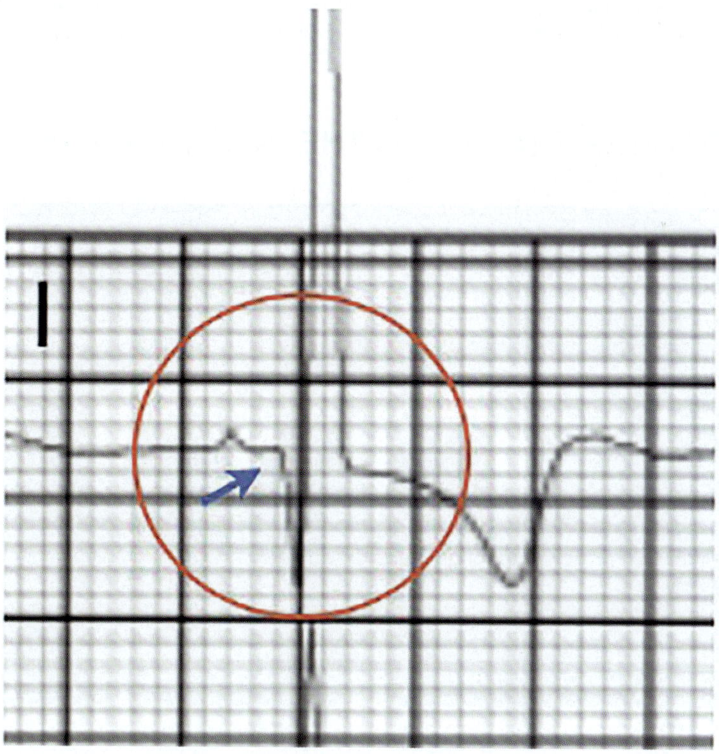

FIGURE 2.44 The striking initial forces in lead I show a very large abnormal Q wave or abnormal initial forces mimicking the pattern of myocardial infarction.

THE VENTRICULOGRAM

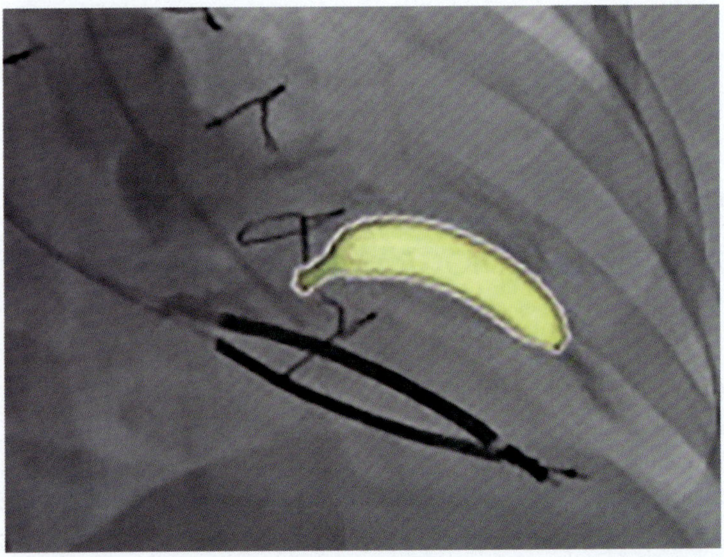

FIGURE 2.45 During systole, the left ventricle is small and has a crescent or *banana shape*. The small left ventricular cavity often makes it difficult to find a stable position of the catheter for measurement of intracavitary gradients.

THE DAGGER SHAPE AND THE VALSALVA MANEUVER

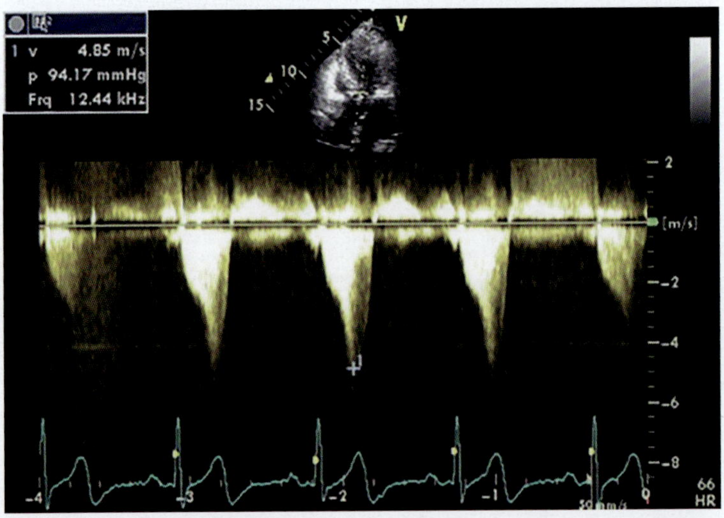

FIGURE 2.46 The provoked gradient with Valsalva maneuver showing an increased gradient up to 94 mm Hg. The Doppler curve has a late systolic peak and is shaped like a dagger.

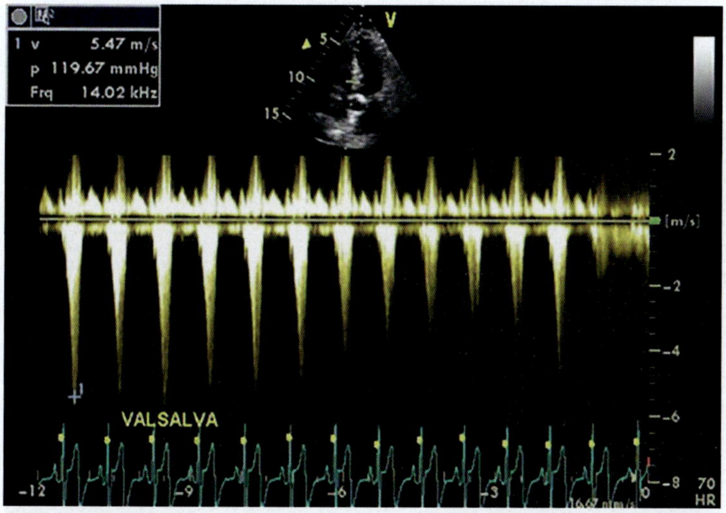

FIGURE 2.47 Releasing the Valsalva maneuver and observing the gradient declining from the 120 mm Hg range to 50 mm Hg range.

APICAL HYPERTROPHY (YAMAGUCHI SYNDROME)

In this entity, apical HCM or Yamaguchi syndrome, the hypertrophy is localized to the apex, or it is generalized and most prominent at the apex. Small pouch-like aneurysms develop at the apex. Early on, it has a generally good prognosis; however, as the process evolves and more hypertrophy occurs, scarring and diastolic dysfunction develop, and arrhythmias occur, the overall situation changes to a more unfavorable state. Initially, the EKG may not show more than changes of left ventricular hypertrophy as is seen in one of the examples; however, later on the characteristic changes of very prominent voltage, dramatic ST changes with elevation in the lateral precordial leads, prolonged QT interval, and "giant negative T waves" as first described by Yamaguchi[60] appear in the precordial leads leading to the diagnosis. The electrocardiographic, echocardiographic, and CMRI findings in the cardiac catheterization laboratory are illustrated in the following panels.

THE ECHOCARDIOGRAM, THE ELECTROCARDIOGRAM, AND THE CARDIAC MAGNETIC RESONANCE IMAGE

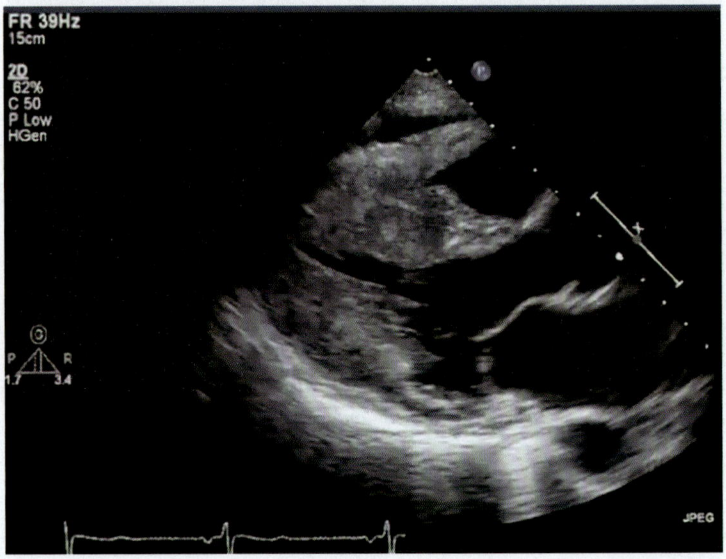

FIGURE 2.48 Apical hypertrophic cardiomyopathy is shown with cavity obliteration at the apex and extremely thick walls. The right ventricle also has apical hypertrophy. TTE, PLX view.

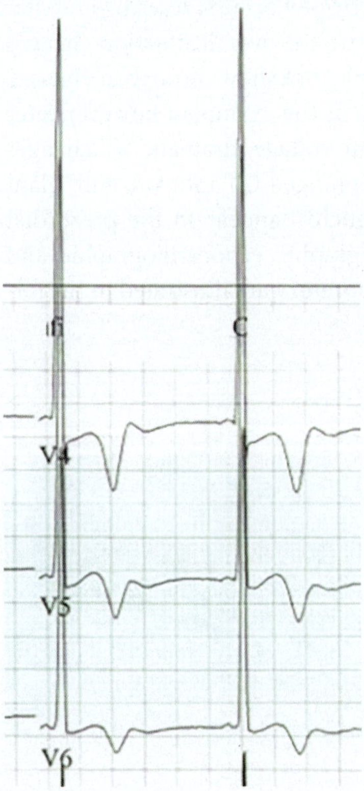

FIGURE 2.49 ECG shows tremendous voltage and unusual ST and T changes in the inferior and lateral precordial leads consisting of upsloping ST elevation and associated T-wave inversion. The T vector is toward the right shoulder, yet the ST vector is downward. In classic LVH, the ST and T vectors both point toward aVR together.

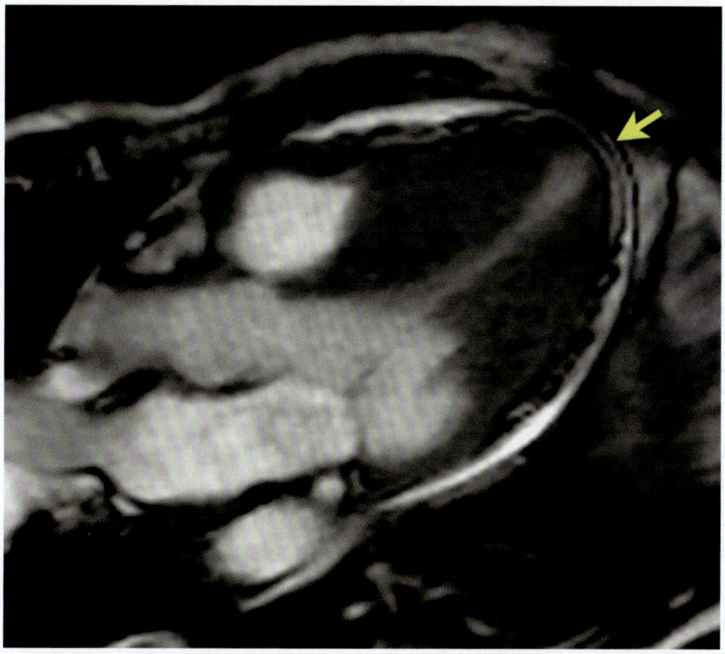

FIGURE 2.50 Inflow view of the left ventricle that demonstrates no significant systolic anterior motion of the mitral valve and cavity obliteration at the apices. There is a small pouchlike area at the apex (*yellow arrow*) as is sometimes seen in this disease process.

TREATMENT OF HYPERTROPHIC OBSTRUCTIVE CARDIOMYOPATHY

Several categories of treatment of HCM are currently available. Medical treatment with agents that have a negative inotropic effect includes beta-blockers, calcium channel blockers, and disopyramide.[50,58,61,62] In past years, pacemakers have been used to alter the sequence of contraction of the interventricular septum and therefore decrease the left ventricular outflow gradient. Surgery has been performed to remove the portion of the hypertrophic myocardium that is part of the obstruction (Morrow procedure). Additionally, the mitral valve has been replaced in order to remove the component of obstruction that was offered by the anterior leaflet of the mitral valve. Alcohol septal ablation of the appropriated septal perforator supplying the interventricular septum also has had suggest in relieving left ventricular outflow gradients.

Important findings that suggest that intensive treatment is needed:

- Symptoms of shortness of breath on exertion, light-headedness, or chest pain
- History of syncope or cardiac arrest
- Failure to increase BP with exercise or a >20 mm drop in BP with exercise
- Ventricular tachycardia documented on ambulatory monitoring
- Resting or provoked LVOT gradient of >50 mm Hg
- Adverse family history
- >30-mm thickness of the interventricular septum or any segment of the left ventricle

ALCOHOL SEPTAL ABLATION

Alcohol septal ablation (ASA) is a technique that utilizes the effects of isopropyl alcohol on the myocardium when injected directly into the vessel of interest. In the case of HCM, an appropriate septal perforator is chosen at the time of the coronary arteriogram that is localized in the hypertrophic area. Echocardiography is used to locate the appropriate perforator. This vessel is wired and cannulated with a small catheter followed by injection of echo contrast. In the cath lab using transthoracic echo, the corresponding myocardium to the septal perforator becomes bright. This should match the area of concern at the mitral-septal contact point. Once the appropriate location is identified, absolute alcohol is injected and the vessel becomes occluded and the myocardium is injured. A controlled myocardial infarction occurs.[1,59]

With proper selection, this process results in a gradual decrease in the gradient at this specific point while being observed in the cardiac catherization laboratory. Hemodynamic and echocardiographic monitoring follows over the short period after injection looking for the desired effect. Monitoring of the cardiac rhythm is also necessary since occasionally these individuals develop complete AV block that requires a permanent pacemaker. Temporary pacing is in place during the procedure for use if needed.[63,64]

ASA is indicated in older individuals who are not acceptable surgical candidates. Early outcomes may be similar in these two techniques; however, the longer-term results may be influenced by arrhythmias from ventricular scarring that are yet to be defined. Surgery is the first line of treatment in younger individuals because of these factors. In addition, ASA in individuals with septal thickness of >30 mm is of questionable benefit.[62]

HYPERTROPHIC CARDIOMYOPATHY, IMAGES IN THE CARDIAC CATHETERIZATION LABORATORY

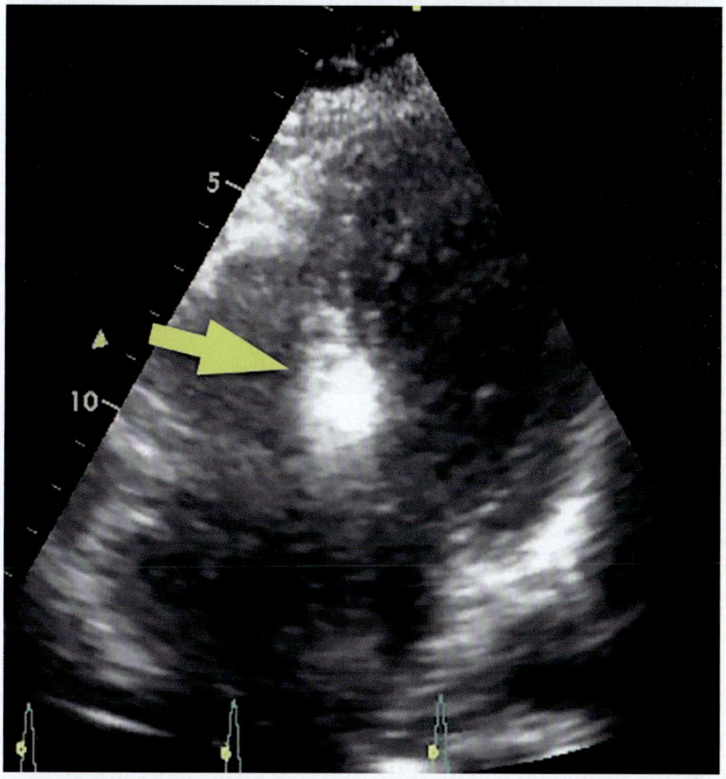

FIGURE 2.51 A septal perforator has been selected and contrast has been injected. The location is appropriate and alcohol injection follows.

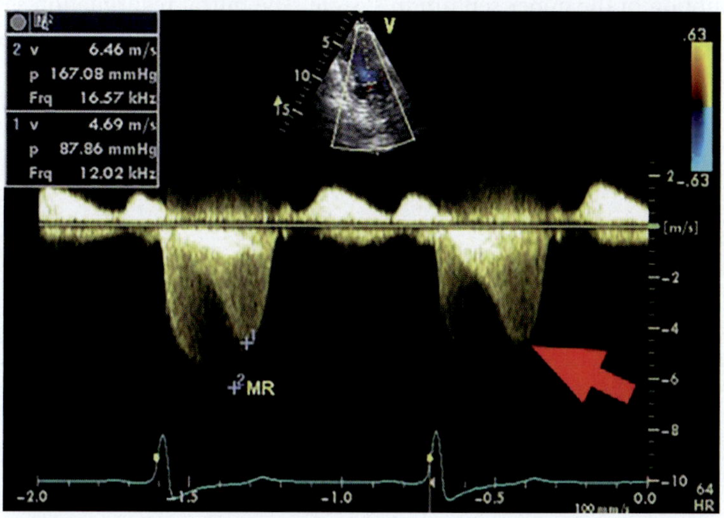

FIGURE 2.52 Before alcohol septal ablation, the late peaking gradient in the left ventricular outflow region measures 88 mm Hg (*red arrow*). The MR jet has an earlier peak and a longer duration and is usually a much higher velocity. The "dagger"-shaped velocity profile is the appropriate profile for the outflow obstruction gradient calculation.

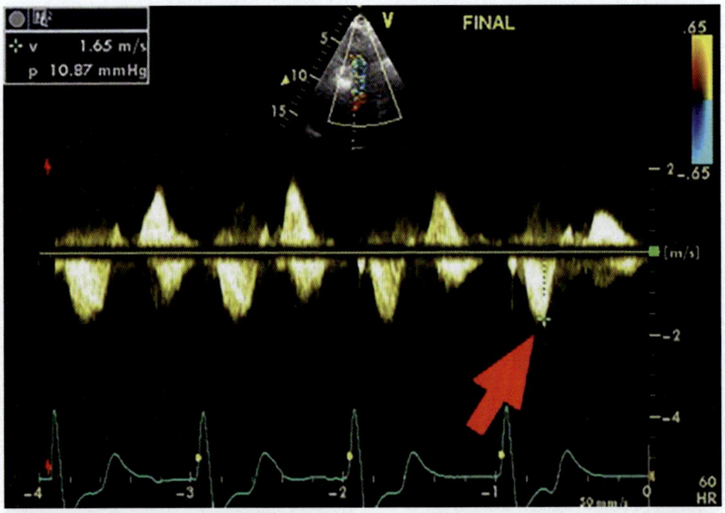

FIGURE 2.53 Final gradients are obtained from the apex with transthoracic Doppler and noted to be acceptable in the 11 mm Hg range (*red arrow*). These are also checked from a hemodynamic standpoint.

SURGICAL TREATMENT: THE "MORROW PROCEDURE"

Surgery is the treatment of choice in individuals who are suitable candidates for this procedure. The procedure consists of a transaortic approach and resection of a rectangular-shaped segment of the hypertrophy from the base of the right coronary cusp to ~1 cm below the anterior mitral leaflet/septal contact point. Transesophageal monitoring can aid in determining the septal thickness and defining the depth and length of the resected area. Care must be taken to avoid creating a ventricular septal defect or high-grade AV block. Left bundle-branch block often follows this procedure, which in itself can be helpful as it changes the motion of the upper septum in systole. The mitral regurgitation seen associated with HOCM usually improves with surgical resection of the hypertrophic region.[65-67]

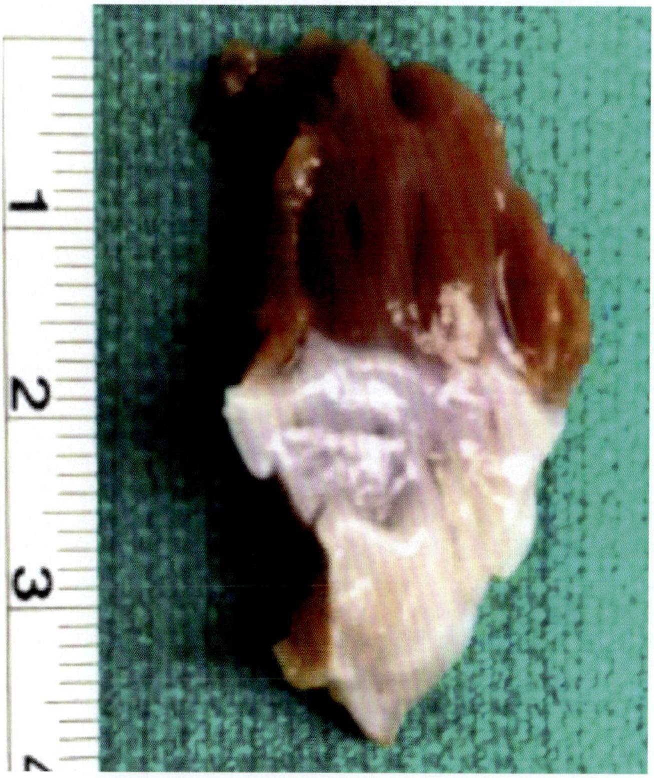

FIGURE 2.54 A surgical specimen from a Morrow procedure showing the endocardium and excised segment of the basal septum that has been removed from the left ventricular outflow tract.

GROSS AND MICROSCOPIC FINDINGS IN HYPERTROPHIC

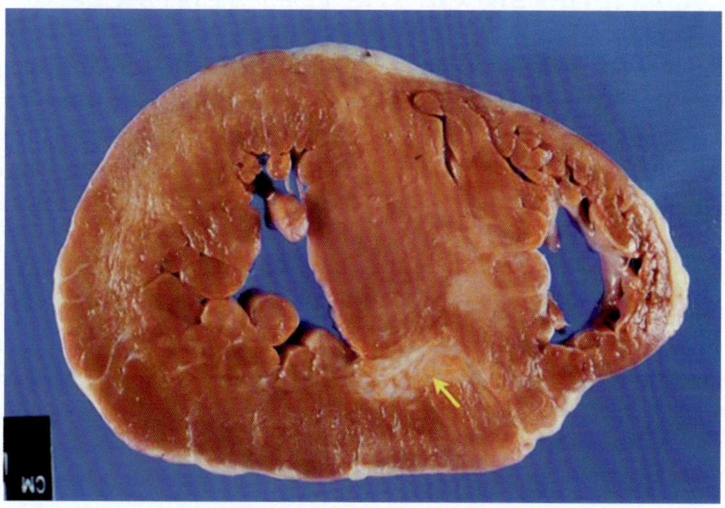

FIGURE 2.55 Cross section of a gross specimen in an individual with hypertrophic cardiomyopathy with severe asymmetric septal hypertrophy and scarring. *Yellow arrows* indicate scarring. This scarring has arrhythmia potential (ventricular tachycardia) and further worsens systolic and diastolic function. Scar is known to be located at the junction of the free wall of the left and right ventricle and the inter ventricular septum.[50,68] Courtesy of Dr. Michael Gravanis.

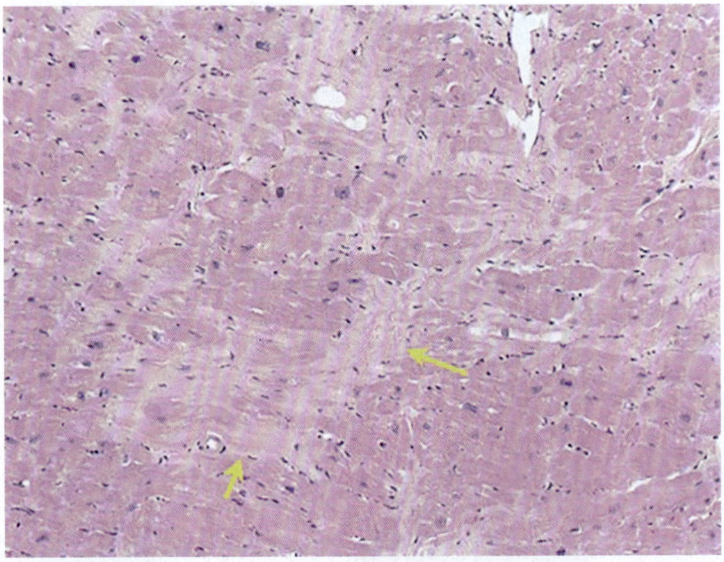

FIGURE 2.56 Myocardial fiber disarray (from a myomectomy specimen) in another patient with hypertrophic cardiomyopathy—fibers coursing in various directions and significant scarring are present (*yellow arrows*). Small intramural vessels in these areas have intimal dysplasia, which is thought to play a role in the pathogenesis of scar.[50,68]

SECTION 9

LEFT VENTRICULAR ANEURYSM

DEFINITIONS OF TRUE ANEURYSM AND PSEUDOANEURYSM OF THE LEFT VENTRICLE

A true left ventricular aneurysm is a distortion of the shape of the left ventricular cavity both in systole and diastole. The wall consists of remnants of myocardium in addition to scar. The neck is wide in that the ratio of the neck to the maximum diameter of the cavity is >50%. Often, there is laminated thrombus present. These can be located anywhere that myocardial infarction occurs. The echocardiogram shows the broad neck and the distortion of the left ventricular cavity in addition to various degrees of mural thrombus. The wall of the aneurysm moves dyskinetically in systole. The MRI shows scarred myocardium in the remaining wall. The EKG often shows persistent changes of acute myocardial infarction in which Q waves are present along with persistent ST and T wave changes that have not continued to evolve after the acute event.

A pseudoaneurysm of the left ventricle is the result of a contained rupture of the heart usually in the setting of a prior myocardial infarction. The wall consists of pericardium that is subjected to left ventricular pressure. Pericarditis has often accompanied the infarction. These can be located anywhere that myocardial infarction has occurred. The neck of these pseudoaneurysms is often narrow relative to the diameter of the cavity (>50%), and laminated thrombus is often present. On the echocardiogram and the MRI, the entrance points start abruptly as if there is a disconnect of the walls from each other. This effect is produced by the tear of the wall as the blood has dissected through the acutely injured myocardium.

Although these definitions have been put forth, it is not always possible to categorize these aneurysms accurately. It is important to do so since pseudoaneurysms do progressively enlarge and rupture. In addition, although these examples focus on myocardial infarction as an etiology, occasionally there can be other causes such as congenital disease, trauma, and infection.[69]

TRUE VENTRICULAR ANEURYSM

Ventricular aneurysms may present in many ways. Individuals with ventricular aneurysms may evolve under observation after a large myocardial infarction, or they may present with angina pectoris, symptoms of left ventricular dysfunction, or ventricular arrhythmias some period after infarction. The geometric distortion of the left ventricle produces a mechanical disadvantage and left ventricular dysfunction may occur. Energy ordinarily used for ejection of blood from the left ventricular cavity is used to expand the aneurysm. Adjacent segments of myocardium are placed under extra stress and can become ischemic producing angina pectoris. The junction of scar and viable tissue is a nidus for electrical instability and the generation of ventricular arrhythmias. Therefore, left ventricular dysfunction, myocardial ischemia, and ventricular arrhythmias may accompany ventricular aneurysms. In addition, areas of slow flow and endothelial dysfunction lead to thrombus formation and peripheral embolization may occur. The hallmark of electrocardiographic changes is the persistence of ST and T wave changes. The changes of acute infarction do not undergo the normal evolutionary process.

Anatomically, these aneurysms have a relatively broad neck or entrance region, and the walls have scarred, thinned myocardium. Thrombus may or may not be present. Clinicians are aware of the situation of large dyskinetic areas especially in the anterior wall and apex and frequently give anticoagulants to prevent thrombus formation.

LEFT VENTRICULAR ANEURYSM WITH MURAL THROMBUS

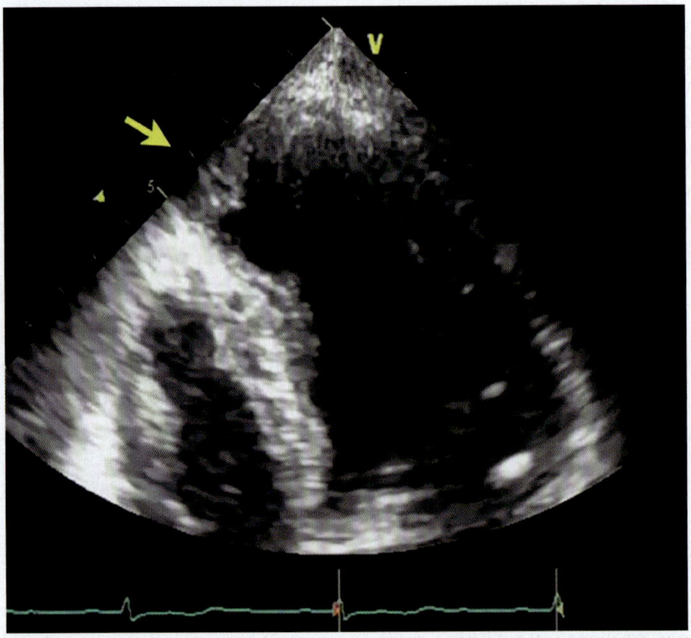

FIGURE 2.57 Left ventricular aneurysm at the apex of the left ventricle that does contain a thrombus (*yellow arrow*). TTE, A4C view.

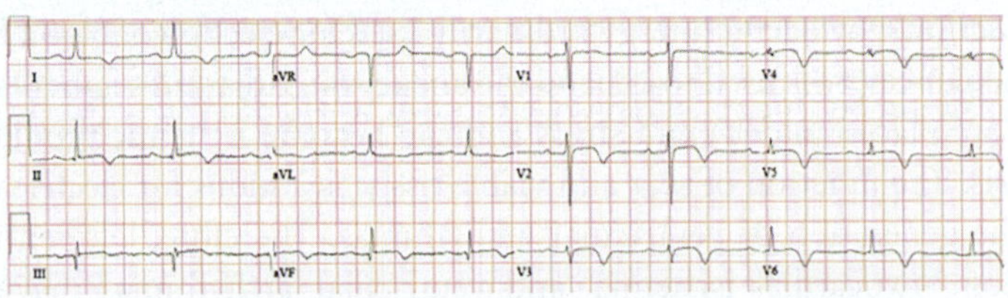

FIGURE 2.58 The EKG in this individual showing anterolateral ST and T changes that are persistent and did not change over several years. There is "persistent ST-segment elevation" in some leads.

VENTRICULAR PSEUDOANEURYSM[69]

Pseudoaneurysm results from rupture or dissection of blood through the myocardial wall. By definition, there is no remaining myocardium. This rupture essentially forms a clot in the pericardial space that becomes organized and contains the rupture. Sometimes it is a small discrete area, and other times it can be extensive. Characteristically, the neck or entrance to the pseudoaneurysm is relatively narrow compared to the aneurysm itself. Generally, these aneurysms progressively enlarge and have the potential to rupture.

If the entrance regions of these pseudoaneurysms are narrow enough, they sometimes can be closed with devices percutaneously. Otherwise, surgery is needed if the clinical situation will permit.

The electrocardiogram in the situation of ventricular pseudoaneurysm is sometimes not diagnostic. Often, this occurs relatively soon after infarction, and there is

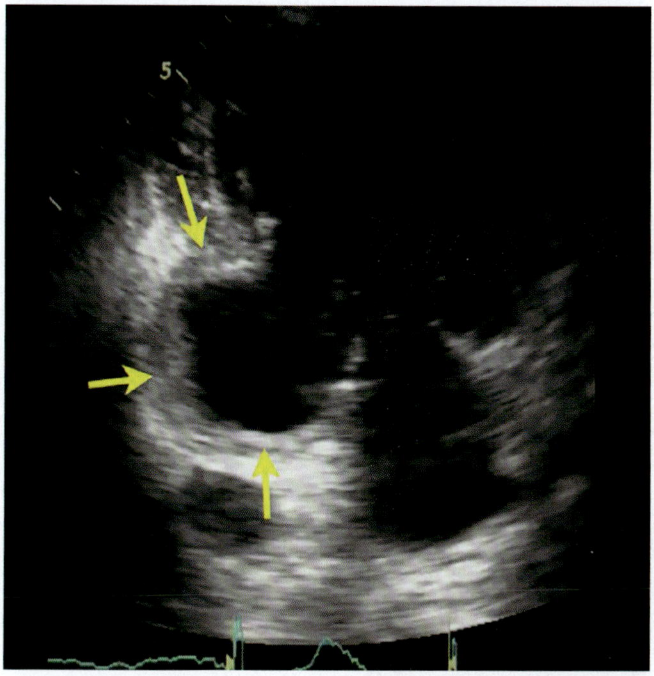

FIGURE 2.59 Basal inferior left ventricular pseudoaneurysm that has a relatively narrow neck and dyskinesis of the entire area. Mural thrombus lines this pseudoaneurysm. The wall does not contain muscle. This basically represents a "contained rupture" of the left ventricle associated with a prior acute myocardial infarction (*yellow arrows*). TEE, A2C view.

a large infarction. On the other hand, it can occur in the setting of a relatively small infarction, and the electrogram may not demonstrate major changes. The echocardiogram is a valuable tool in the postinfarction state and makes the diagnosis.

BASAL POSTERIOR LATERAL PSEUDOANEURYSM DEMONSTRATED ON MAGNETIC RESONANCE IMAGING

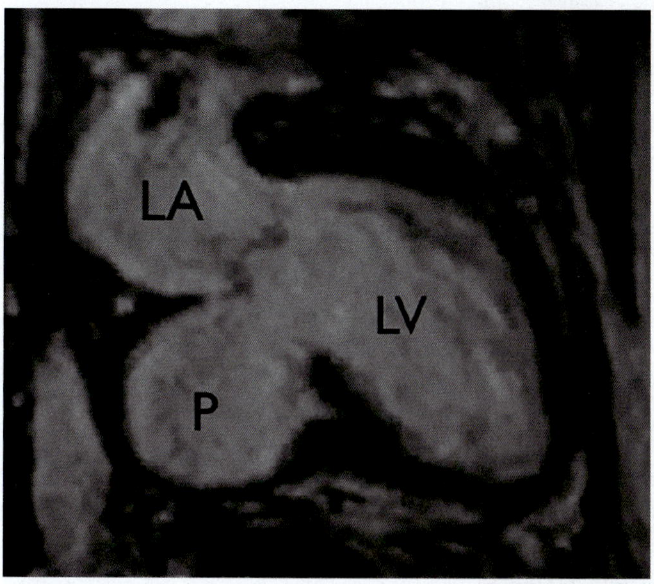

FIGURE 2.60 Still frame in a two-chamber view showing the pseudoaneurysm. LA, left atrium; LV, left ventricle; P, pseudoaneurysm.

SECTION 10

MECHANICAL COMPLICATIONS OF MYOCARDIAL INFARCTION

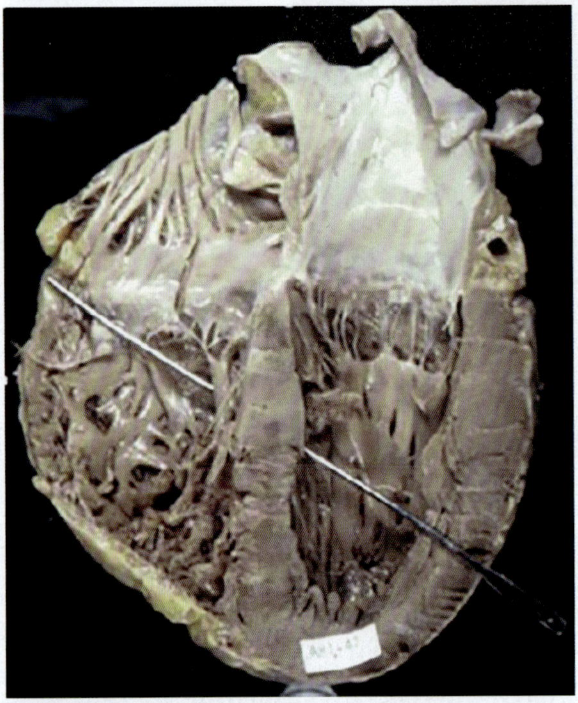

FIGURE 2.61 Ruptured interventricular septum.

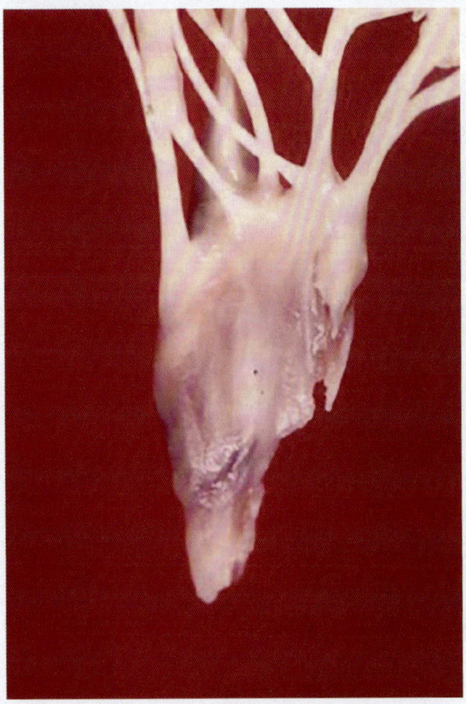

FIGURE 2.62 Ruptured papillary muscle.

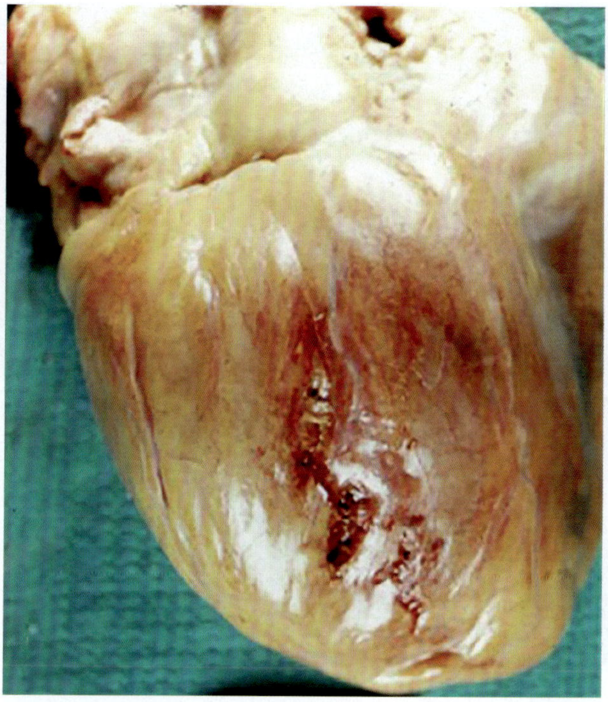

FIGURE 2.63 Ruptured heart.

VENTRICULAR SEPTAL RUPTURE COMPLICATING ACUTE MYOCARDIAL INFARCTION[70]

Ruptured interventricular septum comes in a variety of sizes and shapes. Small defects located at the apex or base result in small shunts and larger defects with larger shunts. The impact of these defects is related to the degree of shunting and also the size of the underlying infarction. The defects at the apex are associated with lesions in the left anterior descending and those at the base are largely associated with the right coronary artery or the distal circumflex when the circulation is dominant left.

The defects are often a tear rather than a round defect. Once the endocardium on the left is disrupted, the effects of pressure dissect through the layers of the damaged myocardium. The size of the underlying infarction is important in that the more the damage, the more the difficulty in dealing with the clinical situation. Sometimes the infarction is relatively small, and at other times there is even aneurysmal formation in the region of rupture.

If the rupture is in the basal region and associated with the right coronary artery, the function of the right ventricle is pivotal in the potential to survive. A proximal right coronary artery occlusion associated with right ventricular infarction and ruptured interventricular septum is not a good combination.

At the bedside, the murmur of ruptured interventricular septum is often loud and holosystolic. If the systolic blood pressure is not at shock levels and there is a significant gradient across the defect from left to right, then a loud murmur will be present. If hemodynamics deteriorate, then the murmur will lessen, not a good sign. As in congenital interventricular defect, the louder the murmur, the smaller the defect, and the larger the defect, the less loud the murmur.

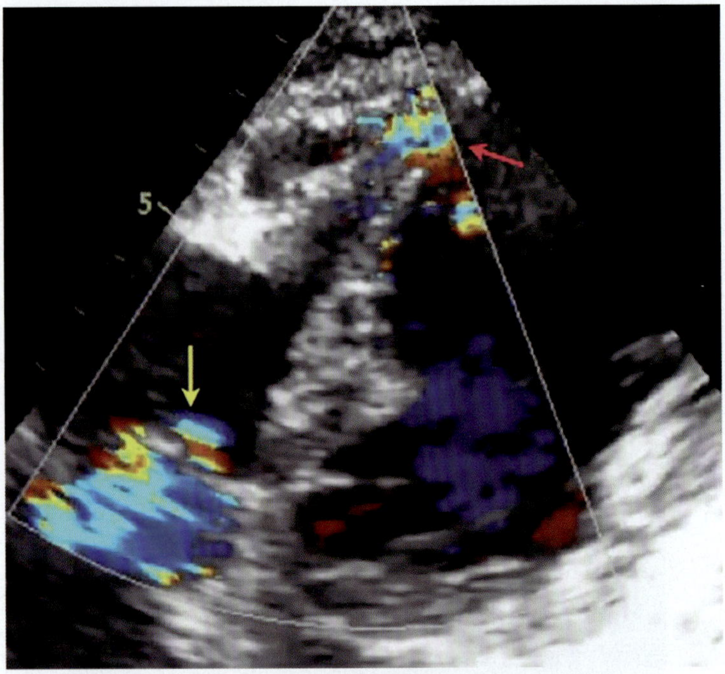

FIGURE 2.64 Color Doppler showing turbulence and PISA (*red arrow*) at the apex coursing through the thinned distal septum and into the apex of the RV. In addition, there is hypokinesis of the distal septum and the right ventricular apex. Tricuspid regurgitation has developed (*yellow arrow*). TTE, A4C view with color Doppler.

PARTIAL RUPTURE OF THE PAPILLARY MUSCLE[71]

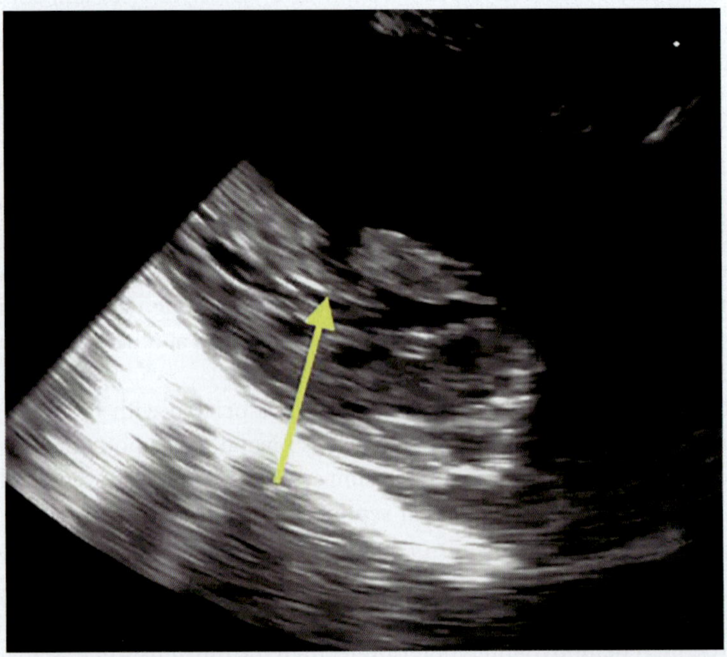

FIGURE 2.65 Partial rupture of the anterolateral papillary muscle is shown (*yellow arrow*). TEE, 89° transgastric view.

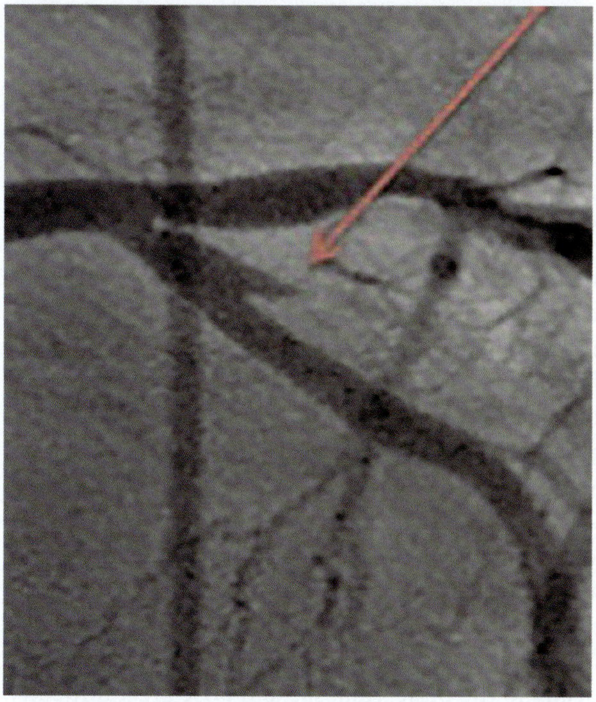

FIGURE 2.66 Coronary arteriogram shows total occlusion of the anterior marginal branch of the circumflex (*red arrow*).

RUPTURED HEART

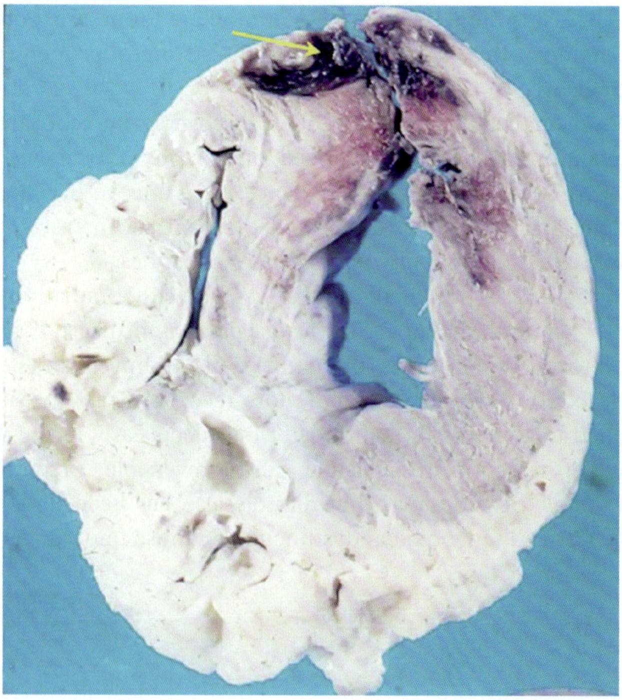

FIGURE 2.67 This ruptured heart was associated with inferior myocardial infarction. These events are often about 7 days out from the acute event; however, sometimes they are earlier or later. The necrotic endocardium loses its integrity, and a rent or tear develops followed by a variable degree of dissection into the wall by pressure forces until it reaches the epicardium. It then ruptures into the pericardium and catastrophe occurs or if contained by thrombus or clot a pseudoaneurysm forms. In the example above, the epicardium could not contain the rupture nor could a clot so the patient expired. The subendocardial injury is more extensive than the subepicardial injury as dictated by the blood supply. In this example, a subepicardial clot formed (*yellow arrow*) that eventually gave way to the intraventricular pressure and the epicardium ruptured into the pericardium. Pathologic specimen courtesy of Dr. HLJ Mario.

SECTION 11

CANCER AND THE LEFT VENTRICLE

Early identification and treatment and longer survival rates in those who have cancer have resulted in cardiac involvement being more noticeable. The most common tumors of the heart are benign (myxoma) and the most common primary malignant tumor of the heart is sarcoma.

Secondary or metastatic tumors spread to the heart in four different pathways: through the blood or the hematogenous route, lymphatic spread, transvenous extension, and direct extension. Hematogenous spread results in myocardial or endocardial metastasis as is seen with melanoma, lymphoma, and sarcoma. Lymphatic spread such as is seen with tumors nearby in the breast or lung results in pericardial and epicardial involvement. Renal and hepatic tumors extend up into the inferior vena cava and extend directly into the right atrium. Mesotheliomas of the pleura, mediastinum, and pericardium arise and extend locally to the pericardial sac and pose great difficulty. Cancer prefers to spread to the pericardium first, to the epicardium and myocardium next, and last to the endocardium. Certain tumors have their tendencies to involve the heart with melanoma being the highest on the list. Lung and breast tumors being more common are found most often, but in the overall scheme of things, melanoma has the strongest propensity to metastasize to the heart.[72,73]

Tumors involving the heart are often discovered by echocardiography, but other modalities—such as computerized tomography (CT) and cardiac magnetic imaging (CMRI)—are used for surveillance, often uncovering cardiac metastasis from malignant tumors. Once discovered, these cardiac metastases often are limiting factors and offer difficulty in treatment modalities.

In addition, cancer treatments themselves with either radiation or chemotherapy or both can result in damage to various parts of the heart. Echocardiography offers monitoring opportunities of the effects of adriamycin and herceptin. Serial ejection fraction measurements and, more recently, strain measurements have been studied in attempts to identify adverse effects early in the disease course. The effects of herceptin in particular can be reversible if identified early. Not only can systole be monitored but diastole also has been under investigation as a marker of early myocardial dysfunction in those undergoing treatment for cancer.

THE LEFT VENTRICLE WITH MYOCARDIAL METASTASIS

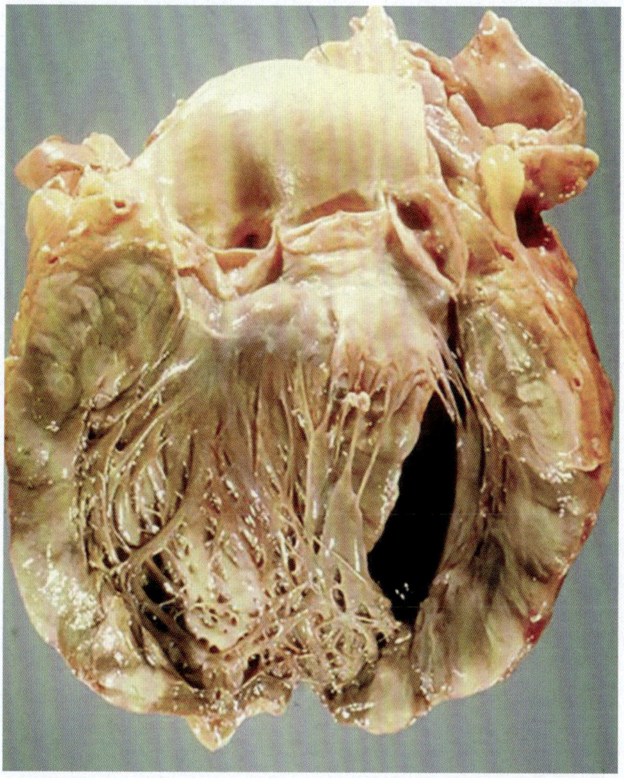

FIGURE 2.68 Histiocytoma metastatic to the left ventricle, hematogenous spread.

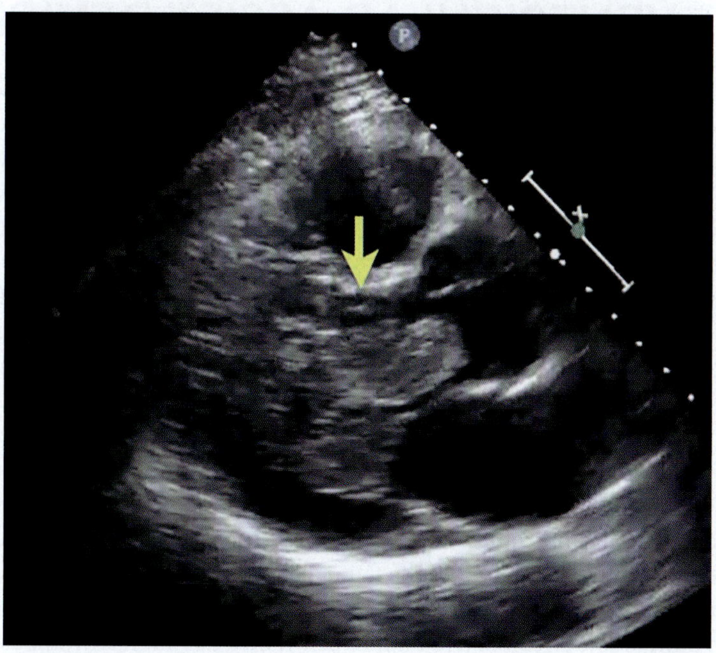

FIGURE 2.69 Metastatic sarcoma noted in the left ventricle and arising from the endocardium, approaching and nearly obstructing the LVOT (*yellow arrow*). There was a 40–mm Hg gradient across the LVOT. From Clements SD, Okene E, Parikh A, Clay MR, Williams BR. Metastatic Sarcoma: A rare Case of left ventricular outflow tract obstruction. *J Heart and Cardiology*. http://www.dx.doi.org/10.15436/2378-691

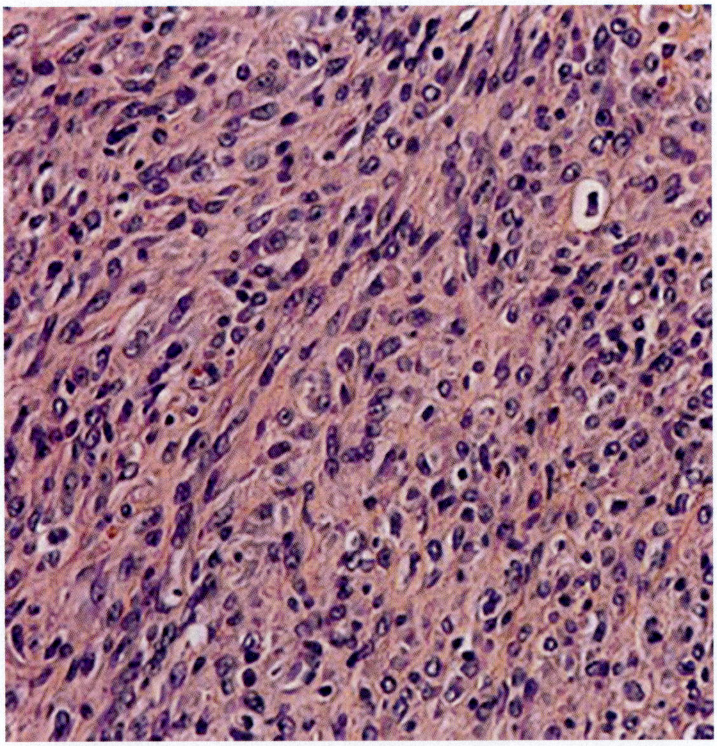

FIGURE 2.70 Micro of the above tumor shows nuclei of multiple types and shapes and chromatin variability.

SECTION 12

LEFT VENTRICULAR ASSIST DEVICE

Left ventricular assist devices have been used more frequently in recent years. They may be used as a bridge to cardiac transplant or as a destination therapy. Much evolution of these devices has taken place since the efforts of Dr. Michael DeBakey in the early 1960s. While historically LVADs generated pulsatile flow, these early devices were prone to mechanical failure and were too large for smaller patients. Modern devices operate with continuous, nonpulsatile flow using either a centrifugal or axial flow pump (Archimedes screw). Blood enters the pump through an inflow cannula at the apex of the left ventricle and exits through a longer outflow graft to the ascending aorta. Output can be varied by changing the speed of the impeller or rotor. Problems can occur in several areas. Thrombi can form in the ventricle in the region of the inlet cannula, in the pump device itself, or in the outflow graft. The outflow graft itself can become kinked or thrombosed.

Echocardiographic evaluation of the heart in the preoperative assessment period is important from several standpoints. Right ventricular function should be adequate to deliver blood to the failing left ventricle. Severe tricuspid regurgitation is undesirable as is severe mitral regurgitation. Aortic regurgitation results in an undesirable circuit of circulation. Left ventricular mural thrombus prohibits placing of the apical cannula, so this area must be clear.[74-76]

In addition to the LVAD devices, an Impella device (Abiomed, Danvers, MA) that is available in the catheterization lab can be inserted percutaneously from the femoral artery. This device crosses the aortic valve and has an entrance port within the left ventricle and an exit port in the aorta and an impella in between. This device has the capability of augmenting the left ventricle output in the range of ~2.5 L/min and is used for a relatively short period of time in situations such as high-risk angioplasty or shock that develops in the cardiac cath lab. Echocardiographic monitoring of the position of the catheter relative to the aortic valve allows for appropriate function.[77]

ASSESSMENT OF THE FUNCTION OF LEFT VENTRICULAR ASSIST DEVICES

An overall survey of the relative size of the cardiac chambers is important as a starting point. The right ventricle should not appear distended and should have adequate systolic function to deliver blood to the assisted left ventricle. Severe right ventricular dysfunction as measured by the standard parameters (TAPSE, TASV, FAC, and longitudinal strain) should be measured as a baseline. The degree of tricuspid regurgitation should be measured along with the calculated RVSP. Severe tricuspid regurgitation hinders forward output of the right ventricle and produces edema and organ congestion. The free wall of the right ventricle to visual exam should be normal or close to normal.

The interventricular septum should generally be in the midline in the apical four-chamber view or shifted slightly toward the right. Significant shifts of the interventricular septum to the right suggest that there may be high pressure or extra volume in the left ventricle and may signal malfunction of the pump. The opposite is true when pump settings are too high and the ventricle collapses and output falls because of resistance to inflow. In this case, the left ventricle is "sucked dry." Decrease in pump settings is the solution to this problem.

Mitral valve regurgitation can hinder blood coming to the intake cannula. In general, inflow velocities should be normal in the 1-2 m/s range and flow propagation should be >50 cm/s. This can be visualized by color Doppler as the "red flow" courses normally toward the apex and less "blue flow" courses toward the LVOT. Small degrees of aortic regurgitation are mixed with these flows and are tolerated when they are minimal.

Flow velocity in the outflow graft should range from 1 to 2 m/s. Imaging of the left ventricular apex for the presence or absence of thrombus is part of the routine examination. The outflow cannula velocity profile can be visualized from the right upper sternal border or the suprasternal notch and should have turbulent systolic and diastolic components that have velocities in the 1-2 m/s range. Higher velocities usually mean that the outflow cannula is kinked in some fashion.

Cardiac tamponade can occur with both chambers being compromised to the point of altering right ventricular function and compromising left ventricular filling. This is usually an event that takes place in the immediate postoperative period.

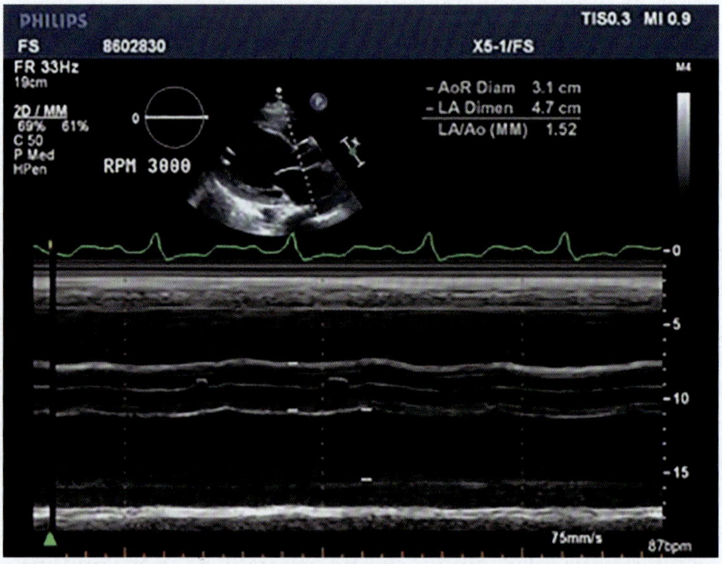

FIGURE 2.71 The desirable status of the aortic valve leaflets. They should open slightly in order to prevent fusion and aortic regurgitation. TTE, PLX view, M-mode.

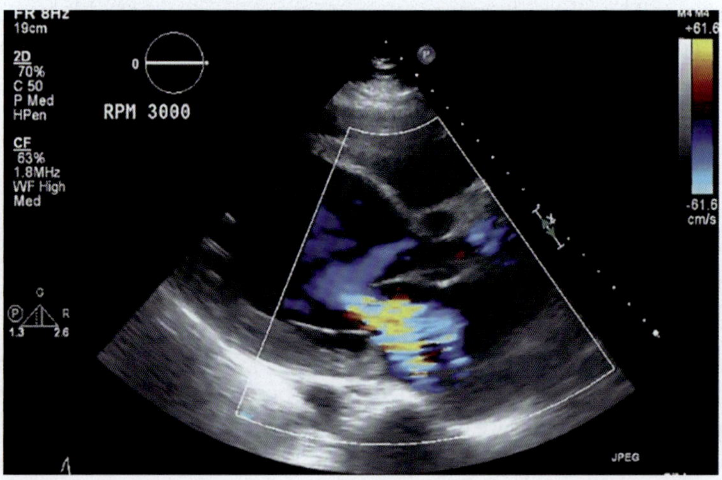

FIGURE 2.72 In this view, the aortic regurgitation exhibits flow throughout the cardiac cycle and a moderate degree of mitral regurgitation is present. Too much mitral regurgitation takes away from the intake of the pump. TTE, PLX view.

"SUCKED DRY"

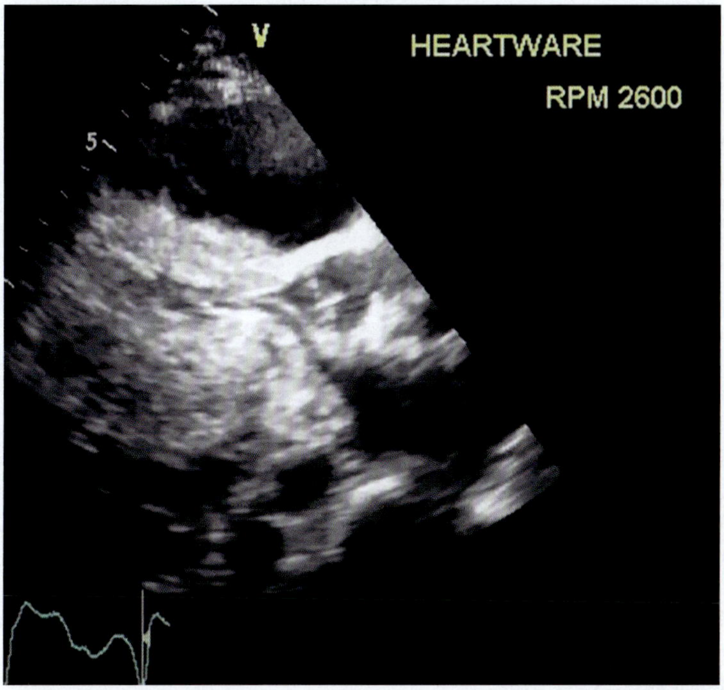

FIGURE 2.73 This image demonstrates the collapsed left ventricle as it appears with pump settings of 260 RPM. Once this image was obtained, the pump setting was immediately reduced to allow filling of the left ventricle. TTE, PLX view.

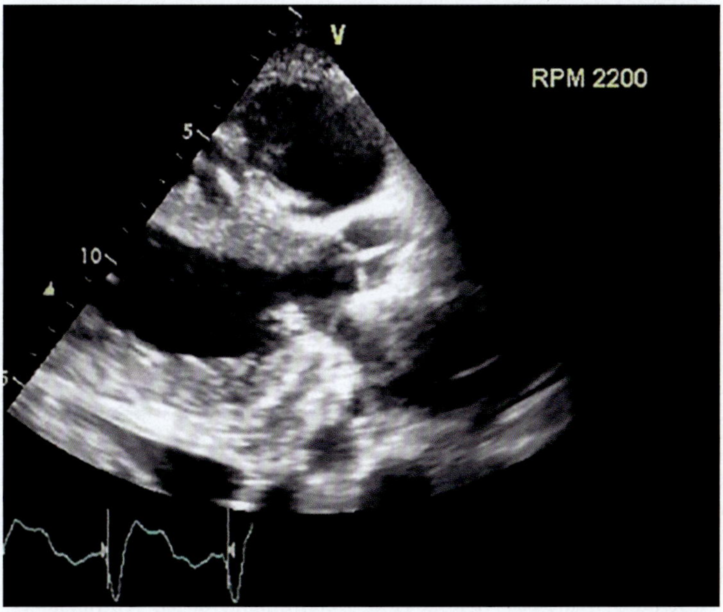

FIGURE 2.74 Images shortly after the pump setting had been reduced from 260 to 2200 RPM such that the heart could behave more like a conduit rather than a resistance vessel.

REFERENCES

1. Popovic ZB, Thomas JD. Left ventricular systolic function: basic principles. *ASE's Comprehensive Echocardiography*. 2nd ed. Philadelphia, PA: Elsevier Sanders; 2016:115-120.
2. Lang RM, Badano LP, Bor-Avi V, et al. Recommendations for cardiac chamber quantification by echocardiography in adults. *J Am Soc Echocardiogr.* 2015;28:1-39.
3. Lang RM, Badano LP, Bor-Avi V, et al. Recommendations for cardiac chamber quantification by echocardiography in adults. *J Am Soc Echocardiogr.* 2015;28:13-16.
4. Holubarsch C, Ruf T, Goldstein DJ, et al. Existence of the Frank-Starling Mechanism in the Failing Human Heart. Investigations on the organ, tissue and sarcomere levels. *Circulation.* 1996;94(4):683.
5. Lang RM, Goldstein SA, Kronzon I, Khandheria BK, Mor-Avi V. *ASE's Comprehensive Echocardiography*. 2nd ed. Philadelphia, PA: Elsevier Sanders; 2015:185.
6. Lang RM, Goldstein SA, Kronzon I, Khandheria BK, Mor-Avi V. *ASE's Comprehensive Echocardiography*. 2nd ed. Philadelphia, PA: Elsevier Sanders; 2016:120-124.
7. Tei C, Ling LH, Hodge DO, et al. New index of combined systolic and diastolic myocardial performance: a simple and reproducible measure of cardiac function—a study in normals and dilated cardiomyopathy. *J Cardiol.* 1995;26:357-366.
8. Oh JK, Seward JB, Tajik AJ. *The Echo Manuel.* 3rd ed. Rochester, NY: Wolters Kluwer/Lippincott Williams & Wilkins; 2007:77.
9. Mor-Avi V, Lang RM, Badano LP, et al. Current and evolving echocardiographic techniques for the quantitative evaluation of cardiac mechanics: ASE/EAE consensus statement on methodology and indications endorsed by the Japanese Society of Echocardiography. *J Am Soc Echocardiogr.* 2011;24:277-313.
10. D'Hooge J, Heimdal A, Jamal F, et al. Regional strain and strain rate measurements by cardiac ultrasound: principles, implementation and limitations. *Eur J Echocardiogr.* 2000;1:154-170.
11. Corsican J, Tanaka H. Echocardiographic assessment of myocardial strain. *J Am Coll Cardiol.* 2011;58(14):1401-1413.
12. Mor-Avi V, Lang RM, Badano L, et al. Current and evolving echocardiographic techniques for the quantitative evaluation of cardiac mechanics: ASE/EAE consensus statement of methodology and indications endorsed by the Japanese Society of Echocardiography. *Eur J Echocardiogr.* 2011;12:167-205.
13. Notomi Y, Srinath G, Shiota T, et al. Maturational and adaptive modulation of left ventricular torsional biomechanics: Doppler tissue imaging observation from infancy to adulthood. *Circulation.* 2006;113:2534-2541.
14. Lang RM, Goldstein SA, Kronzon I, Khandheria BK, Mor-Avi V. *ASE's Comprehensive Echocardiography*. 2nd ed. Philadelphia, PA: Elsevier Sanders; 2016:173-197.
15. Kumar V, Jose J, Jose JJ. L wave in echo Doppler. *Indian Heart J.* 2014;66(3):392-393.
16. Nagueh SF, Appleton CP, Gillegert TC, et al. Recommendations for the evaluation of left ventricular diastolic function by echocardiography. *J Am Soc Echocardiogr.* 2009;22(2):107-133.
17. Nagueh SF, Smiseth OA, Appleton CP, et al. Recommendations for evaluation of left ventricular diastolic function by echocardiography. An update from the American Society of Echocardiography and the European Association of Cardiovascular Imaging. *J Am Soc Echocardiogr.* 2016;29:277-314.
18. Mitter SS, Shah SJ, Thomas JD. A test in context: E/A and E/e′ to assess diastolic dysfunction and LV filling pressure. *J Am Coll Cardiol.* 2017;69(11):1451-1464.
19. Opdahl A, Remme EW, Helle-Valle T, et al. Determinants of left ventricular early-diastolic lengthening velocity: independent contributions from left ventricular relaxation forces and lengthening load. *Circulation.* 2009;119:2578-2586.

20. Yamkado T, Takagi E, Okubo S, et al. Effects of aging on the left ventricular relaxation in humans-analysis of left ventricular isovolumic pressure decay. *Circulation.* 1997;95:917-923.
21. Lang RM, Goldstein SA, Kronzon I, Khandheria BK, Mor-Avi V. *ASE's Comprehensive Echocardiography.* 2nd ed. Philadelphia, PA: Elsevier Sanders; 2016:180-184.
22. Lang RM, Goldstein SA, Kronzon I, Khandheria BK, Mor-Avi V. *ASE's Comprehensive Echocardiography.* 2nd ed. Philadelphia, PA: Elsevier Sanders; 2016:180-181.
23. Lang RM, Goldstein SA, Kronzon I, Khandheria BK, Mor-Avi V. *ASE's Comprehensive Echocardiography.* 2nd ed. Philadelphia, PA: Elsevier Sanders; 2016:182-183.
24. Veress G, Feng D, Oh JK. Echocardiography in pericardial diseases: new developments. *Heart Fail Rev.* 2013;18:267-275.
25. Garcia MJ, Rodrigue L, Ares M, et al. Differentiation of constrictive pericarditis from restrictive cardiomyopathy: assessment of left ventricular diastolic velocities in longitudinal axis by Doppler tissue imaging. *J Am Coll Cardiol.* 1996;27:108-114.
26. Owan TE, Hodge DO, Herges RM, Jacobsen SJ, Roger VL, Redfield MM. Trends in prevalence and outcomes of heart failure with preserved ejection fraction. *N Engl J Med.* 2006;355:251-259.
27. Abhayaratna WP, Marwick TH, Smith WT, Becker NG. Characteristics of the left ventricular diastolic dysfunction in the community: an echocardiographic survey. *Heart.* 2006;92(9):1259-1264.
28. Lang RM, Goldstein SA, Kronzon I, Khandheria BK, Mor-Avi V. *ASE's Comprehensive Echocardiography.* 2nd ed. Philadelphia, PA: Elsevier Sanders; 2016:180.
29. Mitter SS, Shah SJ, Thomas JD. A test in contest: E/A and E/e′ to assess diastolic dysfunction and LV filling pressures. *J Am Coll Cardiol.* 2017;69:1452-1464.
30. Richardson P, McKenna W, Bristow M, et al. Report of the 1995 World Health Organization/International Society and Federation of Cardiology Task Force on the Definition and Classification of Cardiomyopathies. *Circulation.* 1996;93:841-842.
31. Maron BJ, Towbin JA, Thiene G, et al. Contemporary definitions and classification of the cardiomyopathies: an American Heart Association Statement from the Council on Clinical Cardiology, Heart Failure and Transplantation Subcommittee; Quality of Care and Outcomes Research and Functional Genomics and Translational Biology Interdisciplinary Working Groups: and Council on Epidemiology and Prevention. *Circulation.* 2006;113:1807-1816.
32. Elliott P, Andersson B, Argustini E, et al. Classification of the cardiomyopathies: a position statement from the European Society of Cardiology Working Group on myocardial and pericardial diseases. *Eur Heart J.* 2008;29(2):270-276, ISSN 0195-668x.
33. Haugland JM, Asinger RW, Mikell FL, Elsperger J, Hodges M. Embolic potential of left ventricular thrombi detected by two-dimensional echocardiography. *Circulation.* 1984;70(4):588-598.
34. Delwi R, Zijlstra F, Piek JJ. Left ventricular thrombus formation after acute myocardial infarction. *Heart.* 2012;98:1743-1749.
35. Nair A, Sealove B, Halpern JL, Webber G, Fuster V. Anticoagulation in patients with heart failure: who, when and why? *Eur Heart J.* 2006;8(suppl):32-38.
36. Homma S, Thompson JLP, Pullicino MD, et al. Warfarin and aspirin in patients with heart failure and sinus rhythm. *N Engl J Med.* 2012;366:1859-1869.
37. Lang RM, Goldstein SA, Kronzon I, Khandheria BK, Mor-Avi V. *ASE's Comprehensive Echocardiography.* 2nd ed. Philadelphia, PA: Elsevier Sanders; 2016:341.
38. Virchow R. Zur-cellulose-Frage. *Virchow Archiv A Pathol Anat Histol.* 1854;6:416-426.
39. Falk RH. Diagnosis and management of cardiac amyloidosis. *Circulation.* 2005;112:2047-2060.
40. Katzmann JA, Abraham RS, Dispenzeri A, Lust JA, Kyle RA. Diagnostic performance of quantitative kappa and lambda free light chains assays in clinical practice. *Clin Chem.* 2005;51:878-881.
41. Loeffler W. Endocarditis parietalis fibroplastica mit Blut-eosinophilie, ein enginartiges Krankheitshield. *Schweiz Med Wochenschr.* 1936;66:817-820.
42. Solley GO, Maldonado JE, Gleich GJ, et al. Endomyocardiopathy with eosinophilia. *Mayo Clin Proc.* 1976;51(11):697-708.

43. Olsen EG, Spry CJ. Relation between eosinophilia and endomyocardial disease. *Prog Cardiovasc Dis.* 1985;27(4):241-545.
44. Tai PC, Ackerman SJ, Spry CJ, et al. Deposits of eosinophil granule proteins in cardiac tissues of patients with eosinophilic endomyocardial disease. *Lancet.* 1987;1(8534):643-647.
45. Spry CJ, Fai PC, Davies J. The cardiotoxicity of eosinophils. *Postgrad Med J.* 1983;59(689):147-153.
46. Gleich GJ, Frigas E, Loegering DA, et al. Cytotoxic properties of the eosinophil major basic protein. *J Immunol.* 1979;123(6):2925-2927.
47. Slungaard A, Vercollotti GM, Tran T, et al. Eosinophil cationic granule proteins impair thrombomodulin function. A potential mechanism for thromboembolism in hypereosinophilic heart disease. *J Clin Invest.* 1993;91(4):1721-1730.
48. Cunningham D, Davies RA, Catchling J, Veinot JP. Pathologic quiz case: a young woman with eosinophilia and heart failure. Primary hypereosinophilic syndrome with Loeffler endocarditis. *Arch Pathol Lab Med.* 2005;129(1):e29-e30.
49. Priglinger U, Drach J, Ulrich R. Idiopathic eosinophilic endomyocarditis in the absence of peripheral eosinophilia. *Leuk Lymphoma.* 2002;43(1):215-218.
50. Gersh BJ, Maron BJ, Bonow RO, et al. 2011 ACCF/AHA guideline for the diagnosis and treatment of hypertrophic cardiomyopathy. *J Am Coll Cardiol.* 2011;58(25):e212-e260.
51. Chowdhury L, Mahrholdt H, Wagner J, et al. Myocardial scarring and asymptomatic or mildly symptomatic patients with hypertrophic cardiomyopathy. *J Am Coll Cardiol.* 2002;40:2156-2164.
52. Kuribayashi T, Roberts WC. Myocardial disarray at the junction of ventricular septum and the left and right ventricular free walls in hypertrophic cardiomyopathy. *Am J Cardiol.* 1992;70:1333-1340.
53. Spirito P, Bellone P, Harris KM, Bernabo P, Baron BJ. Magnitude of left ventricular hypertrophy and risk of sudden death in hypertrophic cardiomyopathy. *N Engl J Med.* 2000;342:1778-1785.
54. Maron BJ, Epstein SE, Roberts WC. Hypertrophic cardiomyopathy and transmural myocardial infarction without significant atherosclerosis of the extramural coronary arteries. *Am J Cardiol.* 1979;43:1086-1102.
55. Maron BJ, Rowin EJ, Maron MS, Braunwald E. Nonobstructive cardiomyopathy out of the shadows: known from the beginning but larger ignored… until now. *Am J Med.* 2017;130:119-123.
56. Silbiger JJ. Abnormalities of the mitral apparatus in hypertrophic cardiomyopathy: echocardiographic, pathophysiologic, and surgical insights. *J Am Soc Echocardiogr.* 2016;29:622-639.
57. Morrow AG, Reitz BA, Epstein SE, et al. Operative treatment in hypertrophic sub aortic stenosis. Techniques and the results of pre and postoperative assessments in 83 patients. *Circulation.* 1975;52(1):88-102.
58. Sigwart U. Non-surgical myocardial reduction for hypertrophic cardiomyopathy. *Lancet.* 1995;346:211-214.
59. Maron BJ. Role of alcohol septal ablation in treatment of obstructive hypertrophic cardiomyopathy. *Lancet.* 2000;355:425-426.
60. Yamaguchi H, Ishimura T, Nishiyama S, et al. Hypertrophic non-obstructive cardiomyopathy with giant negative T waves (apical hypertrophy): ventriculographic and echocardiographic features in 30 patients. *Am J Cardiol.* 1979;44:401-412.
61. Maron MS, Rowin EJ, Olivetti I, et al. Contemporary natural history and management of nonobstructive hypertrophic cardiomyopathy. *J Am Coll Cardiol.* 2016;67:1399-1409.
62. Gersh BJ, Maron BJ, Bonow RO, et al. 2011 ACCF/AHA guideline for the diagnosis and treatment of hypertrophic cardiomyopathy: a report of the American College of Cardiology Foundation/American Heart Association Task Force on Practice Guidelines. *Circulation.* 2011;124:e783-e831.
63. Gars JB, Maron BJ, Bonow RO, et al. 2011 ACC/AHA Guideline for the diagnosis and treatment of hypertrophic cardiomyopathy. *J Am Coll Cardiol.* 2011;58(25):e212-e260.

64. Sorajja P, Omen SR, Holmes DR, et al. Survival after alcohol septal ablation for obstructive hypertrophic cardiomyopathy. *Circulation.* 2012;126:2374-2380.
65. Morrow AG, Reitz BA, Epstein SE, et al. Operative treatment in hypertrophic sub aortic stenosis. Techniques and the results of pre and postoperative assessments in 83 patients. *Circulation.* 1975;52(1):88-102.
66. Nagged SF, Bierig SM, Budoff MJ, et al. American Society of Echocardiography clinical recommendations for multimodality cardiovascular imaging of patients with hypertrophic cardiomyopathy. *J Am Soc Echocardiogr.* 2011;24:473-498.
67. Desai MY, Bhonsale A, Smedira NG, et al. Predictors of long-term outcomes in symptomatic hypertrophic cardiomyopathy patients undergoing surgical relief of left ventricular outflow obstruction. *Circulation.* 2013;128:209-216.
68. Kwon DH, Smedira NC, Rodriguez ER, Tan C. Cardiac magnetic resonance detection of myocardial scarring in hypertrophic cardiomyopathy. Correlation with histopathology and prevalence of ventricular tachycardia. *J Am Coll Cardiol.* 2009;54:242-249.
69. Zoffoli G, Mangino D, Vetturini A, et al. Diagnosing left ventricular aneurysm from pseudoaneurysm: a case report and review in literature. *J Cardiothorac Surg.* 2009;4:11-16.
70. Jones BM, Kapadia SR, Smedira NG, et al. Ventricular septal rupture complicating acute myocardial infarction: a contemporary review. *Eur Heart J.* 2014;35:2060-2068.
71. Flueckiger PB, Cheng AC, Patton JM, Clements SD. Partial papillary muscle rupture: a cause of acute mitral regurgitation. *Am J Med Sci.* 2013;345(6):478-481.
72. Goldberg AD, Blankstein R, Padera RF. Tumors metastatic to the heart. *Circulation.* 2013;128:1790-1794.
73. Bussani R, De-Giorgio F, Abbate A, Silvestri F. Cardiac metastasis. *J Clin Pathol.* 2007;60(1):27-34.
74. Lee S, Fukamachi K, Golding L, Monazami N, Starling RC. Left ventricular assist devices: from the bench to the clinic. *Cardiology.* 2013;125:1-12.
75. Kirkland JK, Naftel DC, Kormos RL, et al. Taire INTERMACS annual report: the evolution of destination therapy in the United States. *J Heart Lung Transplant.* 2011;30(2):115-123.
76. Ammar KA, Umland MM, Kramer C, et al. The ABCs of left ventricular assist device echocardiography: a systemic approach. *Eur Heart J Cardiovasc Imaging.* 2012;13:855-899.
77. Jones HA, Kalisetti DR, Gaba M, McCormick DJ, Goldberg S. Left ventricular assist for high-risk percutaneous intervention. *J Invasive Cardiol.* 2012;24(10):544-550.

3

The Mitral Valve Apparatus

SECTION 1

CLASSIFICATION OF MITRAL VALVE DISORDERS

The mitral valve apparatus has several amazing functions. The leaflets act as a one-way door in diastole allowing blood to enter from the left atrium to the left ventricle with very little resistance to flow. The leaflets also direct blood to the lateral and apical regions of the left ventricle allowing it to course around the apex and line up in the direction of the left ventricular outflow tract (LVOT) then being ready for ejection. As part of the doorlike function, the leaflets close at the beginning of systole under the influence of changing pressures. Coaptation regions are sealed to the degree of not letting any blood back into the atrium during systolic contraction of the heart. During systole, the anterior mitral leaflet acts a baffle and directs blood into the LVOT for ejection. During this baffle function, the papillary muscles and chordal structures hold the leaflets in place. All of this occurs in the normal heart while preserving laminar flow and allowing for expenditure of minimal energy along the directional pathway of blood coursing through the left side of the heart.

The components of the mitral valve apparatus begin with the walls of the left atrium and end with the anchoring walls of the left ventricle. The left atrium can have an effect on the mitral valve by dilating to such a degree that it retracts or places tension, thus distorting the annulus area and everting the leaflets not allowing proper coaptation of the leaflets. In this situation, mitral regurgitation is already present and begets more mitral regurgitation. The mitral annulus can dilate, calcify, and become abscessed compromising the function of the mitral leaflets. The annulus can calcify to the point of altering the orifice and can result in resistance to flow across that area. One of the hallmarks of mitral valve prolapse is a dilated, enlarged, sometimes calcified mitral annulus that loses its saddle shape and becomes more flattened. Repair of such valves requires an annular ring to resize and reshape the mitral orifice as defined by the mitral annulus. The leaflets themselves can be involved by many processes that result in abnormal function to include infection, myxomatous processes, fibroelastic deficiency, trauma, rheumatic disease, radiation, and various other inflammatory processes. The processes that affect the leaflets can affect the chordal structures in a similar fashion. The papillary muscles can be affected by ischemia, scarring, as well as infection. The left ventricle can remodel, and the papillary muscles and chordal structures can be displaced and tether the leaflets altering coaptation and resulting in mitral regurgitation.

Classification of disorders of the mitral valve can be grouped into primary abnormalities such as degenerative, rheumatic, congenital, infective, marantic, annular calcification, trauma, valve tumors and others. Secondary abnormalities that alter the mitral valve apparatus are idiopathic dilated cardiomyopathy, hypertrophic cardiomyopathy, and myocardial infiltrative diseases.[1,2] Guidelines for quantitation have been updated and offer general concepts in addition to quantitative methods.[3]

Illustrations of these problems are demonstrated in the following displays.

CLASSIFICATION OF MITRAL VALVE DISORDERS

- Primary Mitral Valve Disorders
  - Degenerative
    - Myxomatous degeneration
    - Fibroelastic deficiency
  - Rheumatic
  - Endocarditis (infective and marantic)
  - Congenital (cleft mitral valve)
  - Mitral annular calcification
  - Valvular tumors
- Secondary Mitral Valve Disorders
  - Functional

- Dilated cardiomyopathy
- Ischemic
- Hypertrophic cardiomyopathy
- Myocardial infiltrative diseases

SECTION 2

DEGENERATIVE MITRAL VALVE DISORDERS

The degenerative category of mitral valve diseases is a primary disorder of the mitral valve that results in mitral regurgitation. It is the most common of the disorders of the mitral valve encountered today. This category has been studied in detail, and knowledge of this process has led to the understanding of the natural history and to surgical repair. Surgeons such as Carpentier, the father of modern mitral valve repair, have made major contributions to our understandings of these processes. Carpentier emphasized the importance of defining the etiology of the disease, the lesion that resulted from the disease, and the dysfunction that was created by the disease. This is referred to as the "pathophysiologic triad" described by Carpentier in the early 1980s and remains useful today. The repair technique of Carpentier that follows this analysis of the pathophysiology and pathoanatomy is referred to as the "French Correction."[4,5]

The subcategories of degenerative valves fall into two major types of abnormalities. The first category is myxomatous degeneration resulting in thickened, structurally weakened, redundant leaflets that prolapse toward the left atrium in systole. These valves have come to be known as "Barlow valves." They are thickened, stretched, and redundant due to myxomatous infiltration and weakening of the fibrous structure of the leaflets and chords. Another category in the degenerative group is fibroelastic deficiency valves in which the leaflets are not so thickened but have weakened collagenous components resulting in more regional changes and regional areas of prolapse, usually in the P2 area. These individuals with fibroelastic changes may progress slowly but have the potential to develop severe acute mitral regurgitation when a chord ruptures. Some of these processes that have stretched redundant leaflets are seen in certain inherited connective tissue disorders such as Marfan syndrome and others (see next page). Further understanding of these processes in the future may lead to molecular alterations that could be beneficial from the clinical standpoint.[2,6-8]

These abnormalities will be illustrated in the sections that follow.

BARLOW SYNDROME AND THE BARLOW VALVE

Interest in the mid systolic click and late systolic murmur from the clinical standpoint started with Barlow and Reid. They developed the concept that the origin of the click was from the mitral apparatus and not from what previously was thought to be from an extracardiac source. Their conceptual understanding of the origin of this sound still holds today. The sound of the mid to late systolic click comes from the process of the mitral leaflets shifting position in mid to late systole producing abrupt tension in the valve and chordal structures. These events result in the sound. This process is associated with valves that have myxomatous changes within their microscopic structure. Sometimes this process is advanced to the point of producing very redundant leaflets with various degrees of hooding, redundancy, chordal stretching, and even chordal rupture.[9-11]

Interestingly, Dr. Barlow submitted his work initially for publication in *Circulation*, and it was rejected. Later he visited Dr. Victor McKusick at Johns Hopkins University where his work was discussed, and he was subsequently invited to publish his work in the *Journal of Chronic Disease*. At Hopkins he met a young resident Dr. Michael Criley who had termed the syndrome "mitral valve prolapse" when catheterization laboratory angiographic observations were made of the valve prolapsing up into the left atrium in systole. Barlow did not like the term prolapse and continued to refer to the valve as billowing. Dr. Tsung Cheng relates that Dr. Barlow often said that he thought that the syndrome should be referred to as the Barlow-Cheng syndrome since Cheng had described the late systolic murmur of papillary muscle dysfunction a few years later.[12,13]

The myxomatous mitral valve under the microscope shows infiltration of myxomatous material and weakening and disruption of the integrity of the supporting collagen tissue. The four-layered architecture of the valve (the atrialis, spongiosa, fibrosa, and ventricularis) is abnormal with loose collagen in the fibrous, expanded spongiosa containing excessive proteoglycans and disrupted elastin in the atrialis.[14] This leads to elongation and nodular thickening of chords and hooding of leaflets and can lead to chordal rupture, severe mitral regurgitation, heart failure, and even sudden death. Endocarditis can become superimposed on these valves and hasten chordal rupture and even cause perforation.

Individuals who have this abnormality are identified earlier in life than are those with fibroelastic deficiency. As Barlow and Reid discovered, they have midsystolic clicks and late systolic murmurs. Clinicians make this discovery with the stethoscope and then confirm and quantitate the problem with echocardiography. It has many clinical variants and a variable prognosis. In addition, individuals with certain inherited connective tissue disorders are predisposed to these abnormalities earlier in life as part of their clinical syndrome.[15-17]

The Carpentier Classification

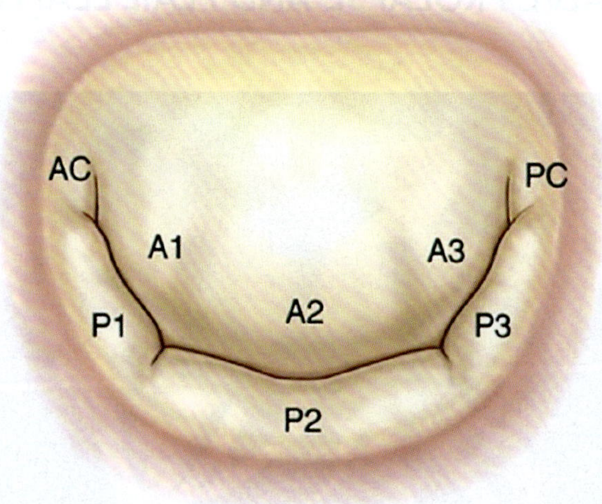

FIGURE 3.1 Carpentier defined the mitral valve as having eight regions. Three posterior leaflet regions separated by commissures and three anterior leaflet regions and two commissural regions. These are best identified by viewing the valve from the "surgeon's view" or placing the mitral aortic curtain at 12 o'clock. (From Carpentier A, Adams DH, Filsoufi F. *Carpentier's Reconstructive Valve Surgery. From Valve Analysis to Valve Reconstruction.* Philadelphia, PA: Elsevier; 2010.)

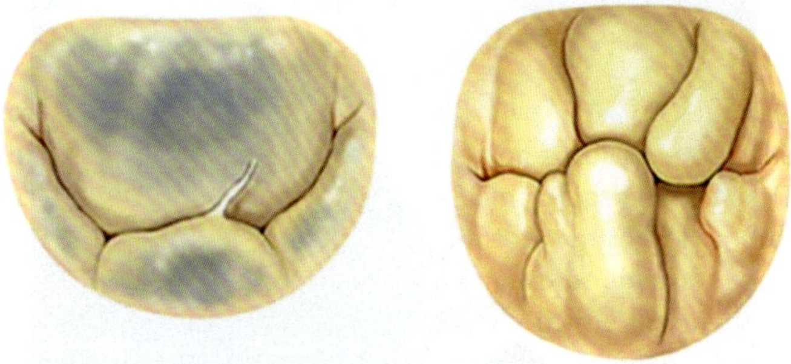

FIGURE 3.2 Degenerative mitral valve disease. **Left:** fibroelastic deficiency. **Right:** Barlow disease.

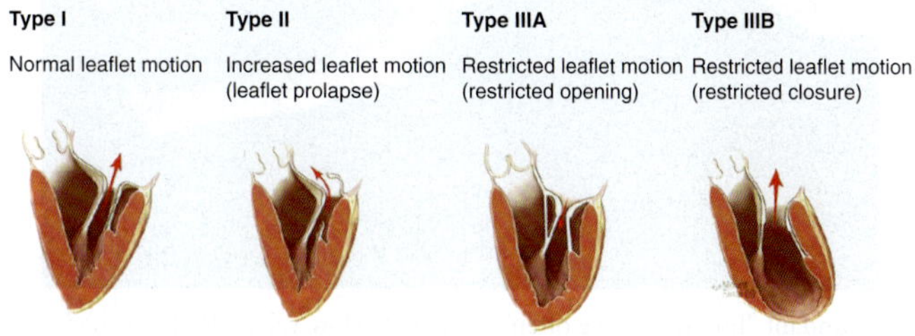

FIGURE 3.3 The triad of types of valve abnormalities falls into three categories according to leaflet motion. Type I is seen in abnormalities such as perforations from endocarditis or long-standing atrial fibrillation and a dilated annulus. Type II is seen with abnormalities such as degenerative valves that have myxomatous changes or fibroelastic deficiency where leaflet motion is excessive. Type IIIA includes mitral stenosis and carcinoid syndrome. Type IIIB includes tethered valves as seen with dilated cardiomyopathy or alterations associated with hypertrophic cardiomyopathy. Carpentier's classification of valve abnormalities according to leaflet motion has stood the test of time and is used frequently when considering mitral valve abnormalities. Carpentier used his techniques to repair valves that have fibroelastic deficiency and P2 segment prolapse, classified as Type II abnormalities. This is the most common type of valve dysfunction that lends itself to valve repair. (Modified from Carpentier A. Cardiac valve surgery—the "French correction". *J Thorac Cardiovasc Surg* 1983;86(3):323-337; Carpentier AF, Lessana A, Relland JY, et al. The "physio-ring" an advanced concept in mitral valve annuloplasty. *Ann Thorac Surg.* 1995;60:1177-1185.)

INHERITED CONNECTIVE TISSUE DISORDERS ASSOCIATED WITH MITRAL VALVE LEAFLET THICKENING AND PROLAPSE[17]

- Marfan syndrome
- Ehlers-Danlos syndrome
- Osteogenesis imperfecta
- Pseudoxanthoma elasticum
- Turner syndrome

ECHOCARDIOGRAPHIC FEATURES OF DEGENERATIVE MITRAL VALVE DISEASE, BARLOW SYNDROME, AND FIBROELASTIC DEFICIENCY

From studies at the bedside of individuals with a click and murmur by Barlow and Reid, our understanding of these entities has come far. It was a landmark clarification when the issue of the etiology of a midsystolic click was investigated. Previously, it was thought to have originated somewhere in the chest wall or pericardium. The variability of the timing of the midsystolic click and the duration of the late systolic murmur with maneuvers such as standing as documented on phonocardiogram put the entity of mitral valve prolapse on the radar screen.[10,11]

From the initial echocardiographic M-mode studies, mitral valve prolapse was probably overdiagnosed. Our understanding of the saddle shape of the mitral annulus and 2D and 3D studies have further clarified the anatomy and physiology of this entity and have increased the accuracy of the diagnosis. Interest in surgical repair and analyses at the operating table allowed further understanding of mitral valve abnormalities. Three-dimensional echocardiography with parametric imaging has further defined coaptation points, leaflet billowing, gaps in coaptation, and their relationships to the normal or distorted mitral valve annulus. Surgeons have been involved in this process, and correlations of the imaging findings and those in the operating room have confirmed the accuracy of these techniques.[15]

Examples of these imaging techniques are illustrated on the following pages.

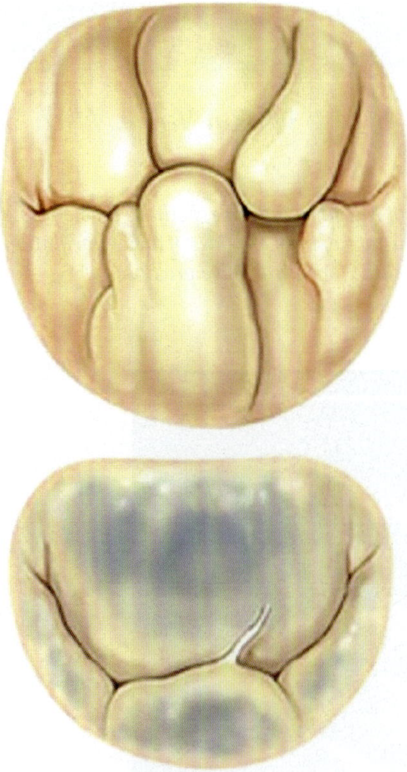

FIGURE 3.5 Degenerative mitral valve disease. **Top:** Barlow disease; **Bottom:** fibroelastic deficiency. (Adapted from Carpentier A, Adams DH, Filsoufi F. *Carpentier's Reconstructive Valve Surgery. From Valve Analysis to Valve Reconstruction*. Philadelphia, PA: Elsevier; 2010.)

PRIMARY MITRAL VALVE DISORDERS WITH MYXOMATOUS DEGENERATION, "BARLOW DISEASE," OR "BARLOW VALVE"

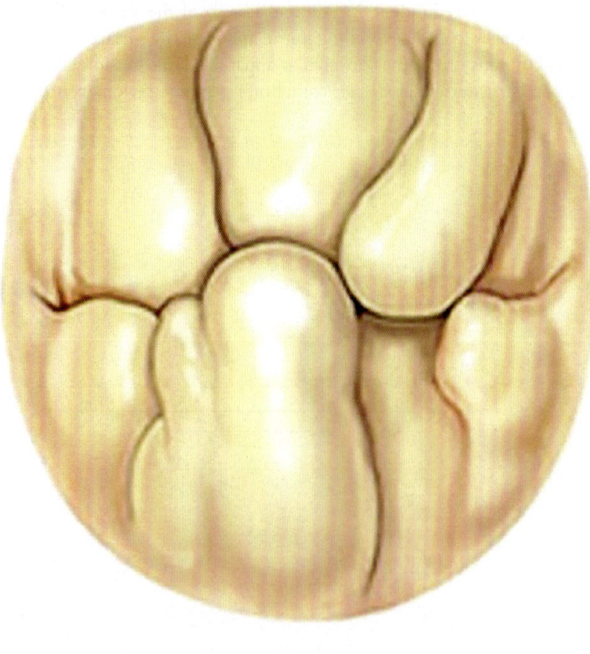

FIGURE 3.6 Examples of various degrees of involvement. (Adapted from Carpentier A, Adams DH, Filsoufi F. *Carpentier's Reconstructive Valve Surgery. From Valve Analysis to Valve Reconstruction*. Philadelphia, PA: Elsevier; 2010.)

CASE PRESENTATION

Severe Myxomatous Degeneration of the Mitral Valve With Only Mild Mitral Regurgitation

A 23-year-old man who is said to have a variant of Marfan syndrome, perhaps forme fruste. He had normal exercise tolerance but did have a history of brief episodes of atrial fibrillation. He had been followed in the pediatric cardiology clinic for mitral valve prolapse.

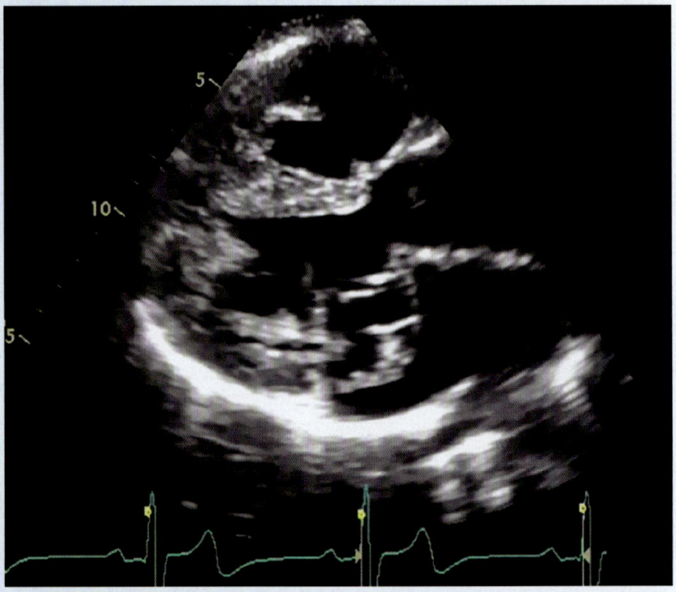

FIGURE 3.7 Severe mitral valve prolapse with very redundant AMVL and less so of the PMVL—the very redundant AMVL overshoots the PMVL and prolapses to and beyond the mitral annulus. The surface area of the anterior leaflet is much increased and places extra tension on the subvalvular apparatus. This tension generated by the expanding leaflets "tugging" on the papillary muscle areas can sometimes generate serious ventricular arrhythmias. TTE, PLX view.

PRIMARY MITRAL VALVE DISEASE WITH MYXOMATOUS CHANGES INVOLVING BOTH LEAFLETS, RUPTURED CHORDS TO THE ANTERIOR MITRAL VALVE LEAFLET, AND SEVERE MITRAL REGURGITATION

2D and 3D Images

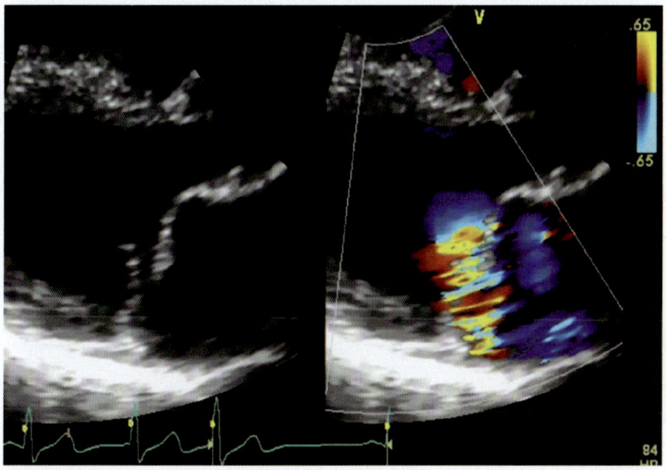

FIGURE 3.8 Ruptured chords to the mid portion of the AMVL resulting in severe mitral regurgitation with a posterior radiating jet. The direction of the radiation of the jet is an index to the most involved segment of the leaflets. TTE, PLA view.

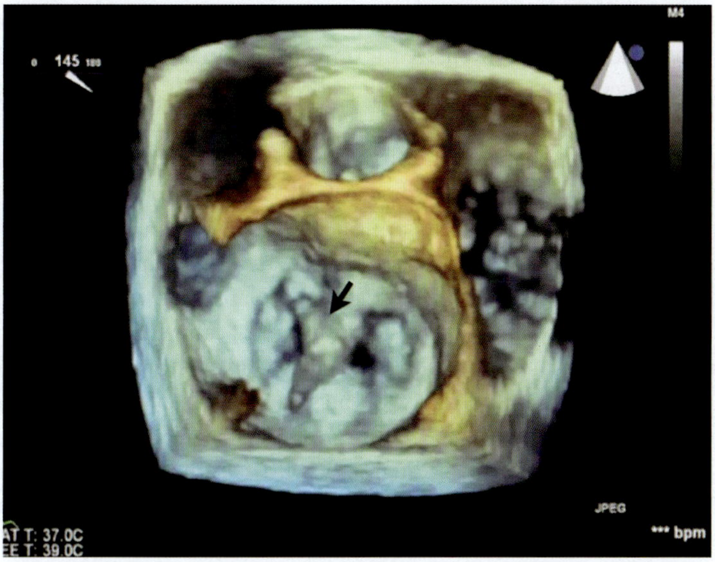

FIGURE 3.9 Flail segment of the AMVL prolapsing above the plane of the MV annulus (*black arrow*) and resulting in severe MR. 3D TEE, 145° view (the "surgeon's view").

PRIMARY MITRAL VALVE DISORDER DUE TO FIBROELASTIC DEFICIENCY AND MITRAL REGURGITATION

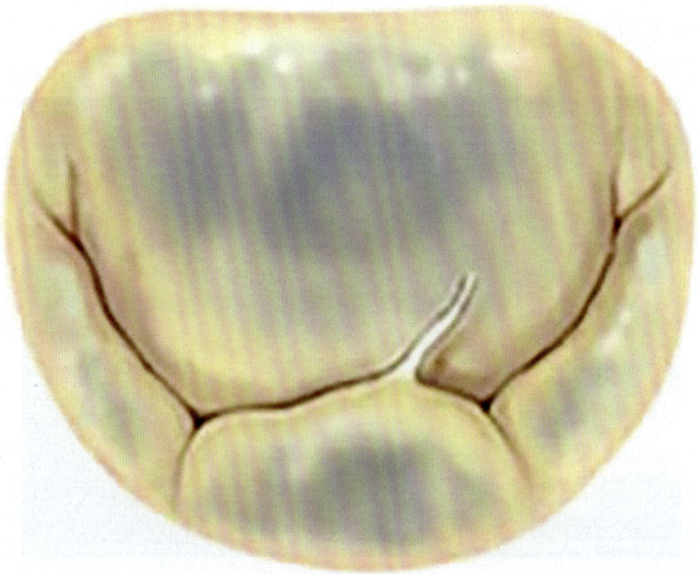

FIGURE 3.10 Fibroelastic deficiency. (Adapted from Carpentier A, Adams DH, Filsoufi F. *Carpentier's Reconstructive Valve Surgery. From Valve Analysis to Valve Reconstruction*. Philadelphia, PA: Elsevier; 2010.)

Individuals who have primary mitral valve disease due to fibroelastic deficiency commonly do not have extensive myxomatous changes in the valve leaflets. They do have degenerative changes in the fibrous integrity of the leaflets, and this most commonly involves the posterior leaflet. As this leaflet stretches and loses its usual anatomic shape, additional tension is placed on this segment and the corresponding supporting chords can lead to chordal rupture. The regionality of this problem lends itself to surgical resection, repair, and reconstruction of the annulus with a ring. The most common area to be involved is the P2 region of the posterior leaflet where flail or severe prolapsed valve segments are present and lend themselves to repair. The anterior mitral can be involved, and repair can be more difficult or not possible. The Barlow valve with myxomatous degeneration and billowing and hooding of both valve leaflets represents the most difficult valve to repair and requires special surgical talents.[6]

Three-dimensional echocardiography with parametric imaging can demonstrate the billowing segments of the valve, coaptation points, and annular shape. Two-dimensional echocardiographic images along with 3D imaging offer a road map for surgical considerations.

The following sections illustrate these issues.

FIBROELASTIC DEFICIENCY OF THE MITRAL LEAFLETS

Ruptured Chords to the P1 Segment of the Posterior Mitral Leaflet

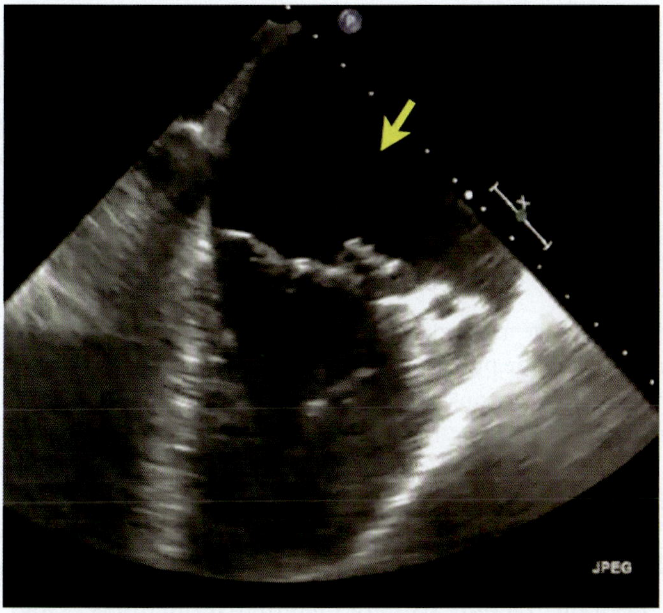

FIGURE 3.11 Ruptured chords to the P1 region of the PMVL—this leaflet prolapses above the plane of the mitral annulus and has its origin in the annulus close to the left atrial appendage and therefore is in the P1 region of the PMVL (*yellow arrow*). TEE, 92° view, 2C view.

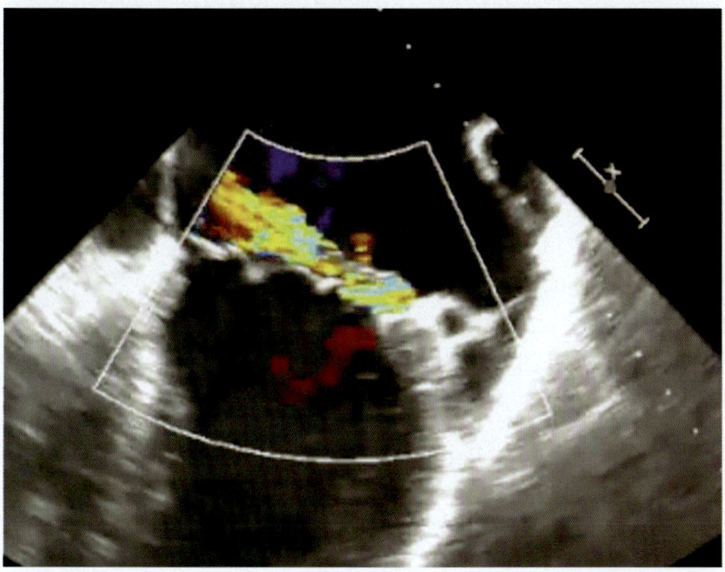

FIGURE 3.12 The same patient from a similar view with color Doppler demonstrating the jet coursing across the mitral orifice away from the left atrial appendage and toward the inter atrial septum. TEE, 65° view.

EVALUATION OF THE SEVERITY OF CHRONIC MITRAL REGURGITATION BY ECHOCARDIOGRAPHY

The 2017 guidelines for evaluation for grading the severity of mitral regurgitation are available for reference.[3] They include an assessment of the structure of the mitral valve, the size of the left atrium, and qualitative, semiquantitative, and quantitative recommendations for grading of severity. For example, a flail leaflet or a very dilated left ventricle with severe tenting would be associated with severe mitral regurgitation. A color flow jet area that is large, eccentric, or coursing around the left atrium or into the pulmonary veins is an eyeball clue to severe mitral regurgitation. A grossly large flow convergence (proximal isovelocity surface area [PISA]) throughout systole or a holosystolic dense CW jet profile suggests that severe mitral regurgitation is present (see table on the following page).

Semiquantitative methods including measurement of the vena contracta width and assessment of the pulmonary vein flow pattern offer quick estimates of severity of mitral regurgitation.

Quantitative methods include effective regurgitant orifice area (EROA) by the PISA method, regurgitant volume, and regurgitant fraction. The 2017 guidelines changed the EROA limits for severe functional mitral regurgitation to >0.40 cm^2 recognizing that sometimes lower numbers are associated with elliptical regurgitant areas in this entity. Regurgitant volume and regurgitant fraction also are quantitative methods. Table 3.1 summarizes the criteria for evaluation of the severity of mitral regurgitation on echocardiography.

TABLE 3.1 CRITERIA FOR EVALUATION OF THE SEVERITY OF MITRAL REGURGITATION

Structural	Flail leaflet or severe tenting Dilated left atrium
Qualitative	Large jet Large flow convergence Holosystolic dense jet that is triangular
Semiqualitative	Wide vena contracta Systolic flow reversal Dominant E-wave
Quantitative	Large EROA > 0.4 cm^2 Large regurgitant volume > 60 mL Regurgitant fraction > 50%

Grading of Chronic Mitral Regurgitation, the 2017 Guidelines[3]

	MR severity[*]			
	Mild	**Moderate**		**Severe**
Structural				
MV morphology	**None or mild leaflet abnormality** (e.g., mild thickening, calcifications or prolapse, mild tenting)	Moderate leaflet abnormality or moderate tenting		**Severe valve lesions** (primary: flail leaflet, ruptured papillary muscle, severe retraction, large perforation; secondary: severe tenting, poor leaflet coaptation)
LV and LA size[†]	Usually normal	Normal or mild dilated		Dilated[‡]
Qualitative Doppler				
Color flow jet area[§]	**Small, central, narrow, often brief**	Variable		Large central jet (>50% of LA) or eccentric wall-impinging jet of variable size
Flow convergence[‖]	**Not visible, transient or small**	Intermediate in size and duration		**Large throughout systole**
CWD jet	Faint/partial/parabolic	Dense but partial or parabolic		Holosystolic/dense/**triangular**
Semiquantitative				
VCW (cm)	<0.3	Intermediate		≥0.7 (>0.8) for biplane)[¶]
Pulmonary vein flow[#]	**Systolic dominance** (may be blunted in LV dysfunction or AF)	Normal or systolic blunting[#]		Minimal to no systolic flow/ **systolic flow reversal**
Mitral inflow[**]	**A-wave dominant**	Variable		E-wave dominant (>1.2 m/sec)
Quantitative[††,‡‡]				
EROA, 2D PISA (cm^2)	<0.20	0.20-0.29	0.30-0.39	≥0.40 (may be lower in secondary MR with elliptical ROA)
RVol (mL)	<30	30-44	45-59[††]	≥ 60 (may be lower in flow conditions)
RF (%)	<30	30-39	40-49	≥50

ROA, Regurgitant orifice area.
Bolded qualitative and semiquantitative signs are considered specific for their MR grade.
[*]All parameters have limitations, and an integrated approach must be used that weights the strength of each echocardiographic measurement. All signs and measures should be interpreted in an individualized manner that account for body size, sex, and all other patient characteristics.
[†]This pertains mostly to patients with primary MR.
[‡]LV and LA can be within the "normal" range for patients with acute severe MR or with chronic severe MR who have small body size, particularly women, or with small LV size preceding the occurrence of MR.
[§]With Nyquist limit 50-70 cm/sec.
[‖]Small flow convergence is usually <0.3 cm, and large is 1 cm at a Nyquist limit of 30-40 cm/sec.
[¶]For average between apical two- and four-chamber views.
[#]Influenced by many other factors (LV diastolic function, atrial fibrillation, LA pressure).
[**]Most valid patients >50 years old and is influenced by other causes of elevated LA pressure.
[††]Discrepancies among EROA, RF, and RVol may arise in the setting of low or high flow states.
[‡‡]Quantitative parameters can help subclassify the moderate regurgitation group.

FIGURE 3.13 These 2017 guideiines offer parameters for determining the severity of chronic mitral regurgitation. Source: Zohgbi WA, Adams D, Ronow RO, et al. Recommendations for Noninvasive Evaluation of Native Valvular Regurgitation. A report from the American Society of Echocardiography Developed in Collaboration with the Society for Cardiovascular Magnetic Resonance. *J Am Soc Echocardiogr.* 2017;30(4):303-371.

Imaging and Calculations Obtained From the Principle of the Proximal Isovelocity Surface Area

- An apical view should be chosen that identifies the PISA as a hemisphere and is in an axis that is as parallel as possible to the Doppler beam. This is most accurately done when there is one jet.
- The scale should be turned down in the direction of flow such that the PISA radius is as well defined as possible (usually in the 20-30 cm/s range).
- The PISA radius should be measured from the base of the hemisphere to the outer aliased limit. One can sometimes measure the vena contracta when these settings are made.
- Next, the CW Doppler should be used to find the complete envelope of the MR jet, and this should be traced to obtain the maximum velocity and the velocity time integral (VTI) of the velocity profile.
- The surface area of a sphere is $4\pi r^2$ and that of a hemisphere is $2\pi r^2$. The continuity equation can be rearranged such that the effective orifice area (ERO) equals $2\pi r^2$ × the ratio of the aliasing velocity to the maximum MR velocity (not the VTI).

- In order to calculate the regurgitant fraction, one has to measure the velocity-time integral of the LVOT using pulsed wave Doppler, the LVOT diameter, and from these calculate the volume per beat. The MR volume is equal to the ERO × the VTI of the MR velocity profile. The regurgitant fraction (%) is the MR volume divided by the stroke volume × 100.

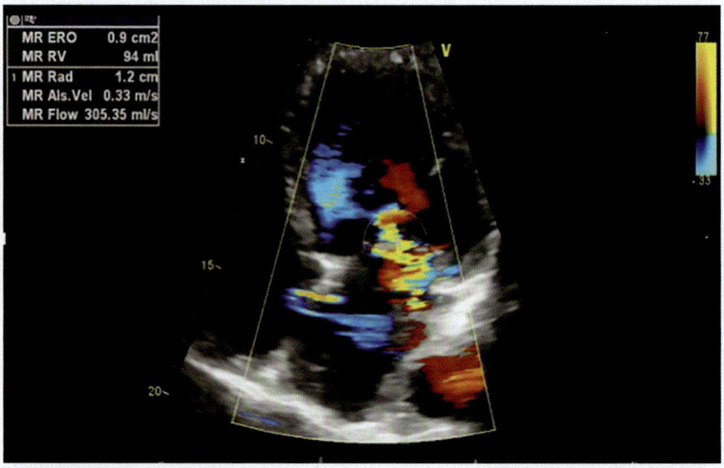

FIGURE 3.14 PISA radius = 1.2 cm
MR Max velocity = 335 cm/s
Aliasing velocity = 33 cm/s
MR ERO = 0.9 cm²
MR volume = 94 mL
MR VTI = 103.6 cm.

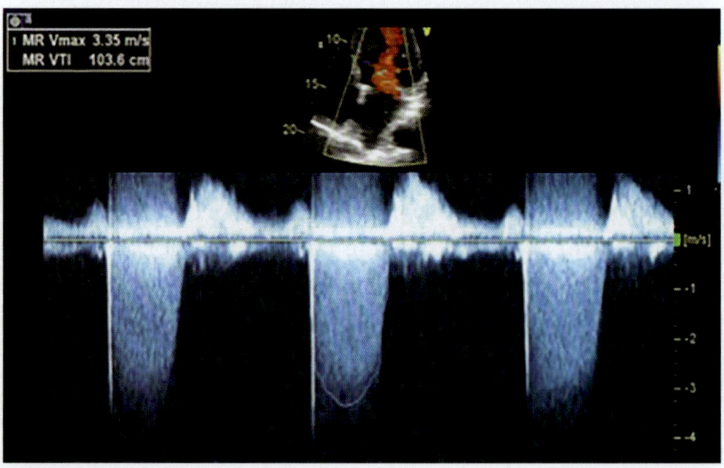

FIGURE 3.15 ERO = 6.28 × $(1.2)^2$ × 33/335 = 0.9 cm²
MR volume = 0.9 × 103.6 = 94 m.

CALCULATION OF THE ERO AND THE REGURGITANT VOLUME BY THE PISA METHOD

PISA radius = 1.2 cm
MR Max velocity = 335 cm/s
Aliasing velocity = 33 cm/s
MR ERO = 0.9 cm^2
MR volume = 94 mL
MR VTI = 103.6 cm

$$\text{ERO} = 2\pi r_{\text{PISA}^2} \times \frac{\text{Aliasing velocity}}{\text{max MR velocity}}$$

$$\text{ERO} = 6.28 \times (1.2)^2 \times \frac{33}{335} = 0.9 \text{ cm}^2$$

$$\text{MR volume} = \text{ERO} \times \text{VTI}_{\text{MR}}$$

$$\text{MR volume} = 0.9 \times 103.6 = 94 \text{mL}$$

PITFALLS IN QUANTIFICATION OF MITRAL REGURGITATION

This method assumes that the shape of the isovelocity region is hemispheric (surface area = $2\pi r^2$). This may not be true, and at times there are two regurgitant jets or a different shape associated with an EROA of an unusual shape. The PISA may vary in shape depending on the type of disease process that is present and the timing of the regurgitant jet. For example, in late systolic mitral regurgitation, the PISA may be the largest during the latter part of systole and care must be taken to choose the largest hemispheric radius. In addition, in the case of functional mitral regurgitation, the vena contracta may be long and narrow and not a perfect circle. The vena contracta may not be well defined. If the proximal flow acceleration field is constrained by ventricular walls and the area of convergence does not have a flat base, then an angle correction should be made. For example, if the angle is constrained to 160°, then a factor of 160/180 should be applied to the PISA equation.[19]

Three-dimensional echocardiographic imaging along with parametric analysis can offer more accurate assessment of the actual EROA, annular shape and size, and leaflet position.[18]

SEMIQUANTITATIVE METHODS

Practically in the setting of a procedure such as a MitraClip in the catheterization laboratory, an assessment of the degree of mitral regurgitation must be done quickly for reference and then for comparison after the procedure. In different settings, more time is available for more detailed assessment of mitral regurgitation for quantity, anatomy, and feasibility for repair or replacement.

For example, in the catheterization laboratory, a visual assessment of the size of the regurgitant jet relative to the left atrial area, the direction of the jet, and the influence of the mitral regurgitation on the pattern of pulmonary vein inflow pattern can be coupled with information from the catheterization table such as the V wave height in the LA pressure tracing or pulmonary capillary wedge pressure to quickly assess baseline information and postintervention information. Eccentric jets are often underestimated, the Coanda effect.[20] At this point, the question about the adequacy of the result must be answered. If a clip has been applied and these assessments indicate incomplete result, then another might be needed.

The above-mentioned quantitative and semiquantitative methods will be illustrated.

MitraClip Procedure

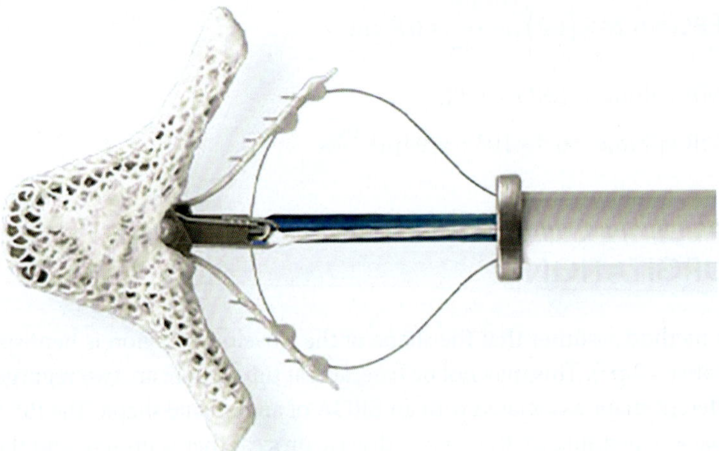

FIGURE 3.16 The distal end of the clip device is shown above. The clip itself is covered with polyester and is made of chromium and cobalt alloy. It has "grippers" that have small teeth that pin the leaflet down. The "grippers" are controlled by small coaxial wires allowing them to be moved down toward the clip at the correct time. Control of the clip itself is dome by a coaxial system and allows them to be opened and closed and even everted if necessary.

The MitraClip repair is a procedure that uses the above device to clip the anterior and posterior mitral leaflets in the region of the malcoaptation. This clip is delivered from a transvenous catheter that is advanced from the inferior vena cava to the right atrium. After choosing an appropriate location in the interatrial septum as guided by transesophageal echo, a puncture is made followed by advancement of a larger delivery catheter into the left atrium. The device is then positioned above the appropriate location on the mitral orifice, oriented in the anteroposterior position, and advanced into the left ventricle. After pulling up the wings toward the leaflets such as to trap the anterior and posterior leaflets, the grippers are dropped and the leaflets captured. A 3D echo is used to appropriately orient the device, and the 2D images from the grasping view and its orthogonal view are used to locate and guide the grasp. After grasping, assessment is made with echo using analysis of flow disturbance in the pulmonary veins and left atrial appendage (LAA). Color Doppler analysis of the mitral regurgitation jet gives

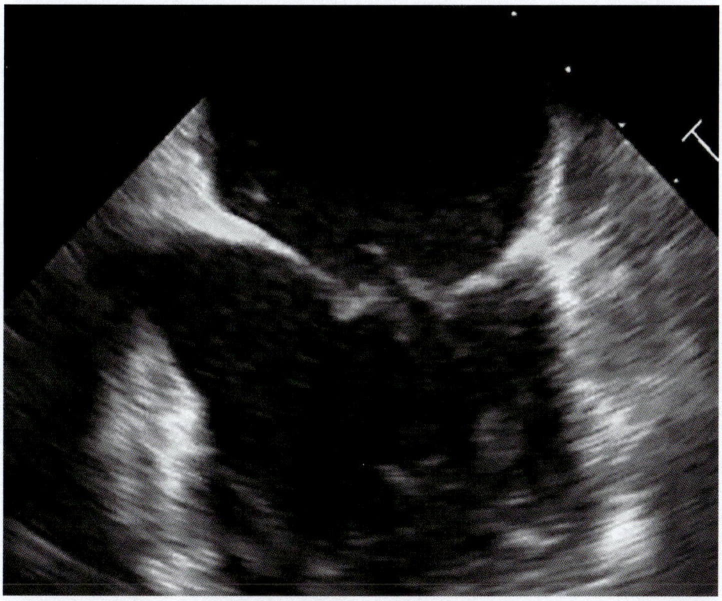

FIGURE 3.17 This view of the mitral valve in a long axis view shows the target ruptured chord to the posterior leaflet, the site of the problem and the source of the severe mitral regurgitation. TEE, 20° view.

immediate information of the jet also. If adequate reduction of the mitral regurgitation is deemed present, the procedure is complete; if it is less than desired, then another clip is guided into place on one or other side of the first device.

These steps are illustrated in the sections that follow.

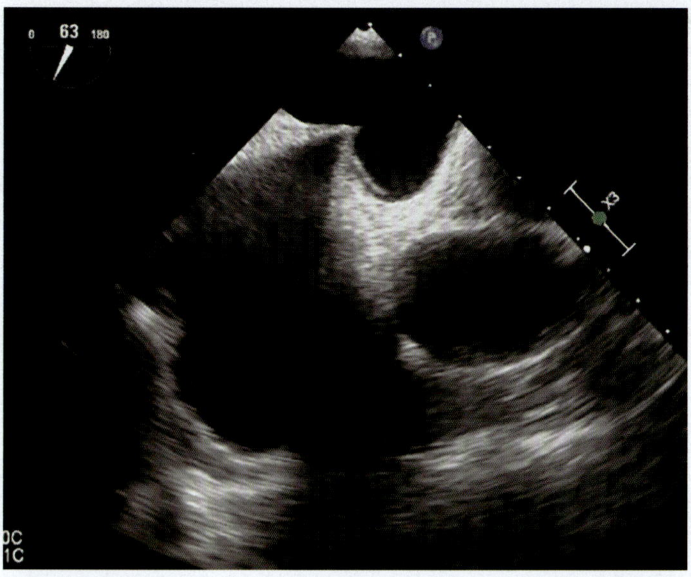

FIGURE 3.18 Transesophageal echo is used for guidance of the transseptal puncture. The desirable location for the puncture is within the fossa ovalis and well away from the aorta. Once the puncture is made, the delivery catheter can be introduced and preparations for clip delivery can be started. TEE, 63°, the short axis view to include the aorta.

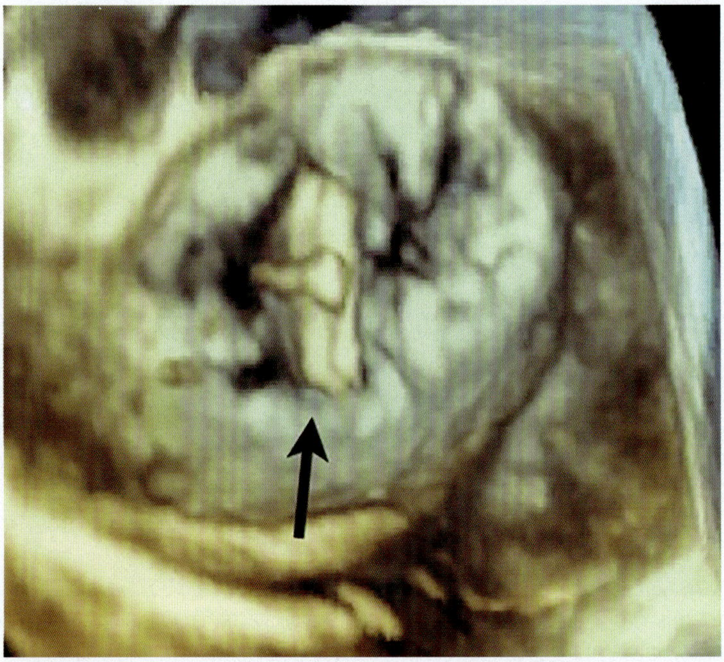

FIGURE 3.19 3D assessment of the position of the open-winged clip (*black arrow*) is performed, noting that it is located close to the A1/P1 region from the surgeon's view.

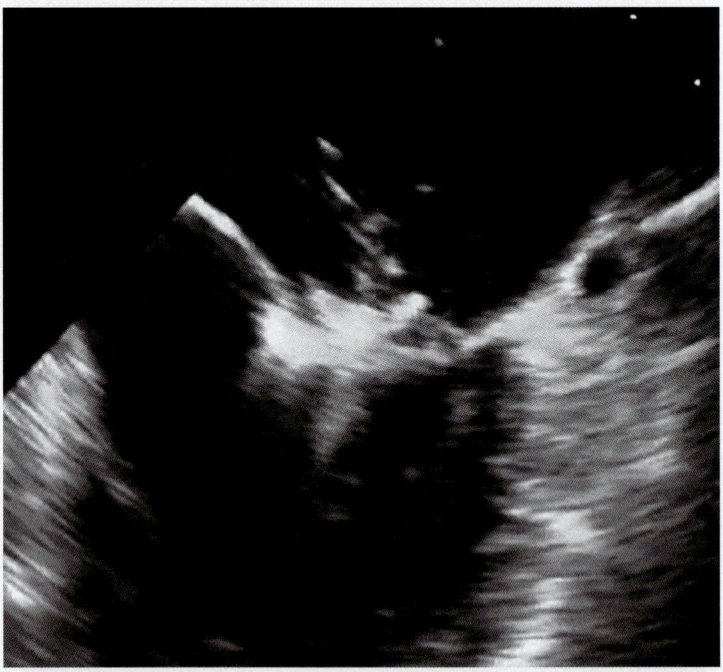

FIGURE 3.20 The clip with wings open has been advanced through the mitral valve, and the grippers are up and in place to be closed at the appropriate time. The location in other views is confirmed. The relationship of the clip to the vena contracta of the jet is also assessed. TEE, 20° view.

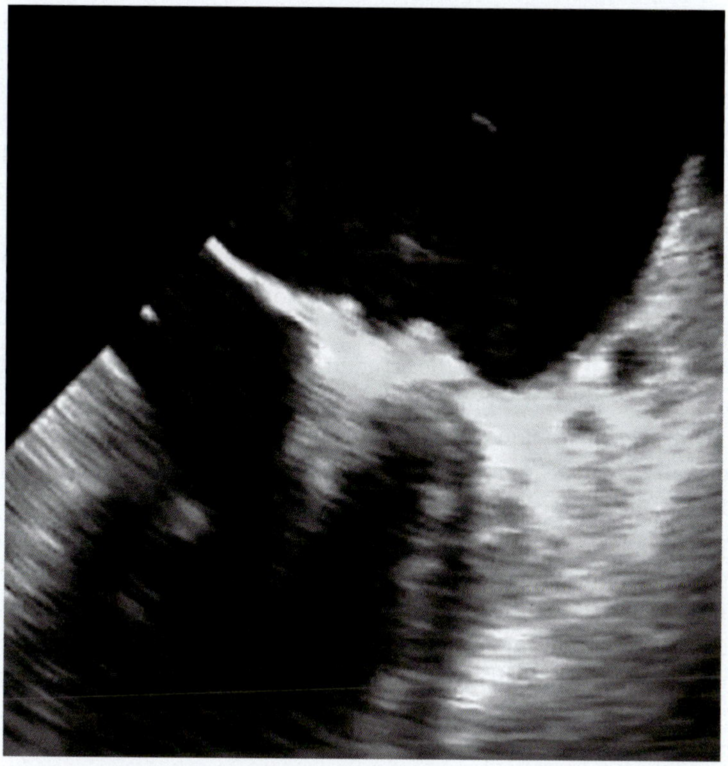

FIGURE 3.21 The grippers have been dropped, and the flail segment of the posterior leaflet has been grasped. Both anterior and posterior leaflets are within the grippers.

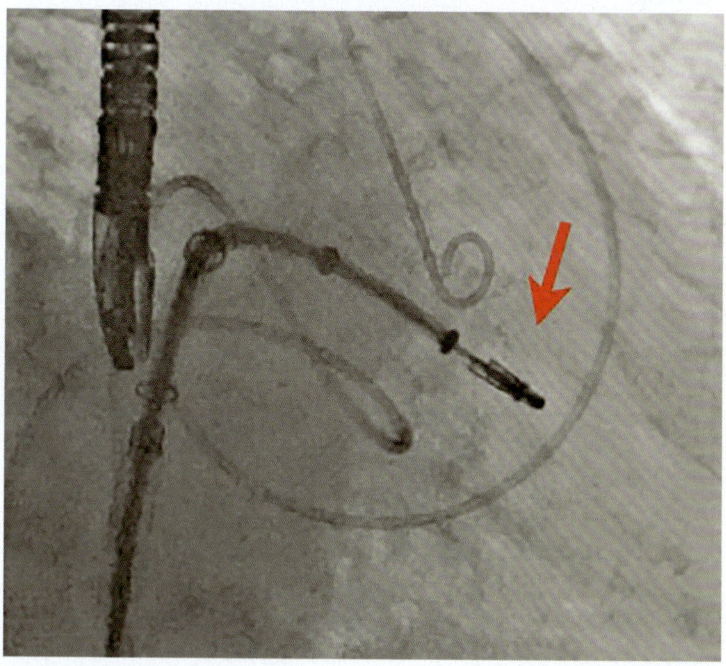

FIGURE 3.22 From the right anterior oblique view in the catheterization laboratory, the clip is in place and preparations for release are made. Clip indicated by *red arrow*.

The above sequence is from the initial transseptal puncture to the deployment of the clip. Transseptal puncture is guided using echo from the short axis 60° view to assess the position relative to the aorta and the 90° view to assess the superoinferior orientation. The puncture site can then be assessed from the apical four-chamber view to determine the height above the mitral annulus, which ideally is in the 4.5-cm range from a perpendicular dropped from a line parallel to the annulus at the level of the puncture.

Position of the clip above the targeted area and monitoring of the position of the clip in addition to determining the location of the leaflets within the grippers are performed before the moment of "dropping the grippers."

Throughout this process, the structural interventionalist is making observations on fluoroscopy, making sure from that standpoint all is in position. From the right anterior oblique (RAO) view on fluoroscopy, these structures usually have a familiar appearance, and both modalities should be in agreement before "dropping the grippers." Once these two modalities come together, the postclip assessment of the result begins with analysis of the MR jet on color Doppler, the status of pulmonary vein flow patterns, and the 3D visualization of the positioning of the clips. From the four-chamber views, a figure-of-8 configuration of the mitral leaflets should be present, and assessment of the gradients through each orifice is made. Once all is satisfactory, the catheters are removed and a final assessment from the imaging and hemodynamic standpoint is made of the cardiac status to include the presence or absence of pericardial effusion.

The V Wave in the Catheterization Laboratory Before and After the Clip

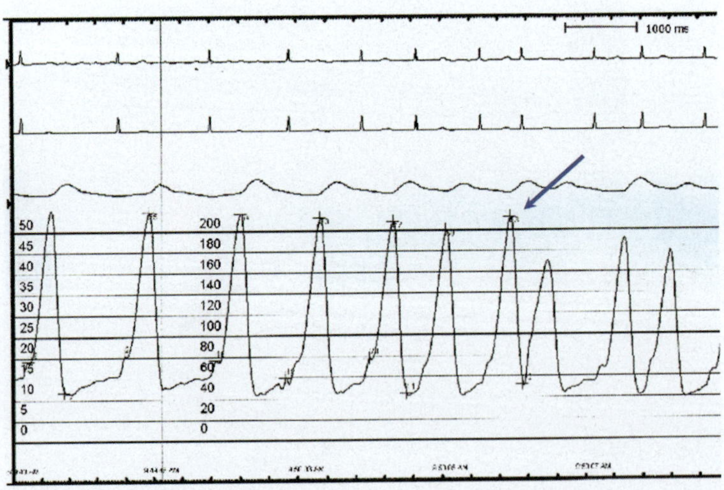

FIGURE 3.23 The V wave peaks out above 50 mm Hg when directly measured in the left atrium recorded just after the transseptal puncture (*blue arrow*). Atrial fibrillation is present; note the late systolic peak of the V wave.

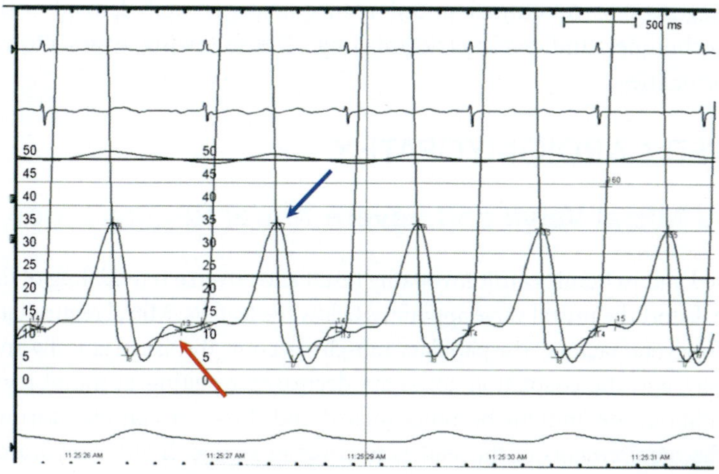

FIGURE 3.24 The V wave measured directly from the left atrium just after the application of the clip. In this tracing, the left ventricular tracing is recorded at the same scale. Note that the peak V wave (*blue arrow*) occurs on the downslope of the left ventricular pressure curve and that it peaks out at 35 mm Hg. Note also that there is no significant diastolic gradient (*red arrow*).

SECTION 3

FUNCTIONAL MITRAL REGURGITATION

Functional mitral regurgitation is a type of secondary mitral regurgitation in which the leaflets themselves are normal. The abnormality is present because the left ventricle is dilated and the papillary muscles are displaced from their central axis and pulled downward into the left ventricle. This tethers the mitral leaflets, pulling apart the coaptation areas, and results in mitral regurgitation. The jet of this type of regurgitation is usually centrally directed in contrast to that of degenerative disease of the mitral valve, which produces jets of mitral regurgitation that are usually directed eccentrically either to an anterior or a posterior direction depending on which leaflet is involved. The exception is the functional mitral regurgitation seen in the setting of inferior myocardial infarction and the tethering that occurs results in a posterior-directed jet of mitral regurgitation.[21]

Intervention in functional mitral regurgitation requires risk-benefit analysis since the underlying myocardial disease is a significant factor and manipulations such as pump runs are compromising in themselves.[21,22] Surgical repair with mitral rings is not ideal since the problem is in the ventricle and not with redundant, prolapsing leaflets. MitraClip procedures are possible if the opposing leaflets lend themselves to the clip. Another factor is that the left ventricle is afterloaded and the mitral regurgitation is a "pop off" for the compromised left ventricle. The ejection fraction may not fully reflect the systolic function of the left ventricle.

Hypertrophic cardiomyopathy also is associated with a type of function mitral regurgitation in which there is abnormal orientation of papillary muscles, elongated leaflets, and abnormal coaptation that all occurs within the left ventricle and not in a prolapsed position.[23]

Diagnosis of functional mitral regurgitation is well defined with 2D and 3D techniques and parametric imaging. The following pages illustrate these abnormalities.

DILATED CARDIOMYOPATHY

Tethered Mitral Valve and Severe Mitral Regurgitation

Dilated and ischemic cardiomyopathy result and adverse remodeling of the left ventricle distort the mitral valve apparatus below the leaflets. Mitral regurgitation results due to several factors. The papillary muscles become displaced apically and posterolaterally, and the coaptation zones are decreased resulting in mitral regurgitation. In addition, the annulus becomes dilated and does not contract, further increasing the requirements of the leaflets to cover in systole. Inferior myocardial infarction results in a regional wall motion abnormality that displaces the posterolateral papillary muscle downward, tethering the medial aspect of the mitral apparatus in an asymmetric fashion. Previously this was thought to be due to papillary muscle dysfunction; however, more recently, the tethering concept has clarified this issue.

Two-dimensional echocardiography has been used to analyze the annular dimension, leaflet length, coaptation depth, and tethering area. Three-dimensional echocardiography has further clarified these issues and made measurements that quantitate the above parameters.[21,24-26]

MECHANISMS OF MITRAL REGURGITATION

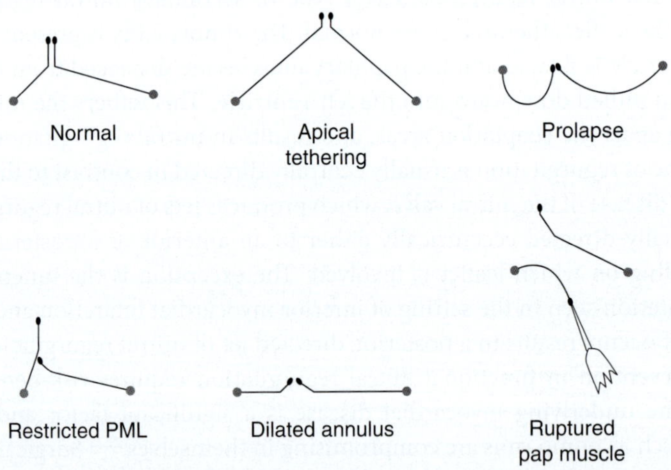

FIGURE 3.25 In this diagram, note the line of coaptation of the normal valve, which is usually ~1 cm and in general allows for a perfect seal in systole. In prolapse, there is billowing as described by Dr. Barlow and the coaptation point is at or above the line of the annulus in the parasternal long axis view of the echocardiogram. The billowing can be demonstrated well with parametric imaging. In the case of dilated cardiomyopathy, the leaflets are pulled apart and the line of coaptation goes to zero and mitral regurgitation occurs. In inferior myocardial infarction, the posterior mitral leaflet is pulled down and leaves the anterior leaflet behind losing the line of coaptation, and regurgitation follows. Not in this diagram is hypertrophic cardiomyopathy in which the anterior leaflet is elongated and in a more anterior position, and when the posterior leaflet is relatively short, then coaptation is lost and mitral regurgitation occurs, especially when the anterior leaflet is pulled toward the interventricular septum. (Source: Dal-Bianco JP, Levine RA, Goldstein SA. *ASE's Comprehensive Echocardiography*. 2nd ed. Philadelphia, PA: Elsevier (Sanders); 2016.)

Hypertrophic Cardiomyopathy and Mitral Regurgitation

The mitral regurgitation that is seen with hypertrophic cardiomyopathy has been studied in detail. The systolic anterior motion of the anterior mitral leaflet pulls apart the mitral coaptation zones of the mitral leaflets and results in a variable degree of regurgitation. Often the anterior leaflet of the mitral valve is longer than usual, and coaptation somewhat depends on the length of the corresponding posterior mitral leaflet. Papillary muscle orientation is also abnormal in that the muscles are thicker and are oriented in a direction toward each other and the overall position of the anterior papillary muscle is more toward the interventricular septum than usual. Abnormal and anomalous papillary muscles often aggravate this abnormal systolic orientation of the anterior leaflet further adding to the development of systolic anterior motion of the mitral valve. If the posterior leaflet is relatively short, then during systole when the anterior leaflet assumes a more septal position coaptation is disrupted and mitral regurgitation results. A longer posterior leaflet offers a more favorable opportunity for maintaining coaptation as the anterior leaflet is pulled away by systolic anterior motion. Generally, after intervention with either alcohol septal ablation or surgical myomectomy, the mitral regurgitation decreases. The mechanisms of the mitral regurgitation seen in hypertrophic obstructive cardiomyopathy are outlined in an excellent recent publication by Silbiger.[27]

SECTION 4

MITRAL VALVE ENDOCARDITIS

Endocarditis is a dreaded complication of valve disease. Before the era of antibiotics, endocarditis was almost universally fatal resulting in progressive destruction of the valve and resultant severe regurgitation, embolization, and heart failure. It was termed "malignant endocarditis." Extracardiac manifestations of this illness included embolic lesions to the fingernails, skin, eyes, and brain and glomerulonephritis. Peripheral septic manifestations in the joints to include the back, liver, spleen, and kidneys all indicate advanced disease. Penicillin was a major factor in the treatment of this illness.

Currently, focus has been on prevention and early identification of the illness. The presence of a murmur and fever triggers the need for blood cultures before antibiotics are prescribed and allows for a diagnosis before any of the embolic complications. Unexplained stroke always provokes thoughts about valve lesions, and the echocardiogram has answers to give. In addition, hospitalized patients with bacteremia often need investigation of the heart for vegetations and valve involvement. In this situation, the transesophageal echo has offered another dimension in diagnostic accuracy and is often part of the evaluation of bacteremia. The Duke Criteria are helpful in diagnosing endocarditis.[28,29]

Organisms vary from the indolent *Streptococcus viridans* and HACEK organisms (*Haemophilus* species, *Aggregatibacter* species, *Cardiobacterium hominis*, *Eikenella corrodens*, and *Kingella* species) to aggressive virulent *Staphylococcus* species. Immunocompromised individuals and those on long term antibiotics are predisposed to fungal endocarditis. Fungal vegetations are on top of the list of organisms producing large vegetations.[30-32]

The possibility of endocarditis is always a serious consideration in the presence of a prosthetic valve and requires special attention to the diagnosis and treatment. In native and prosthetic valve endocarditis, transesophageal echocardiography offers better sensitivity in detecting vegetations and extent of involvement than does transthoracic echocardiography.[33,34]

Examples of infective endocarditis and the effects on the heart are illustrated on the following pages.

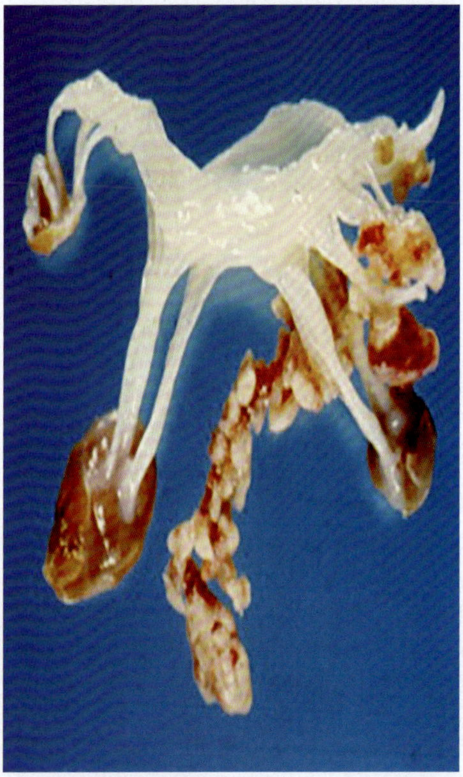

FIGURE 3.26 A long stringlike vegetation attached to the chordal surface of the mitral valve apparatus (*yellow arrow*).

ENTEROCOCCUS FAECALIS ENDOCARDITIS IN A PARAPLEGIC INDIVIDUAL—POST MVA

Enterococcus is an indolent yet destructive organism. It usually has an origin in the gastrointestinal or urinary tract and requires antibiotic adjustments for appropriate sensitivities. Vancomycin-resistant enterococcus is a particularly difficult-to-treat organism but usually does not cause endocarditis as the *faecalis* subspecies does.

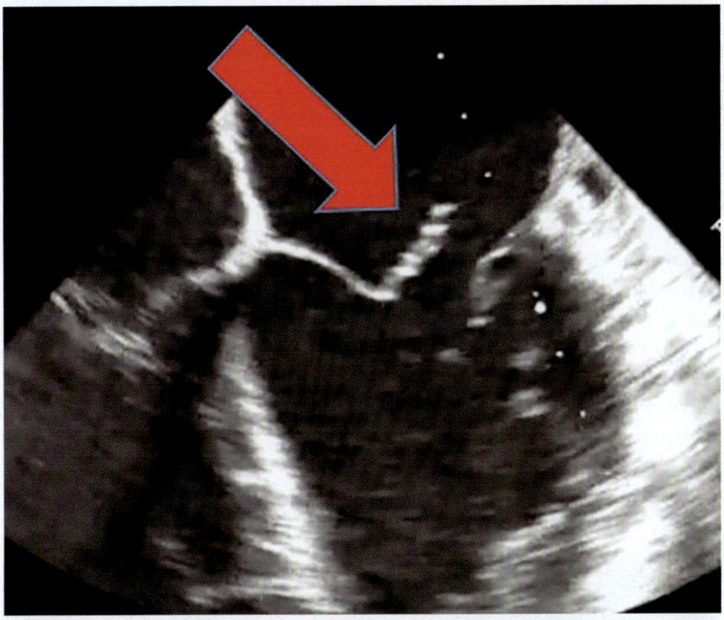

FIGURE 3.27 Mitral anterior leaflet with flail segment. There was a history of *Enterococcus faecalis* sepsis—the infection has destroyed the chordal structure of the AMVL (*red arrow* indicated ruptured chord). TEE, 32°.

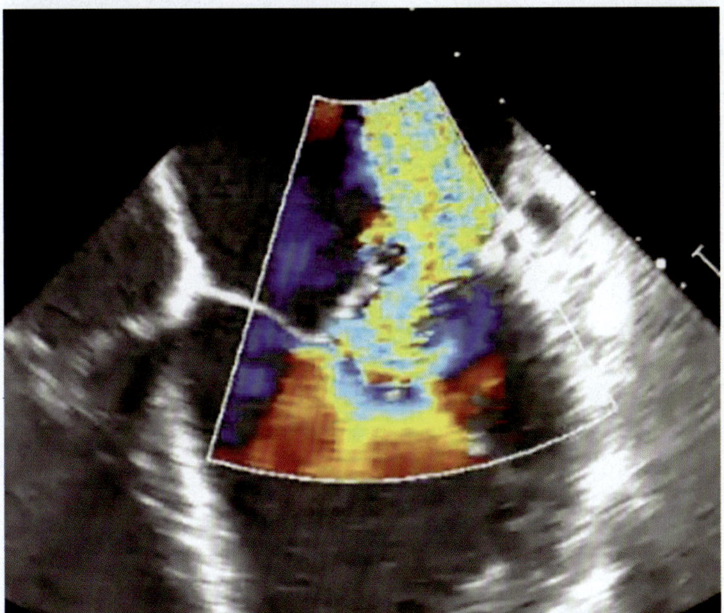

FIGURE 3.28 Severe mitral regurgitation with a large PISA and a wide vena contracta resulting from the flail midsection of the AMVL. TEE, A4C view.

CASE PRESENTATION

Endocarditis With Large Vegetations on the Mitral Valve Due to *Candida Albicans*

Candida albicans and other fungal organisms are responsible for some of the largest vegetations seen on echocardiograms. They have major embolic potential and are often seen in individuals who are immunocompromised.

A 64-year-old gentleman who has had a renal transplant 6 years before. He was immunosuppressed. On presentation, he had experienced emboli to several areas including the brain. The brain involvement was such that cardiopulmonary bypass and anticoagulation were not possible. He expired a few days later.

Fungal vegetations are often large and bulky and tend to embolize. They may not be so destructive to valve tissue, but the embolic consequences can be a major problem as in this clinical situation.

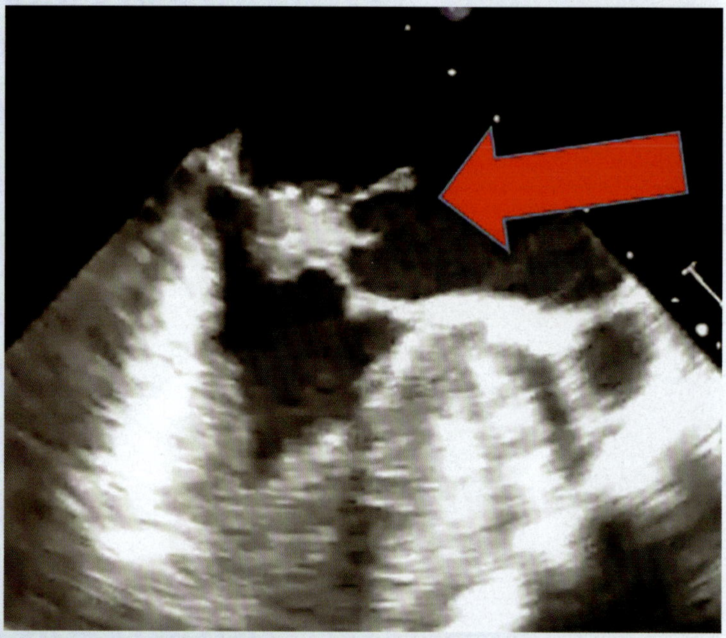

FIGURE 3.29 Large vegetation with complex irregularities (*red arrow*). TEE, 64°.

SECTION 5

MITRAL PROSTHETIC VALVES

Prosthetic valves that are currently available for use in the mitral position fall into two categories. First is that of mechanical valves, which can be ball-in-cage valves, single-leaflet valves, or bileaflet valves. Efforts have been made through the years to develop a valve that has a favorable hemodynamic profile and a minimal tendency to form thrombi. Careful attention to maintaining adequate anticoagulation is imperative to avoid thrombus formation on the valve. Bleeding risks are still present despite excellent control at times when anticoagulation is interrupted or if inadequate for one reason or other. The second category is that of bioprosthetic valves, which are either bovine or porcine. The bovine valves are constructed using bovine pericardium whereas the porcine valves are made from the actual aortic leaflet tissue itself. Mechanical valves have the potential of lasting indefinitely whereas the tissue valves generally have a durability of 10 to 15 years before degenerative changes begin to occur.[35]

Mitral valve repair as developed by Carpentier[5] is the procedure of choice for valves that have degenerative disease. This procedure is commonly used throughout the world. Echocardiography is an integral part of the surgical procedure in determining the etiology of the valve disease, planning the surgical procedure, and determining the adequacy of the repair when coming off the cardiopulmonary bypass. Follow-up echocardiograms offer long-term monitoring of the repair.

Transcatheter valves are on the drawing board and hopefully will have applications to individuals in whom more invasive procedures cannot be tolerated similar to the applications currently in use in the aortic position.

Echocardiography is a vital part of monitoring prosthetic valves both from the hemodynamic standpoint and from the durability standpoint. Echocardiography is the procedure that is used when complications such as thrombosis are suspected.

Illustrations of echocardiographic finding in prosthetic valves are on the following pages.

PROSTHETIC VALVES

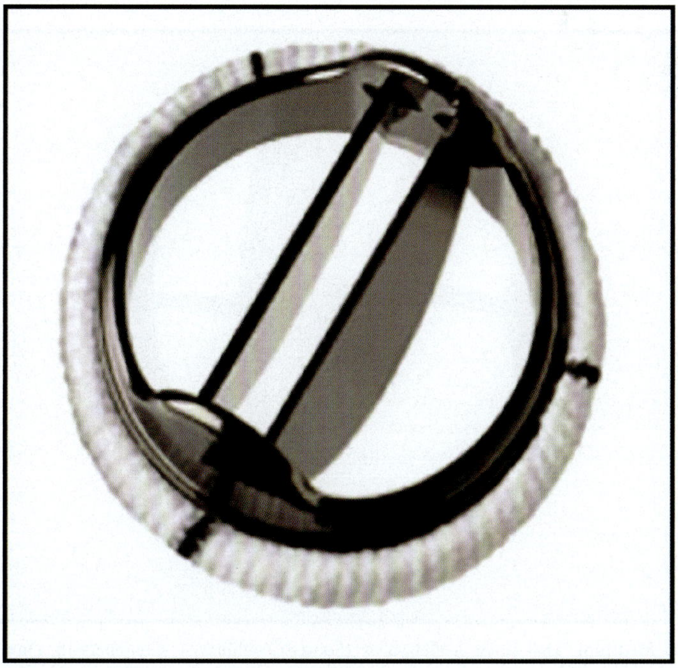

FIGURE 3.30 St Jude Bileaflet Valve. (Source: Zoghbi WA, Chambers JB, Dumesnil JG, et al. Recommendations for evaluation of prosthetic valves with echocardiography and Doppler ultrasound. Guidelines and standards. *J Am Soc Echocardiogr.* 2009;9:975-1014.)

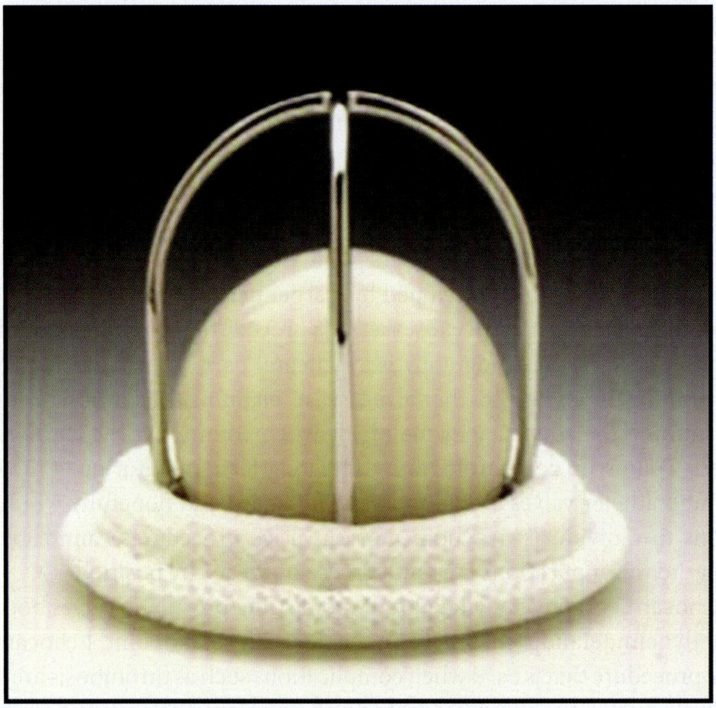

FIGURE 3.31 Starr Edwards ball in cage valve. (Source: Zoghbi WA, Chambers JB, Dumesnil JG, et al. Recommendations for evaluation of prosthetic valves with echocardiography and Doppler ultrasound. Guidelines and standards. *J Am Soc Echocardiogr.* 2009;9:975-1014.)

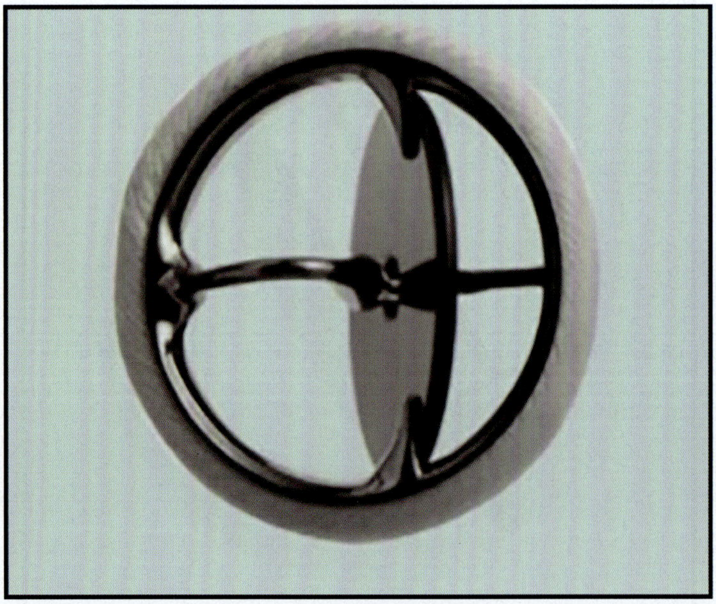

FIGURE 3.32 Medtronic Hall single leaflet valve. (Source: Zoghbi WA, Chambers JB, Dumesnil JG, et al. Recommendations for evaluation of prosthetic valves with echocardiography and Doppler ultrasound. Guidelines and standards. *J Am Soc Echocardiogr.* 2009;9:975-1014.)

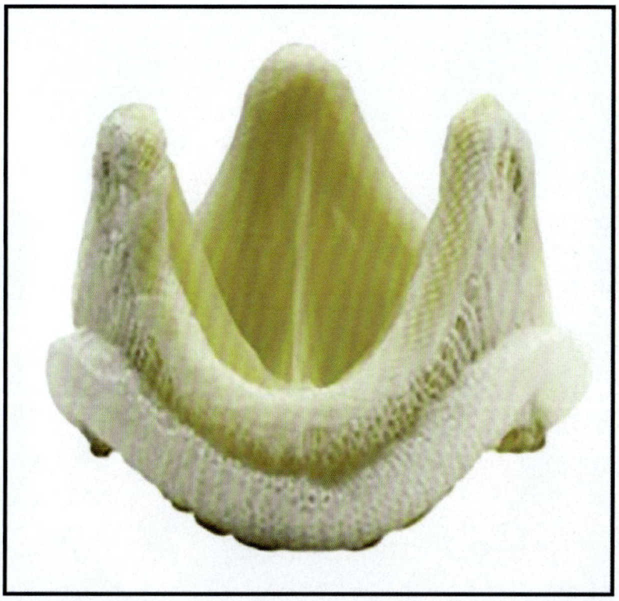

FIGURE 3.33 Porcine bioprosthetic valve. (Source: Zoghbi WA, Chambers JB, Dumesnil JG, et al. Recommendations for evaluation of prosthetic valves with echocardiography and Doppler ultrasound. Guidelines and standards. *J Am Soc Echocardiogr.* 2009;9:975-1014.)

Complications of Bioprosthetic Valves

MECHANISMS OF DEGENERATION OF BIOPROSTHETIC VALVES

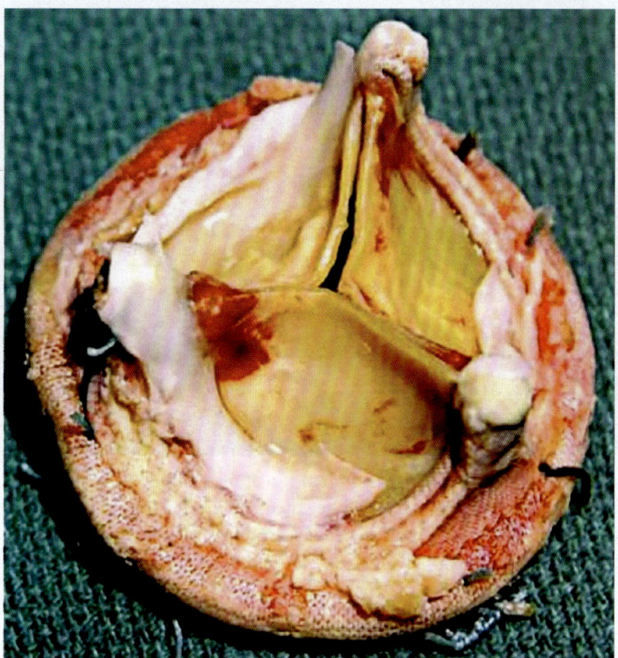

FIGURE 3.34 A pericardial valve that was stiff and stenotic. Although the leaflets appear thin, they were very stiff, and there was a high diastolic gradient across this valve. Pannus is also growing down upon the leaflets.

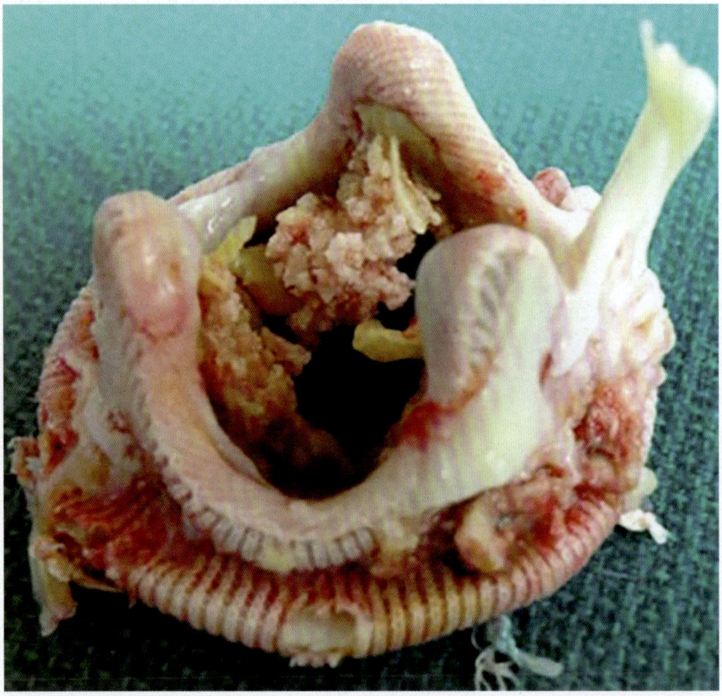

FIGURE 3.35 A calcified stenotic and regurgitant porcine valve.

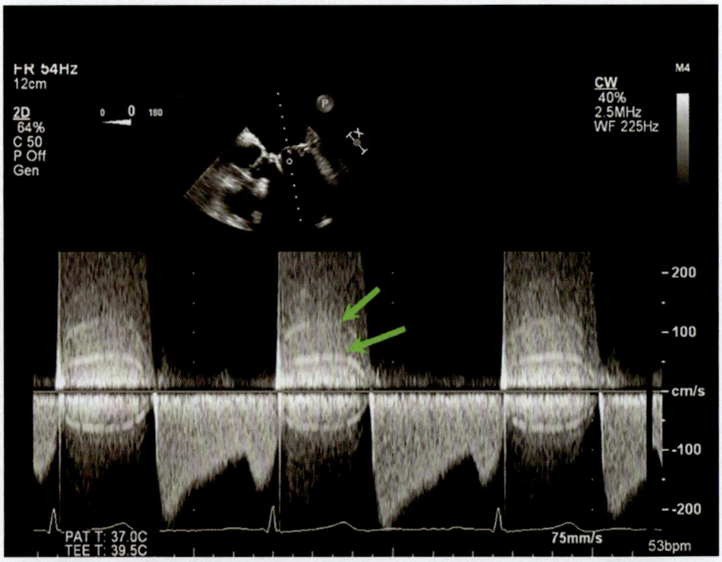

FIGURE 3.36 Sometimes in the setting of a ruptured leaflet of a mitral tissue prosthesis or even a ruptured chord to a native valve, a loud musical murmur will be noted. On CW or PW Doppler, the recordings will show "harmonic" sounds that have clustering of frequencies as seen above. This has been called the "rainbow" effect on the Doppler tracings (*green arrows*).

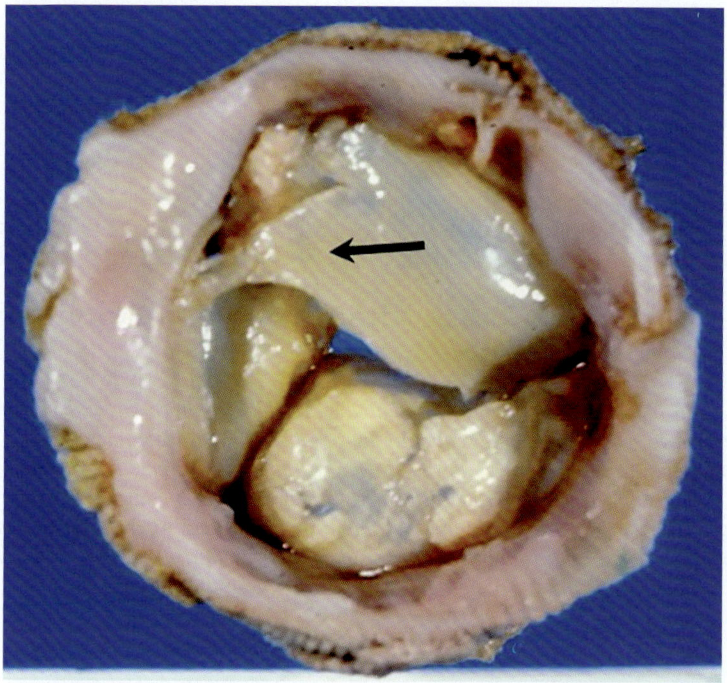

FIGURE 3.37 A bioprosthetic mitral valve that has been removed at surgery. One of the leaflets (*black arrow*) has ruptured, and the commissural area has become disrupted resulting in severe regurgitation. The atrial surface is shown.

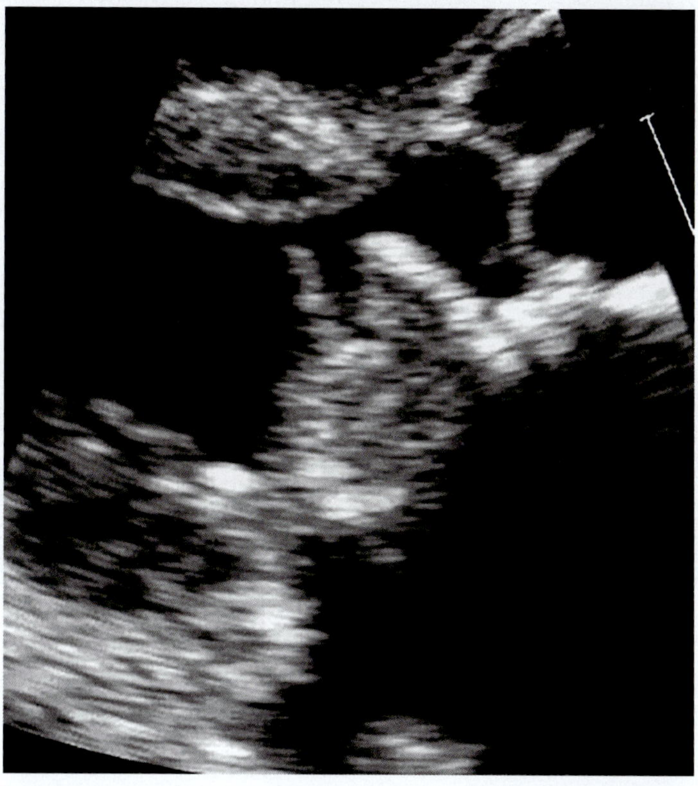

FIGURE 3.38 Endocarditis with large vegetations almost totally obstructed this bioprosthetic valve.

- Tears in the leaflets usually at the commissures
- Calcification of the leaflets
- Thrombosis of the valve
- Infection on the valve

CASE PRESENTATION

An Unusual Clinical Course After Mitral Valve Replacement with a Bioprosthetic Valve

A 60-year-old man who originally presented with alpha streptococcus endocarditis requiring mitral valve replacement. Subsequently he developed a paravalvular leak and had repair through a minimally invasive approach. He then presented 4 years after the original operation with fibrous deposits on the leaflets resulting in stenosis and later requiring replacement of the original prosthetic valve with a second mitral prosthesis. After the second valve and the development again of thrombus and pannus, prolonged anticoagulation resulted in resolution of the process, and the patient has continued to do well.

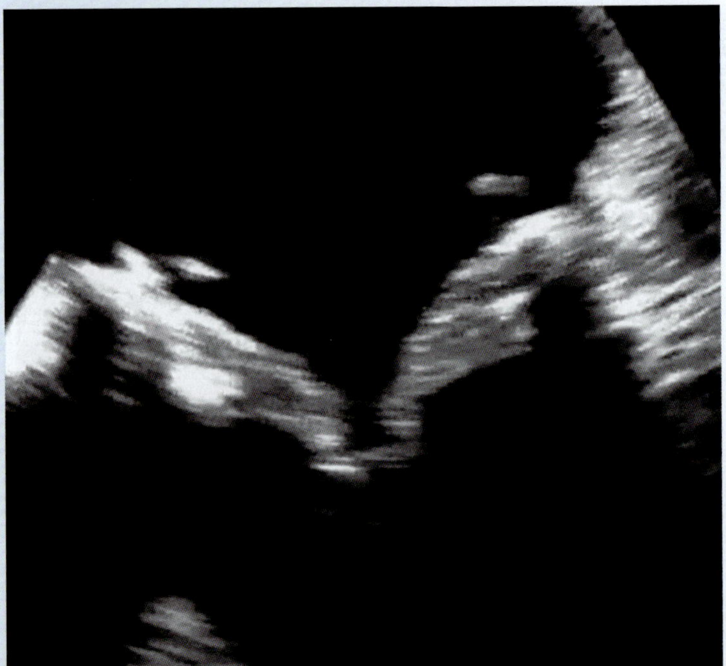

FIGURE 3.39 A diastolic frame on transesophageal echo showing thickening prosthetic leaflets—A4C view.

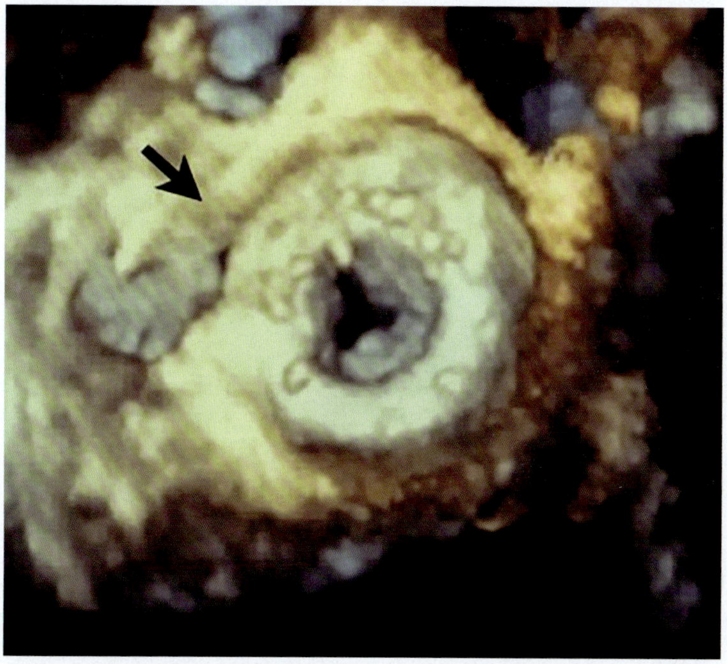

FIGURE 3.40 3D transesophageal echo demonstrating the stenotic MV, the small paravalvular defect (*black arrow*) adjacent to the LAA. TEE, surgeon's view.

BIOPROSTHETIC MITRAL VALVE WITH ENDOCARDITIS AND VEGETATIONS OBSTRUCTING THE VALVE

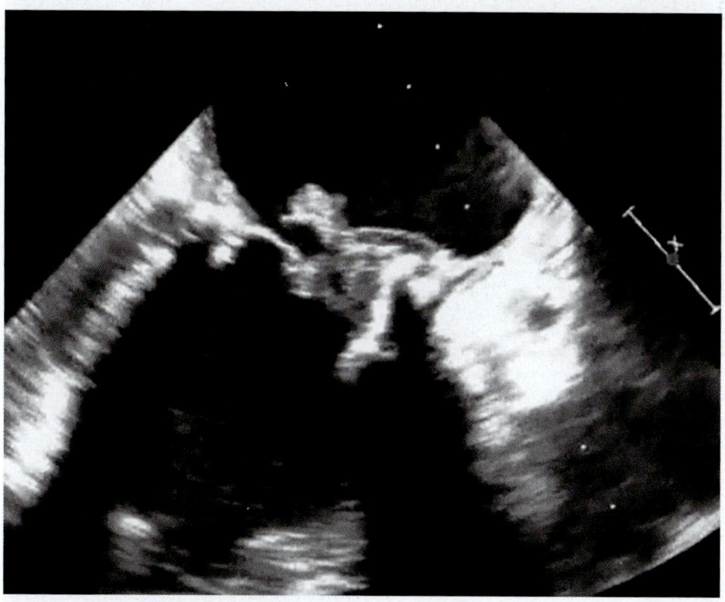

FIGURE 3.41 Another TEE view (89°) showing a large vegetation draped over the annulus prolapsing into the orifice of the prosthesis in diastole.

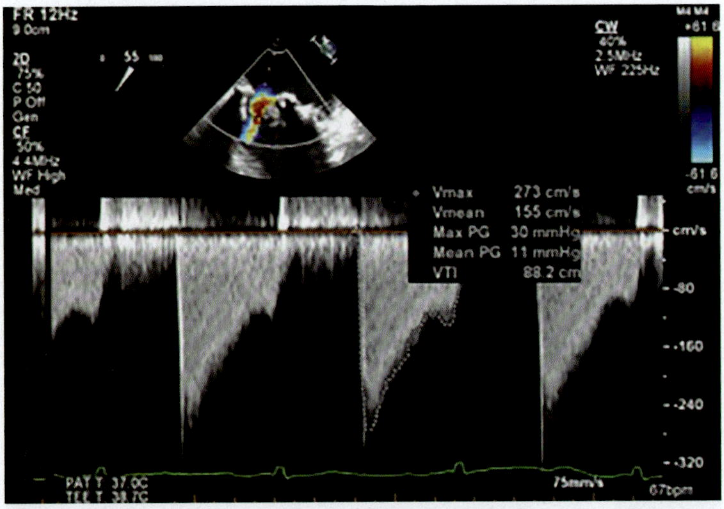

FIGURE 3.42 Another TEE view (89°) showing a large vegetation draped over the annulus prolapsing into the orifice of the prosthesis. The mean diastolic gradient across the valve was 11 mm Hg.

CASE PRESENTATION

Endocarditis on a Mitral Bioprosthetic Valve With Obstruction (*Staphylococcus epidermidis*)

A 70-year-old lady who had MVR and TVR with porcine valves. One year later she presented with positive blood cultures for Staphylococcus epidermidis and the following images.

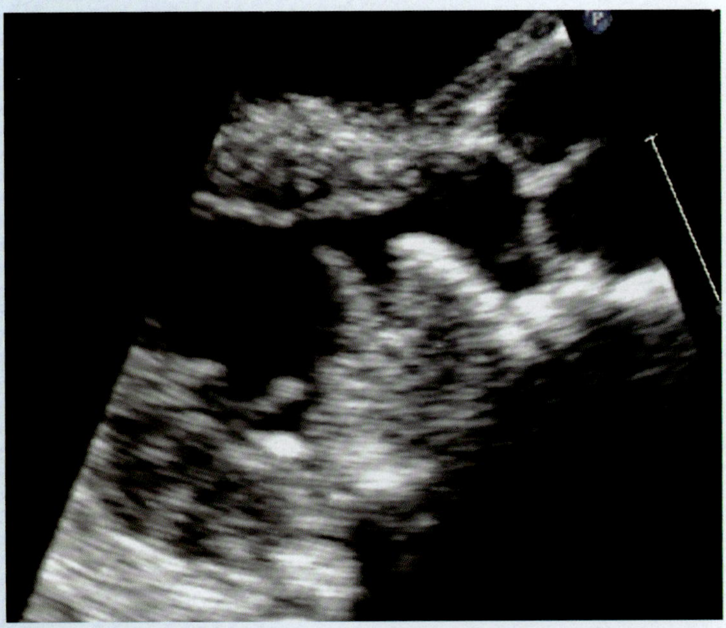

FIGURE 3.43 One year later this echo showing a large vegetation within the prosthetic valve nearly occluding the orifice. Blood cultures positive for *Staphylococcus epidermidis*. TTE, PLX view.

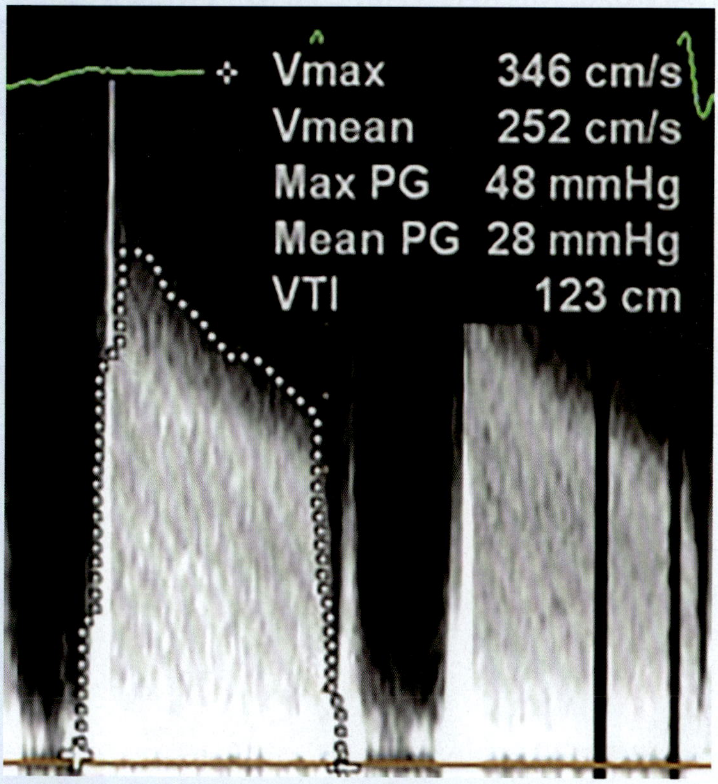

FIGURE 3.44 The CW Doppler tracing through the prosthetic mitral valve showing a mean gradient of 28 mm Hg.

Complications of Mechanical Valves

Thrombosis and obstruction of mechanical valves is a dreaded complication that requires immediate attention. Surgical removal or thrombolysis are the options. In addition, embolization related to the status of anticoagulation is also of major concern. Repeated surgical procedures can also result in leaks around the valves that can be detected by echocardiography. These sometimes lend themselves to transcatheter procedures for "plugging" of the leak.

If individuals with mechanical or bioprosthetic valves are not doing well clinically or if they have anemia due to hemolysis, transesophageal echo should be done searching for a perivalvular leak around the valve is often productive. Acoustic shadowing from these prostheses prevents identification of these leaks, and only indirect evidence is present. Location and degree of regurgitation can be quickly identified with transesophageal echocardiography.

Illustrations of these problems are noted in the pages that follow.

MECHANICAL MITRAL VALVE AND A MEDIAL PARAVALVULAR LEAK—AMPLATZER DEVICES APPLIED

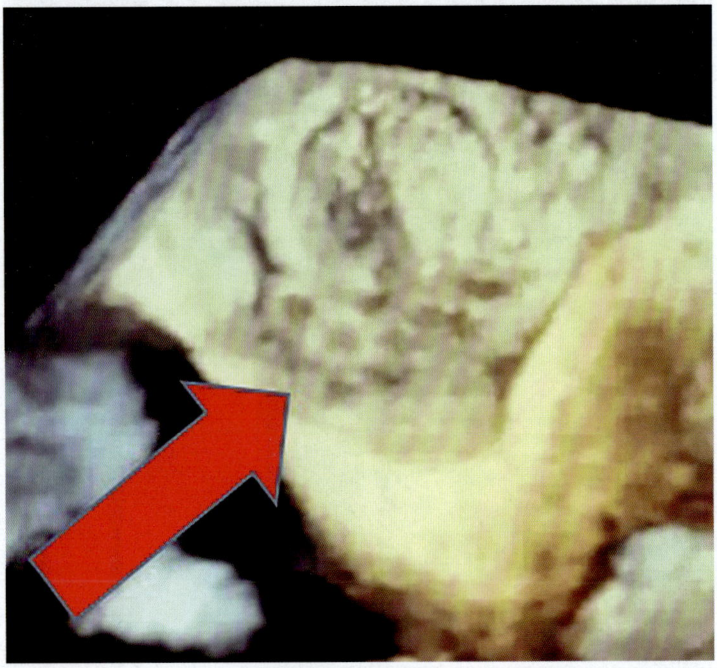

FIGURE 3.45 Posterior and medial Amplatzer plugs (two) applied to the paravalvular leak (*red arrow*). 3D TEE, 60° view.

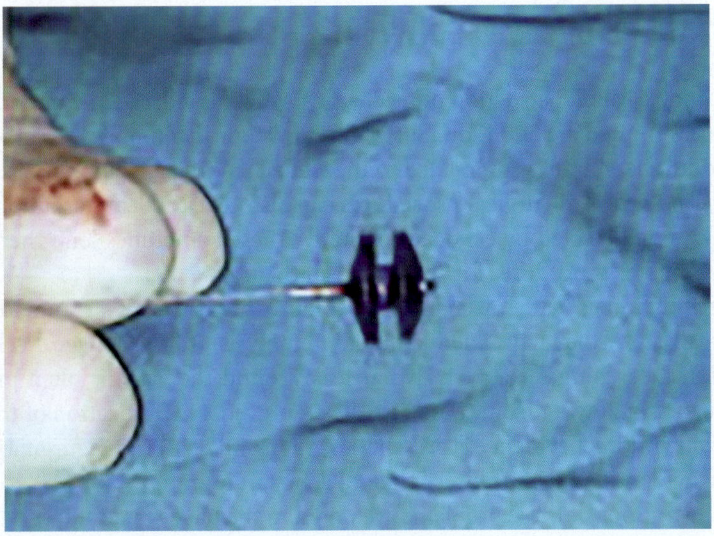

FIGURE 3.46 One of the small Amplatzer devices before placement.

SECTION 6

MITRAL ANNULAR CALCIFICATION

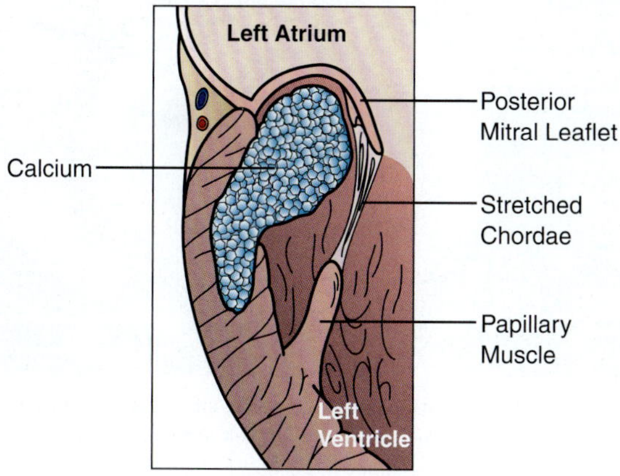

FIGURE 3.47 Drawing of calcified mitral annulus showing the calcification (*blue color*) of the annulus, lifting up the posterior mitral leaflet, and extending down into the posterior wall of the left ventricle. The calcification also encroaches on the orifice size of the mitral annulus and can cause stenosis. Distortion of the leaflets can alter coaptation and result in some degree of mitral regurgitation.

Note that the mitral annular calcification is such that the posterior mitral valve leaflet is on its ventricular side and results in the valve leaflet being draped over the calcification. When the calcification compromises the mitral orifice, it lifts the posterior leaflet up and extends it out into the orifice. This not only compromises the size of the mitral orifice but also can alter the motion of the leaflet. When the edges of the calcification are jagged and sharp, they might even sever chordal structures and result in mitral regurgitation. Calcification can also lift the mitral leaflet to the point of displacing it from the normal coaptation region and also resulting in mitral regurgitation.

Sometimes at surgery annular calcification causes placement of sutures to be difficult, and removal of the calcium has to be done. Surgeons have described this situation as that of the "hostile mitral annulus."[36,37] Manipulation of the mitral annular calcium must be done very carefully since the circumflex coronary artery and the coronary sinus are in this area. The left ventricular lead of biventricular pacers is also in this area. In mitral valve prolapse, the mitral annulus is frequently calcified, and also, it occurs in isolation in older patients and in those who are on hemodialysis.

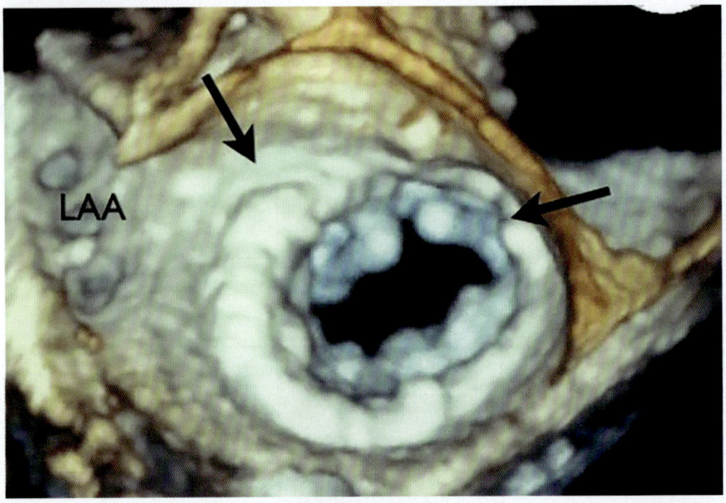

FIGURE 3.48 Calcified mitral annulus forming an incomplete circle extending all around the mitral annulus and sparing the mitral aortic curtain area (*black arrows*). LAA, left atrial appendage. 3D TEE, surgeon's view.

SECTION 7

RHEUMATIC HEART DISEASE

RHEUMATIC MITRAL VALVE DISEASE—ANATOMY

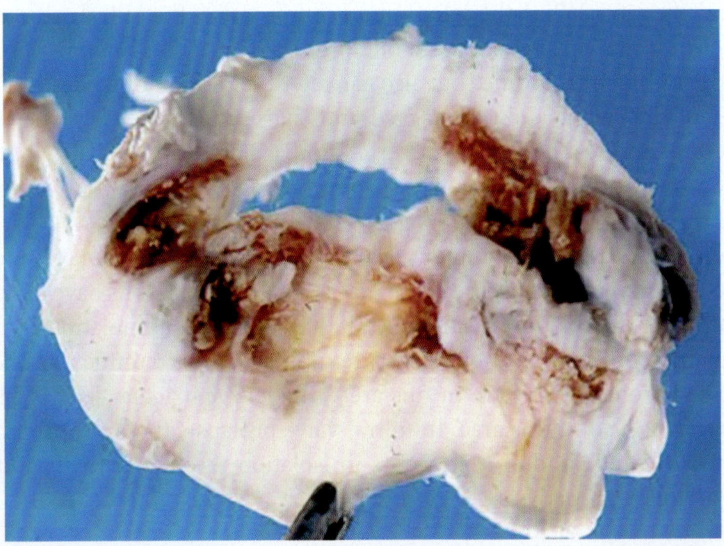

FIGURE 3.49 Severe calcific mitral stenosis with ulceration, commissural fusion, and hemorrhage.

OTHER CAUSES OF MITRAL STENOSIS PHYSIOLOGY

One should remember that mitral stenosis can be caused by conditions other than rheumatic disease. For example, on the left, a bacterial vegetation is completely filling the orifice of the prosthetic valve. Certain drugs can cause the mitral valve to become inflamed, and other conditions can involve the mitral valve such as carcinoid, radiation, and Loeffler syndrome. Cor triatriatum can also be a cause of what appears to be mitral stenosis as can the supravalvular ring as seen in the Shone complex and the arcade abnormality. Even stenosis of the pulmonary veins by procedures such as ablation for atrial fibrillation or sarcoidosis can produce similar syndromes of shortness of breath and pulmonary edema.

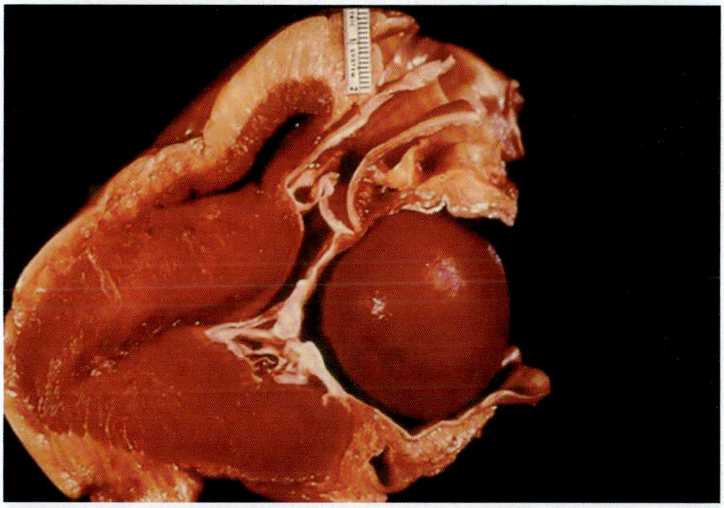

FIGURE 3.50 Ball valve thrombus obstructing an already stenotic mitral valve—pathology specimen. Courtesy of Dr. Michael Gravanis.

CASE PRESENTATION

Rheumatic Mitral Stenosis With a Pliable Mitral Valve and No Calcification

A 39-year-old lady who presented in the first trimester of pregnancy for consultation regarding the risks of continuing pregnancy. There was a history of pulmonary edema previously. The valve was not thought to be suitable for valvuloplasty because of the mitral regurgitation. This pregnancy was not continued because of high risk for mother and fetus, and subsequently the valve was replaced with a tissue valve and she had a successful uncomplicated pregnancy.

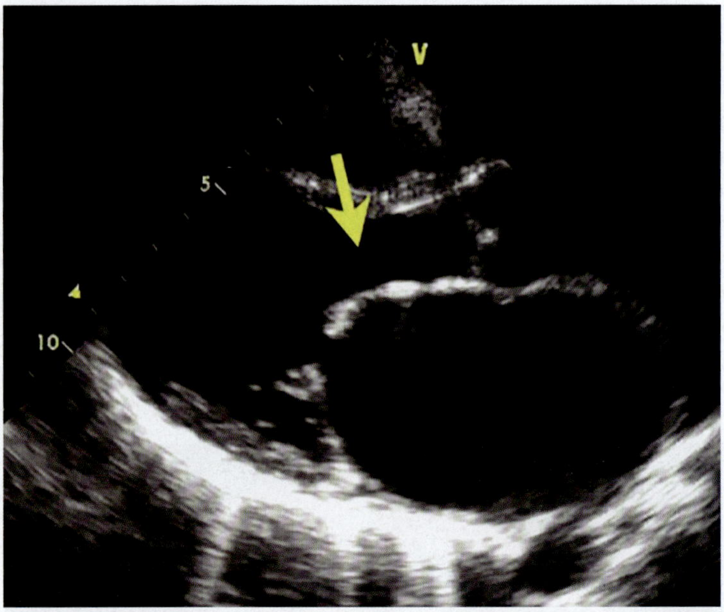

FIGURE 3.51 The "hockey stick" deformity of the AMVL in diastole (*yellow arrow*). No calcification present. TTE, PLX view.

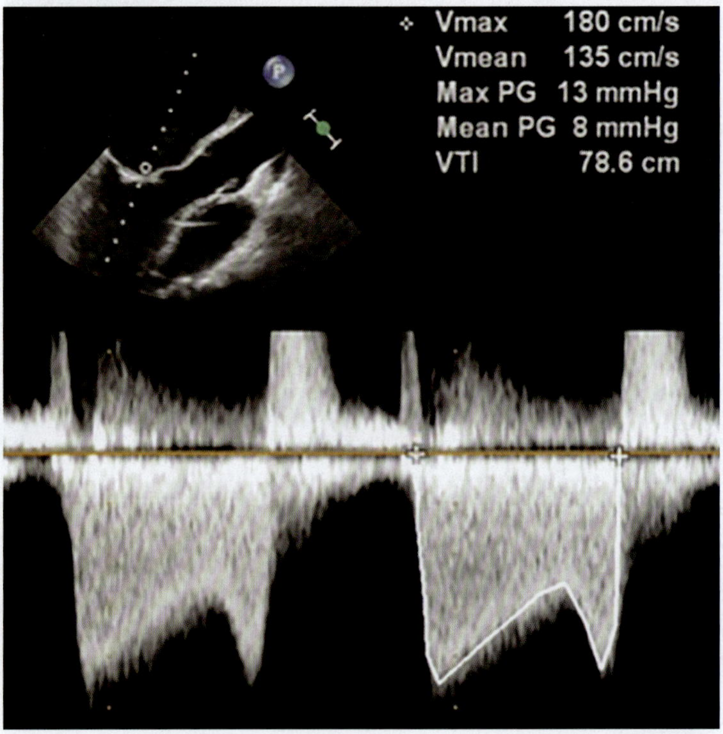

FIGURE 3.52 The mean gradient from the TEE measured at 8 mm Hg. The patient was sedated.

In this individual, the valve area by the pressure half-time method was 0.89 cm^2.

SEVERE MITRAL STENOSIS, TWO- AND THREE-DIMENSIONAL VIEWS AND CALCULATION OF THE MITRAL VALVE AREA: SEVERE RHEUMATIC VALVE STENOSIS

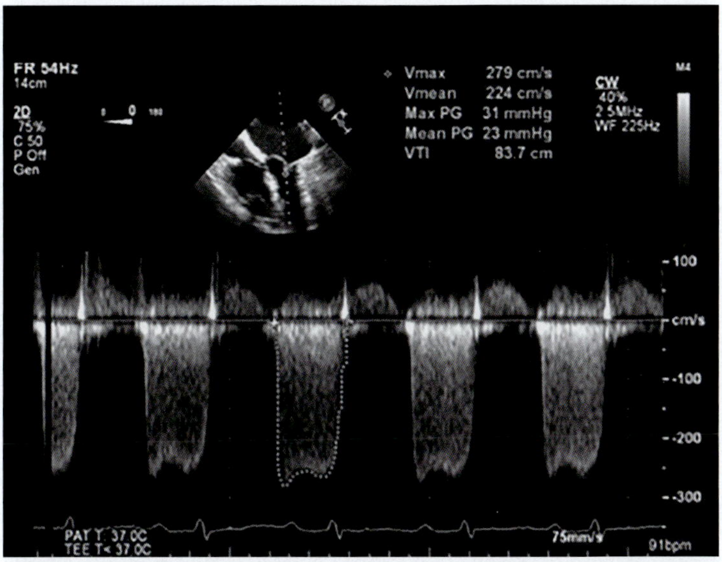

FIGURE 3.53 Continuous wave Doppler velocity profile across the stenotic mitral valve demonstrating a very high velocity, an abnormal deceleration time, and a very high mean gradient of 23 mm Hg. TEE, 4C view.

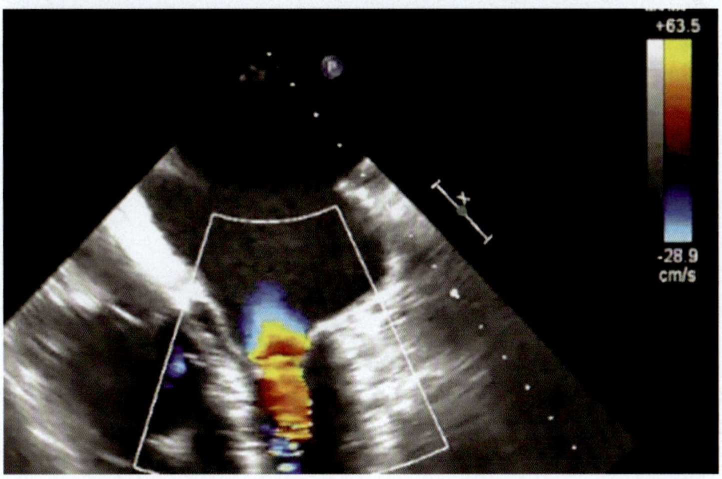

FIGURE 3.54 PISA forming as the aliasing velocity is turned down in the direction of flow and blood gathers at the constricted mitral orifice to enter the left ventricle. TEE, 4C view.

CALCULATION OF THE MITRAL VALVE AREA

$$\text{MVA} = 2\pi r^2 \times \frac{\text{Aliasing velocity}}{\text{Peak mitral velocity}} \times \frac{a}{180}$$

$r = 1.0$ cm
Aliasing velocity = 28.9 cm/s
Peak mitral velocity = 279 cm/s
alpha = 160°

$$\text{MVA} = 2\pi (1.0)^2 \times \frac{28.9}{279} \times \frac{160}{180} = 0.58\ \text{cm}^2$$

VALVULOPLASTY IN THE CATHETERIZATION LABORATORY AND THE INOUE BALLOON[38]

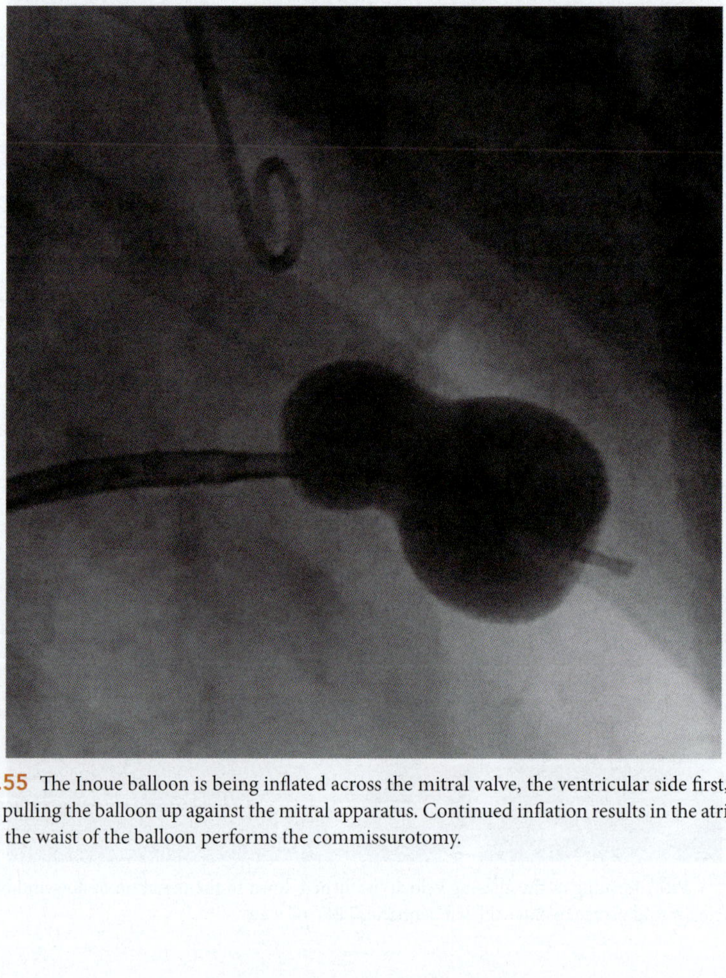

FIGURE 3.55 The Inoue balloon is being inflated across the mitral valve, the ventricular side first, and tension is applied by pulling the balloon up against the mitral apparatus. Continued inflation results in the atrial side being inflated, and the waist of the balloon performs the commissurotomy.

SECTION 8

CONGENITAL MITRAL VALVE DISEASE

CONGENITAL MITRAL STENOSIS—"PARACHUTE MITRAL VALVE"

Abnormalities in the class of congenital mitral stenosis could actually start with "cor triatriatum" and extent into the subvalvular portion of the mitral valve apparatus to include the papillary muscles. Cor triatriatum is illustrated in the section on the LAA and left atrium.[39,40] The supravalvular membrane is part of the Shone complex (supravalvular mitral membrane, parachute mitral valve, subaortic stenosis of either membranous or muscular type, and coarctation of the aorta).[41] Abnormalities of the tensor portion of the mitral valve apparatus or the chordal structures is seen in the arcade or hammock mitral valve in which the papillary muscles are connected directly to the valve leaflets themselves.[42] In the case of the parachute mitral valve in which the valve leaflets resemble the shape of the canopy of a parachute, the abnormality is in the papillary muscles. These in embryologic states fail to separate, and all of the chordal structures attach to one papillary muscle head.[43] There are variations in this abnormality.

An example of the parachute mitral valve follows.

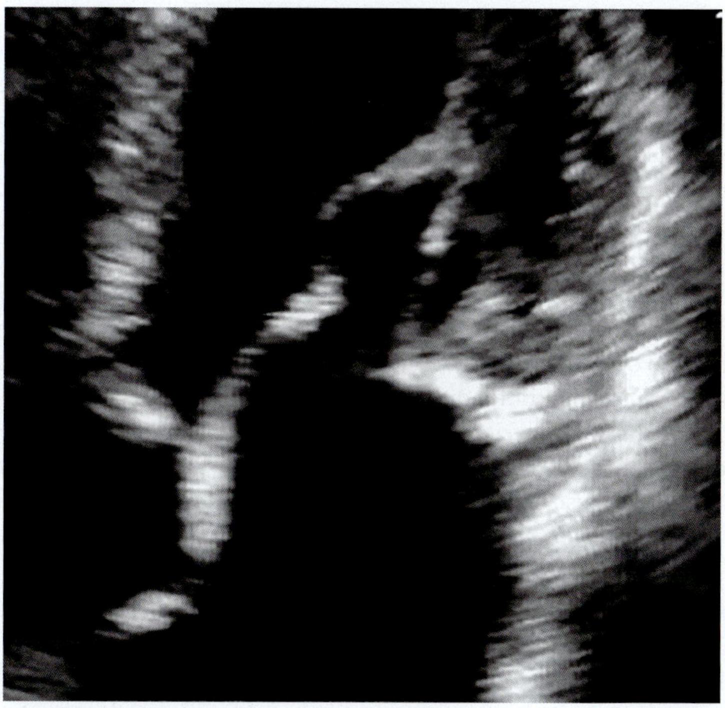

FIGURE 3.56 The stenotic mitral valve tethered by the one papillary muscle and the chordae. The AMVL tends to have a "hockey stick" configuration in diastole. TTE, A5C view.

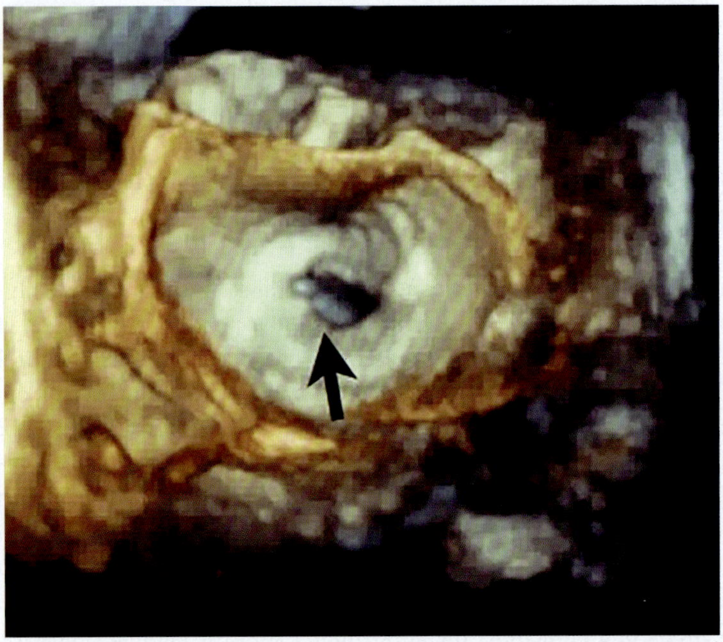

FIGURE 3.57 The stenotic mitral valve on 3D DTEE from the surgeon's view demonstrating the stenotic orifice (*black arrow*). TEE, 10° view.

THE ARCADE MITRAL VALVE

This rare condition was described in 1967 by Layman and Edwards[42] and involves an arrest in development of the chordal structures as they attach to the papillary muscles. Surgical descriptions of this abnormality by Carpentier have described the valve from the atrial side as appearing like a "hammock."[44] The anterior leaflet chords are more involved than are those to the posterior leaflet. As a result, the arcade of chords are not fully separated, remain very short or nonexistent, and pull the anterior mitral leaflet down forming a funnel-like arrangement acting more like a baffle than a leaflet. This prevents closure and also results in stenosis of the apparatus well into the ventricle. The mitral orifice size is usually normal. To outline these four features, they are (1) normal-sized mitral orifices; (2) short, thick and poorly differentiated chordal with direct union to the papillary muscles to the anterior leaflet; (3) narrow or nonexistent spaces between the abnormal chordae; and (4) more differentiated chordal structures to the posterior papillary muscle. These features result in varying degrees of regurgitation and stenosis.[45,46]

This abnormality is illustrated in the following pages.

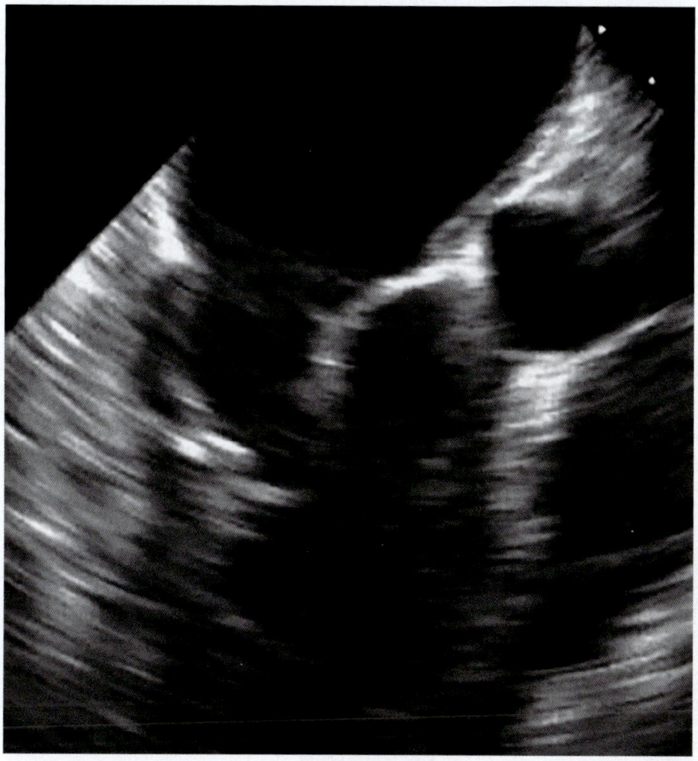

FIGURE 3.58 The arcade mitral valve has shortened or no chordal structures. Those that are present are not differentiated and form a bandlike arrangement. Both mitral leaflets appear to be directly attached to the papillary muscle. TEE, 136° view.

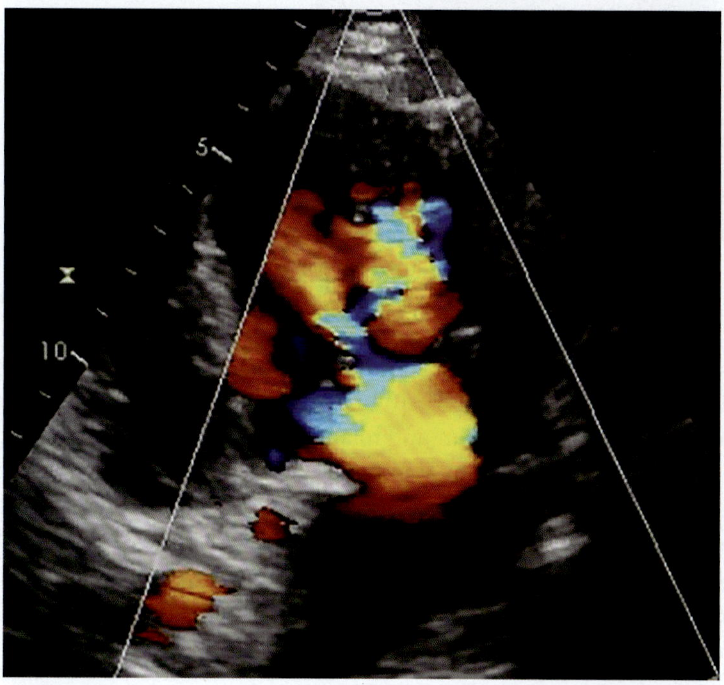

FIGURE 3.59 Color Doppler pattern of inflow shows a PISA well into the ventricle and two jets spraying into the ventricle rather than the single candle flame seen in classic rheumatic mitral stenosis. A4C view with color Doppler.

SECTION 9

CORONARY ATHEROSCLEROTIC HEART DISEASE

COMPLETE AND PARTIAL RUPTURE OF THE PAPILLARY MUSCLE

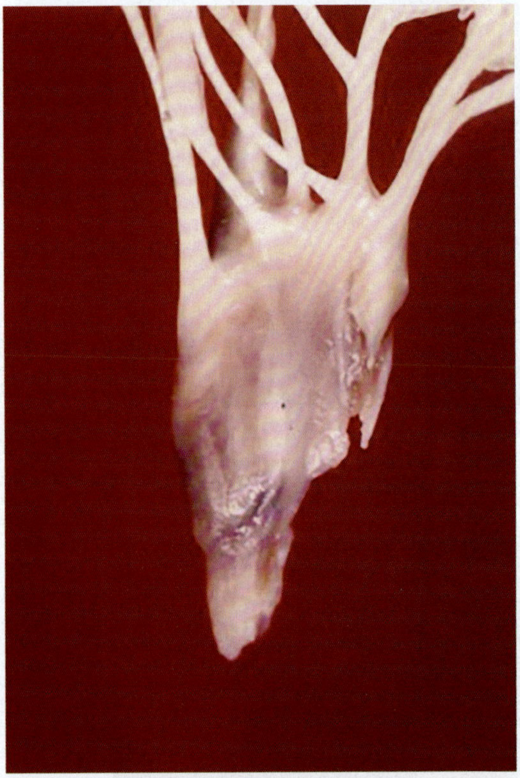

FIGURE 3.60 Complete rupture of the papillary muscle showing the entire body of the papillary muscle being pulled away from the posterior wall. The muscle has a pale appearance from being infarcted.

Rupture of papillary muscle may be secondary to a very small myocardial infarction or part of a larger one. Usually the posterior medial papillary muscle is the most vulnerable because of its blood supply from a single vessel, usually a branch of the right coronary artery. The obtuse marginal branch of the circumflex is a common culprit vessel for an anterolateral papillary muscle. Often, these ruptured papillary muscles occur about the same time as do other mechanical complications of myocardial infarction, ~7 days after the initial episode of chest pain. When complete rupture does occur, it is usually catastrophic leading to pulmonary edema. A partial rupture may cause less catastrophic consequences, but it may be closely followed by complete rupture and more serious clinical events.[47]

PARTIAL RUPTURE OF THE PAPILLARY MUSCLE

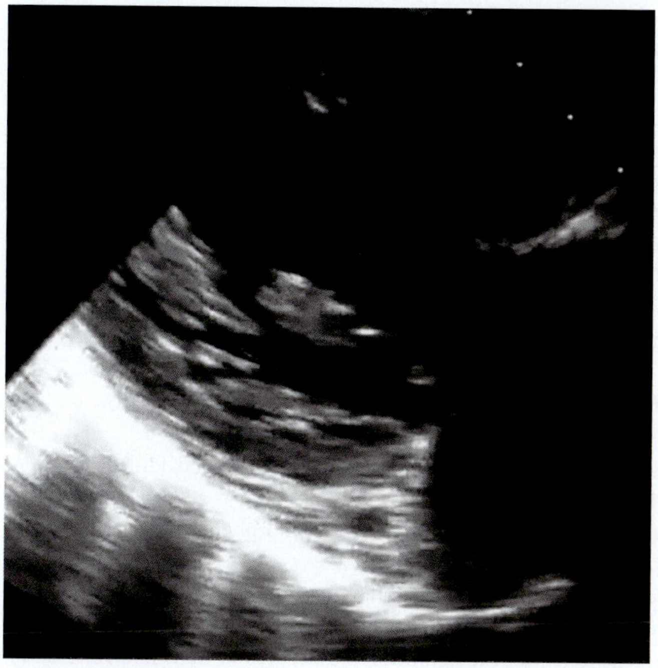

FIGURE 3.61 Partial rupture of the anterolateral papillary muscle viewed from the transgastric view. TEE, 89°, the transgastric view. (From Flueckiger PB, Cheng AC, Patton JM, Clements SD Jr. Partial papillary muscle rupture: a cause of acute mitral regurgitation. *Am J Med Sci.* 2013;345(6):478-481.)

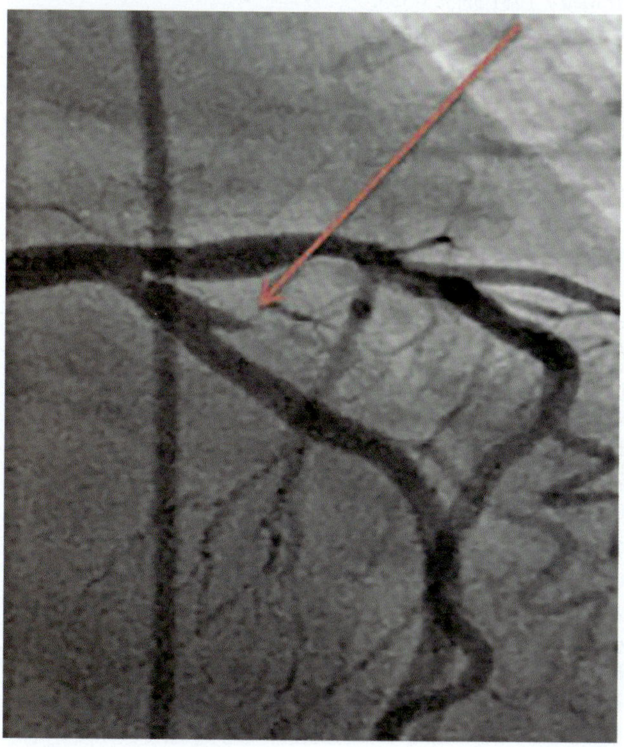

FIGURE 3.62 Coronary arteriogram, RAO view, showing total occlusion of the anterior marginal branch of the circumflex (*red arrow*).

REFERENCES

1. Nishumura RA, Otto CM, Bonow RO, et al. 2014 AHA/ACC Guideline for the Management of Patients with Valvular Heart Disease. A report of the American College of Cardiology/American Heart Association Task Force on Practice Guidelines. *J Am Coll Cardiol.* 2014;63(22):e34-e35.
2. Lang RM, Goldstein SA, Kronzon I, Khandheria BK, Mor-Avi V. *ASE's Comprehensive Echocardiography.* 2nd ed. Elsevier (Saunders); 2016:477-481.
3. Zohgbi WA, Adams D, Ronow RO, et al. Recommendations for Noninvasive Evaluation of Native Valvular Regurgitation. A report from the American Society of Echocardiography Developed in Collaboration with the Society for Cardiovascular Magnetic Resonance. *J Am Soc Echocardiogr.* 2017;30(4):303-371.
4. Carpentier A, Adams DH, Filsoufi F. *Carpentier's Reconstructive Valve Surgery. From Valve Analysis to Valve Reconstruction.* Philadelphia, PA: Elsevier; 2010.
5. Carpentier A. Cardiac valve surgery—the "French correction". *J Thorac Cardiovasc Surg.* 1983;86(3):323-337.
6. Ananou AC, Adams DH. Etiologic classification of degenerative mitral valve disease: Barlow's disease and fibroelastic deficiency. *Semin Thorac Cardiovasc Surg.* 2007;19:90-96.
7. Tsang W, Freed BH, Lang RN. *ASE's Comprehensive Echocardiography.* 2nd ed. Philadelphia, PA: Elsevier (Saunders); 2016:477-484.
8. Living RA, Hagege AA, Judge DP, et al. Mitral valve disease—morphology and mechanisms. *Nat Rev Cardiol.* 2015;12(12):689-710.
9. Barlow JB. Conjoint clinic on the clinical significance of late systolic murmurs and non-ejection systolic clicks. *J Chronic Dis.* 1965;18:665-673.
10. Barlow JB, Pocock WA, Marachand P, et al. The significance of late systolic murmurs. *Am Heart J.* 1963;66:443-452.
11. Reid J. Mid-systolic clicks. *S Afr Med J.* 1961;35:353-355.
12. Cheng TO. John B. Barlow: the man and his syndrome. *Int J Cardiol.* 2014;177(2):311-316.
13. Criley JM, Lewis KB, Humphries JO, et al. Prolapse of the mitral valve: clinical and cineangio-cardiographic findings. *Br Heart J.* 1966;28:488-496.
14. McCarthy KP, Ring L, Rana BS. Anatomy of the mitral valve: understanding the mitral complex in mitral regurgitation. *Eur J Echocardiogr.* 2010;11:i3-i9.
15. Carpentier AF, Lessana A, Relland JY, et al. The "physio-ring" an advanced concept in mitral valve annuloplasty. *Ann Thorac Surg.* 1995;60:1177-1185.
16. Kumar N, Kumar M, Duran CM. A revised terminology for recording surgical findings of the mitral valve. *J Heart Valve Dis.* 1995;4:70-75.
17. Levine RA, Hagege AA, Judge DP, et al. Mitral valve disease—morphology and mechanisms. *Nat Rev Cardiol.* 2015;12(12):689-710.
18. Lancellotti P, Moura L, Pierard LA, et al. European Association of Echocardiography recommendations for the assessment of valvular regurgitation. Part 2: mitral and tricuspid regurgitation (native valve disease). *Eur J Echocardiogr.* 2010;11:307-332.
19. Rodriguez L, Thomas JD, Monterroso V, et al. Validation of the proximal flow convergence method. Calculation of orifice area in patients with mitral stenosis. *Circulation.* 1993;88:1157-1165.
20. Cape EG, Yoganathan AP, Weyman AE, et al. Adjacent solid boundaries alter the size of regurgitant jets on Doppler color flow maps. *J Am Coll Cardiol.* 1991;17:1094-1102.
21. Lang R, Goldstein SA, Kronzon I, Khandheria BK, Mor-Avi V. *ASE's Comprehensive Echocardiography.* 2nd ed. Elsevier (Saunders); 2016:500-509.
22. Nishumura RA, Otto CM, Bonow RO, et al. 2014 AHA/ACC guideline for the management of patients with valvular heart disease. A report of the American College of Cardiology/American Heart Association Task Force on Practice Guidelines. *J Am Coll Cardiol.* 2014;63(22):e57-e185.

23. Silbiger JJ. Abnormalities of the mitral apparatus in hypertrophic cardiomyopathy: echocardiographic, pathophysiologic, and surgical insights. *J Am Soc Echocardiogr.* 2016;29:622-637.
24. Otsuji Y, Handschumaker MD, Schwammenthal E, et al. Insights from three-dimensional echocardiography into the mechanism of functional mitral regurgitation. Direct in vivo demonstration of altered leaflet tethering geometry. *Circulation.* 1997;96:1999-2008.
25. Gogoladze G, Dellis SL, Donning R, et al. Analysis of mitral coaptation zone in normal and functional regurgitant valves. *Ann Thorac Surg.* 2010;89:1158-1162.
26. Saito K, Okura H, Watanabe N, et al. Influence of chronic tethering of the mitral valve on mitral leaflet size and coaptation in functional mitral regurgitation. *JACC Cardiovasc Imaging.* 2012;5:337-345.
27. Silbiger JJ. Abnormalities of the mitral apparatus in hypertrophic cardiomyopathy: echocardiographic, pathophysiologic, and surgical insights. *J Am Soc Echocardiogr.* 2016;29:622-639.
28. Durack DT, Lukes AS, Bright DK. New criteria for diagnosis of infective endocarditis: utilization of specific echocardiographic findings: Duke endocarditis Service. *Am J Med.* 1994;96:200-209.
29. Li JS, Sexton DJ, Mick N, et al. Proposed modification to the Duke criteria for the diagnosis of infective endocarditis. *Clin Infect Dis.* 2000;30(4):633-638.
30. Gilbert HM, Peters ED, Lang SJ, Hartman BJ. Successful treatment of fungal prosthetic valve endocarditis: case report and review. *Clin Infect Dis.* 1994;22:348-354.
31. Chambers ST, Murdock D, Morris A, et al. Infective endocarditis: characteristics and outcomes from a large, multi-national cohort. *PLoS One.* 2013;8(5):e63181.
32. Utley JR, Mills J, Roe BB. The role of valve replacement in the treatment of fungal endocarditis. *J Thorac Cardiovasc Surg.* 1975;69:255-258.
33. Reynolds HR, Jagen MA, Tunik PA, et al. Sensitivity of transthoracic versus transesophageal echocardiography for the detection of native valve vegetations in the modern era. *J Am Soc Echocardiogr.* 2003;16:67-70.
34. Daniel WG, Mugge A, Martin RP, et al. Improvement in the diagnosis of abscesses associated with endocarditis by transesophageal echocardiography. *N Engl J Med.* 1991;324:795-800.
35. Zoghbi WA, Chambers JB, Dumesnil JG, et al. Recommendations for evaluation of prosthetic valves with echocardiography and Doppler ultrasound. Guidelines and standards. *J Am Soc Echocardiogr.* 2009;9:975-1014.
36. Cammack PL, Edie RN, Edmonds LH. Bar calcification of the mitral annulus. A risk factor in mitral valve operations. *J Thorac Cardiovasc Surg.* 1987;94:399-404.
37. Lad VS, Newcomb AE, Davis PJ, Leng CY. Surgical techniques for the management of the "hostile mitral annulus". *Heart Lung Circ.* 2014;23(3):217-223.
38. Inoue K, Owaki T, Nakamura T, Kitamra F, Minamoto N. Clinical application of transvenous mitral commissurotomy by a new balloon catheter. *J Thorac Cardiovasc Surg.* 1984;87(3):394-402.
39. Strickland PT, Peretz MA, Jokhadar M, Hartlage G, Clements S. Cor triatriatum sinister: a patient, a review, and some unique findings. *Echocardiography.* 2014;31(6):790-794.
40. Nassar PN, Hamdan RH. Cor triatriatum sinistrum: classification and imaging modalities. *Eur J Cardiovasc Med.* 2011;1(3):84-87.
41. Shone JD, Sellers RD, Anderson RC, et al. The development complex of "PMV", supravalvular ring of the left atrium, sub aortic stenosis and coarctation of the aorta. *Am J Cardiol.* 1963;11:714-725.
42. Layman TE, Edwards JE. Anomalous mitral arcade. A type of congenital mitral insufficiency. *Circulation.* 1967;35:389-395.
43. Seguela P, Houyel L, Acar P. Congenital malformations of the mitral valve. *Arch Cardiovasc Dis.* 2011;104:465-479.
44. Carpentier A, Bizard CP. Congenital malformations of the mitral valve. In: Stark J, Level M, Tsang V, eds. *Surgery for Congenital Heart Defects.* London, UK: Wiley; 2006:573-590.

45. Rajesh GN, Sajeer K, Nair A, Rajeev CG, Krishna N. Hammock mitral valve: a rare cause of congenital mitral regurgitation—a case report. *Indian Heart J.* 2014;66(3):370-371.
46. Kim SJ, Shin ES, Park MK, Choi SH, Lee SG. Congenital mitral insufficiency caused by anomalous mitral arcade in an elderly patient: use of echocardiography and multi detector computed tomography for diagnosis. *Circ J.* 2005;69:1560-1563.
47. Clements SD, Story WE, Hurst JW, Craver JM, Jones EL. Ruptured papillary muscle, a complication of myocardial infarction: clinical presentation, diagnosis and treatment. *Clin Cardiol.* 1985;8:93-103.
48. Flueckiger PB, Cheng AC, Patton JM, Clements SD Jr. Partial papillary muscle rupture: a cause of acute mitral regurgitation. *Am J Med Sci.* 2013;345(6):478-481.

The Aortic Valve, Ascending Aorta, Aortic Arch, Descending Thoracic and Abdominal Aortas

4

SECTION 1

THE AORTIC VALVE REGION

The aortic valve region includes the subvalvular area or the left ventricular outflow tract, the aortic annulus, and the attached leaflets and their attachments or commissures. The aortic annulus and the sinus of Valsalva area up to the sinotubular junction constitute the "aortic root." The aorta from the sinotubular junction to the innominate artery is termed the ascending aorta.

The aortic valve has three leaflets each attached to the aortic annulus and suspended by commissures. The leaflets themselves consist of a more basal area that is thicker than the upper portion of the leaflets and a more superior portion of the leaflets that is thinner than the basal areas. The crescent-shaped areas on the three leaflets define the junction between the stiffer base and the thin coaptation area. This crescent area is called the "lunula" probably because of the half-moon–like shape. The central portion of the leaflets has a small nodular area named the nodes of Arantius. At coaptation, all three of these nodular areas come together in the center of the aorta along with the thin lunular areas to form a tight area of coaptation that does not leak.[1]

All of these areas are subject to various abnormalities. The subvalvular area can have a thick membranelike area that involves the interventricular septum and also reflects onto the anterior mitral valve leaflet offering obstruction to the left ventricular outflow. The aortic annular area is joined with the mitral annular area forming the mitral aortic curtain. The leaflets are subject to thickening, thinning and disruption all of which have associated functional abnormalities. The aortic root itself can become ectatic, as, for example, in Marfan syndrome, which distorts the commissural areas and results in dysfunction of the valve. The ascending aorta can become ectatic in association with bicuspid aortic valve or dissected in association with cystic medial necrosis. Congenital abnormalities of the aortic valve include the unicuspid aortic valve, the bicuspid aortic valve, and even the quadricuspid aortic valve. The valve leaflets can become thickened, and stenosis can result. Stenosis of the aorta itself can occur at or just above the sinotubular junction as is seen in Williams syndrome.

Endocarditis can occur and involve the leaflet areas or the annulus or the valve leaflet areas, and function abnormalities follow.

Prosthetic valves offer relief from regurgitation and stenosis. They have their own unique appearance and set of abnormalities.

ANATOMIC AND ECHOCARDIOGRAPHIC IMAGES OF THE AORTIC VALVE

Understanding the gross anatomy of the aortic valves makes understanding of imaging techniques easier. Several different anatomic abnormalities are illustrated in the following page. The unicuspid valve has no defined cusp regions and little in the way of raphes. The bicuspid valve has two cusps but usually has some identifiable raphe. The trileaflet calcified aortic valve has dense calcification at the base and less calcification at the tips of the leaflets. The leaflets are not fused as they might be in rheumatic disease. The rare quadricuspid aortic valve is illustrated in live 3D stop frame. The following page illustrates some of these valves.

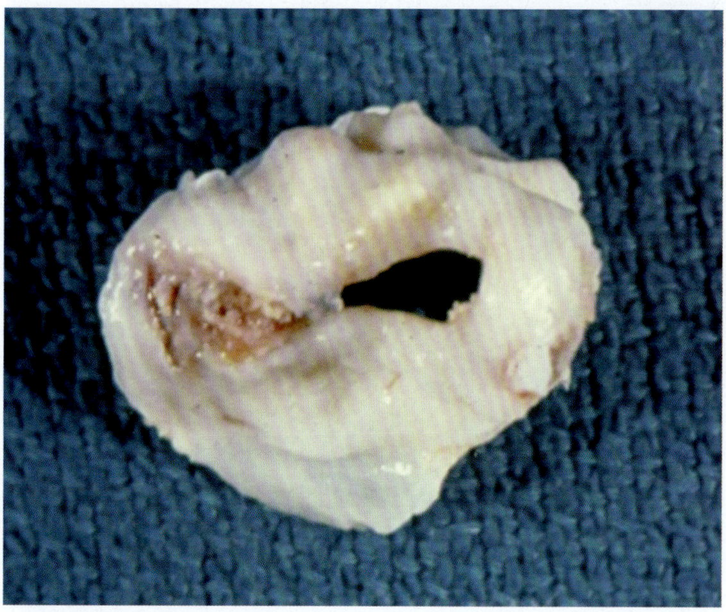

FIGURE 4.1 Calcified unicuspid aortic valve.

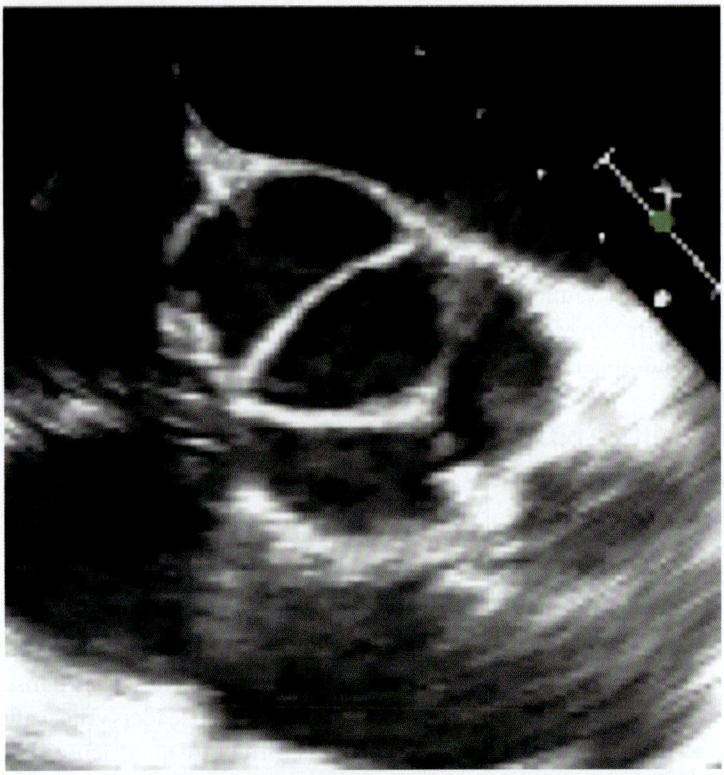

FIGURE 4.2 Bicuspid aortic valve with fusion of the LCC and RCC.

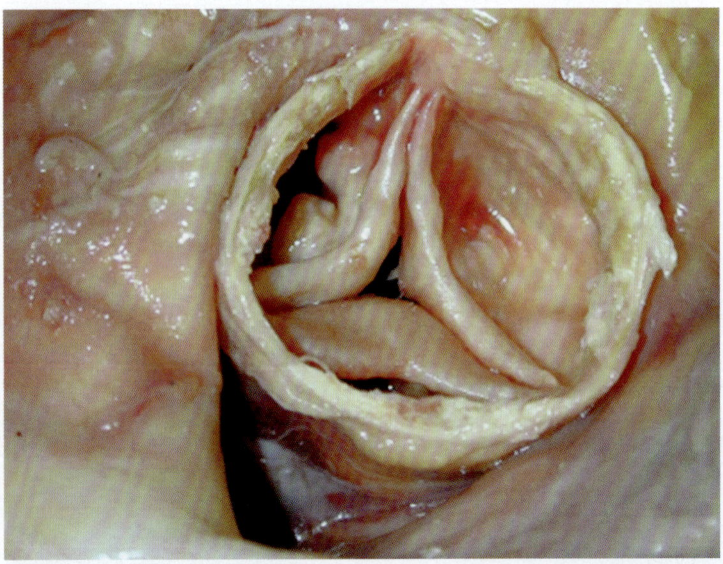

FIGURE 4.3 Calcific aortic stenosis in a tricuspid aortic valve.

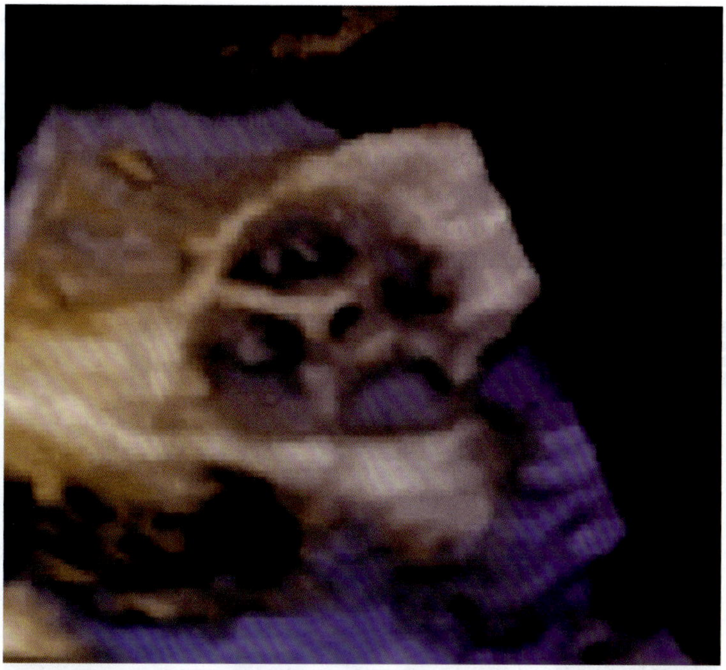

FIGURE 4.4 Quadricuspid aortic valve.

SECTION 2

AORTIC STENOSIS

CLINICAL FEATURES AND NATURAL HISTORY OF AORTIC STENOSIS

Aortic stenosis is a common abnormality in older individuals. The leaflets become sclerotic at their bases and progress to calcification and immobility in the basal portions and thickening above the coaptation line to form a stiff, stenotic valve with a high gradient. Valves with this configuration are usually seen in the seventh decade and higher in contrast to stenosis from a congenital bicuspid valve, which presents in general a decade earlier. Once flow through these trileaflet valves is abnormal, a progressive process develops such that the thickening and calcification begets more of the same.

Symptoms fall onto three categories. Syncope, angina pectoris, and dyspnea are cardinal symptoms that signal a poor prognosis. Symptoms may be subtle in that instead of frank congestive heart failure, simple fatigue or mild shortness of breath may be present. Instead of classic angina pectoris, a complaint of slight chest tightness on exertion may be present. Syncope is never a good sign and may have several causes from atrioventricular block to power failure.[2]

This 76-year-old man who complained of exertional fatigue had on physical exam an ejection murmur that was grade III/VI at the base and audible at the apex. The murmur radiated to the neck and had a late systolic peak and was associated with delayed carotid upstroke. The images of the aortic valve showed that it was trileaflet, was calcified, and had very limited motion of the leaflets. On visual exam and on planimetry, the valve area appeared <1 cm^2. The numbers from the Doppler interrogation included a peak velocity of 4.12 m/s and a mean gradient of 47 mm Hg, echo fit with the clinical story, and the calculated aortic valve of 0.67 cm^2 by the continuity equation. This history and these numbers suggest that definition of coronary anatomy and risk assessment for intervention are indicated. After these considerations, the patient received a TAVR.[3]

THE CONCEPT OF FLOW RESERVE

In individuals who have abnormal left ventricular function and significant aortic stenosis, the question is often asked as to whether the left ventricle can respond by increasing the stroke volume and the cardiac output. In the echo laboratory, flow reserve is assessed by giving dobutamine and measuring surrogates of cardiac output. The velocity time integral (VTI) of the left ventricular outflow tract can be measured, and increase in this parameter suggests that some degree of flow reserve is present. This concept is used for risk stratification in individuals undergoing surgery. Those with low flow reserve do less well than do those who had flow reserve.[4] Flow reserve is defined as an increase in stroke volume (or VTI of the LVOT) by 20% or greater in response to 5 to 20 μg/k/min of dobutamine.

In individuals who have low ejection fraction (<50%) and low mean gradients (<40 mm Hg) and calculated low valve area (<1.0 cm^2, <0.6 cm^2/m^2), evaluation of flow reserve is indicated. In this setting, if an increase in flow is associated with an increase in gradient and the valve area that stays generally the same, severe aortic stenosis is present and flow reserve is present. If stroke volume (VTI of the LVOT) increases by 20%, then flow reserve is present. If an increase flow is associated with only slight increase in gradient and the calculated valve area increases above 1.0 cm^2, then pseudostenosis is present, the problem is low flow reserve, and intervention has high risk and less potential benefit.[5,6]

In addition, there are a group of individuals in whom there is low flow, low gradient, and low valve area and who have normal or preserved EF. These individuals are typically older age, female gender, and associated with systemic arterial hypertension, metabolic syndrome, or diabetes. Concentric remodeling, small cavity size and diastolic dysfunction are also associated with this syndrome. Although the ejection fraction is normal, longitudinal function of the ventricle is abnormal as has been demonstrated by global longitudinal strain.[7]

Much information is available in the literature concerning these issues including recommendations from the guidelines.[8,9]

CASE PRESENTATION

Low-Flow, Low-Gradient Aortic Stenosis With Reduced Left Ventricular Ejection Fraction and Response to Treatment

A 76-year-old man with prior CABG, prior stent to RCA-SVG, and who had ICD and was deemed too high risk for surgery. After these studies, he was evaluated for TAVR and subsequently had the procedure with good success.

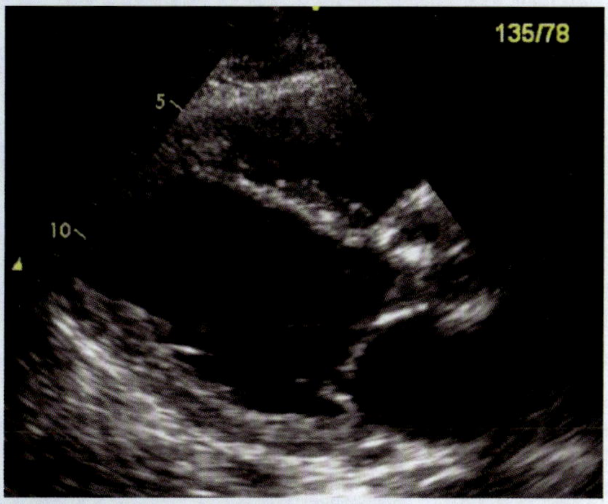

FIGURE 4.7 Very low ejection fraction—15% to 20%.

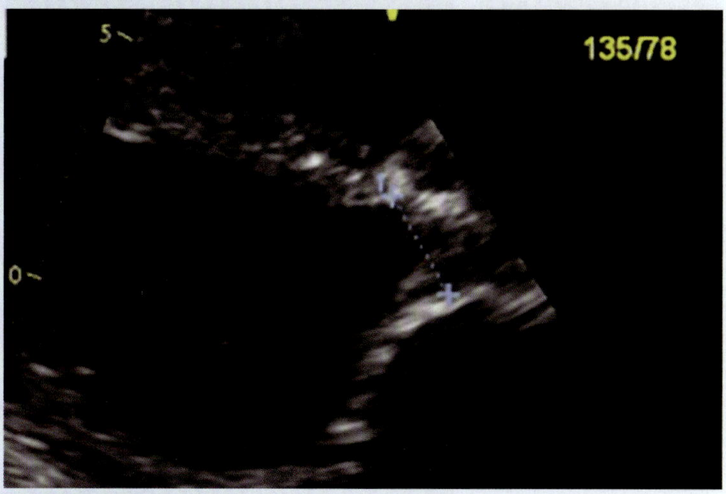

FIGURE 4.8 LVOT diameter = 2.2 cm.

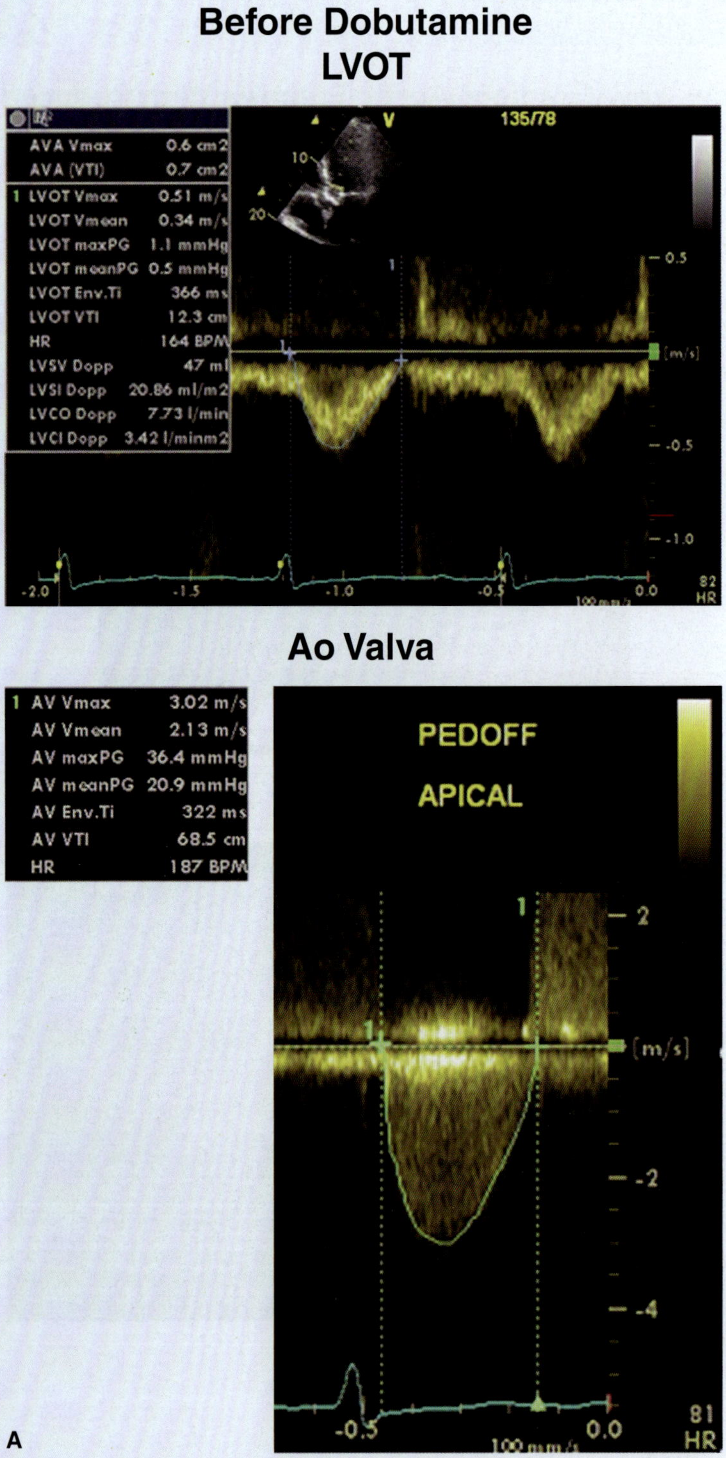

FIGURE 4.9 **A:** Low stroke volume is present with a low VTI of only 12.3 cm. Low gradient from the apex at baseline measured with a Pedoff transducer. The peak gradient was 36.4 mm Hg, and the mean was 20.9 mm Hg.

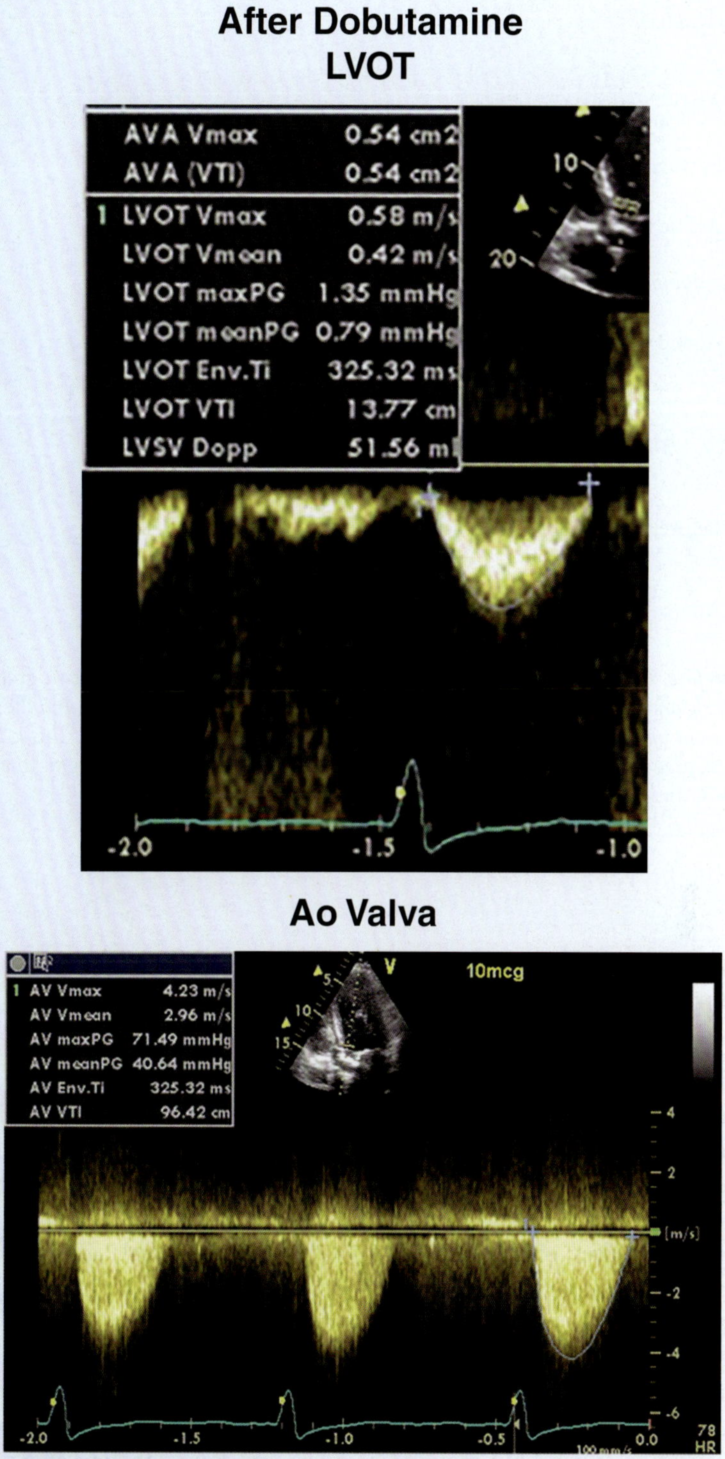

B

FIGURE 4.9 **B:** The VTI of 13.77 cm is demonstrated at maximum dobutamine stimulation. With dobutamine stimulation, LVOT VTI increases from 12.3 to 13.8 (12% change) and the peak gradient increases dramatically (peak at 20 mcg/k/min) from peak of 36.4, mean 20.9 mm Hg, to 72, mean 41 mm Hg. Baseline AVA was 0.7 cm^2 and with dobutamine 0.54 cm^2.

The Calculations

$$A_2 = \frac{\pi}{4} \times d^2 \times \frac{V_1}{V_2}$$

Before dobutamine stress:

$$\text{Aortic valve area} = 0.785 \times (2.2^2) \times \frac{12.3}{68.5} = 0.68 \text{ cm}^2$$

After dobutamine stress:

$$\text{Aortic valve area} = 0.785 \times (2.2^2) \times \frac{13.77}{96.4} = 0.54 \text{ cm}^2$$

Velocity ratios

$$\text{Before: } \frac{12.3}{68.5} = 18\%$$

$$\text{After: } \frac{13.77}{96.4} = 14\%$$

Therefore, this 76-year-old man has a very low ejection and initial mean gradient of 20.9 mm Hg and a calculated valve area of 0.68 cm^2. Dobutamine was given, and the mean gradient went up to 40.6 mm Hg and the calculated valve area was 0.54 cm^2. This is therefore not aortic pseudostenosis, but true aortic stenosis, and there is reserve present. The patient had TAVR, and the result was remarkable.

LOW-FLOW, LOW-GRADIENT SEVERE AORTIC STENOSIS AND PRESERVED LEFT VENTRICULAR SYSTOLIC FUNCTION

There is a group of individuals who have low flow, low gradient, and preserved ejection fraction that has been puzzling. They have calculated aortic valve areas that are <1.0 cm^2 with AVA index <0.6 cm^2/m^2, low-gradient <40 mm Hg peak and low stroke volume index <35 mL/m^2 and EF ≥ 50%. When these findings are present, they often are in older individuals of female gender who have a history of systemic arterial hypertension, diabetes, and metabolic syndrome.[11] Often, centric remodeling is present with left ventricular hypertrophy. It has been shown that although circumferential wall motion is normal, the global longitudinal strain values are not normal.[12,13] Dobutamine stress echo may be helpful in determining whether pseudo-severe aortic stenosis is present.[14,15] The response to intervention is good but may not be great, and transcatheter valve replacement may be a better alternative than surgical treatment.

CASE PRESENTATION

Severe Aortic Stenosis With Low Flow, Low Gradient, Preserved LV Function

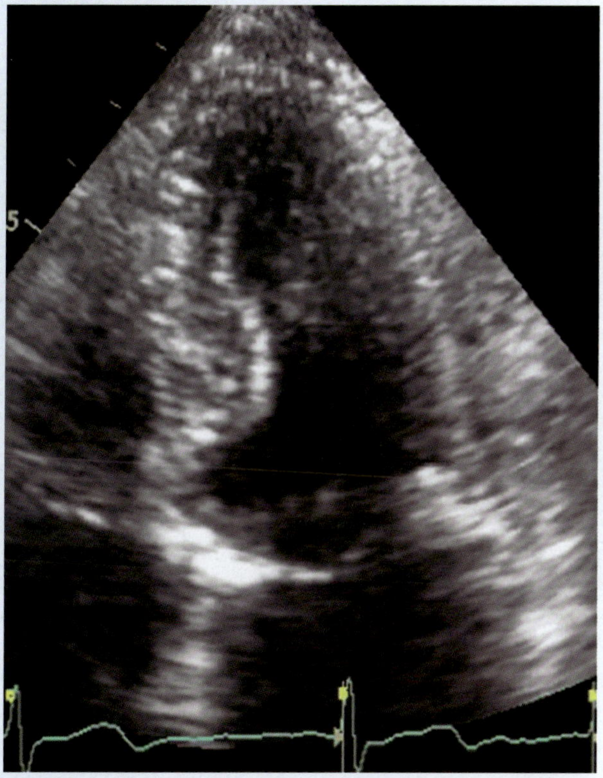

FIGURE 4.10 Systolic frame appears normal with an estimated ejection fraction of ~60%. TTE, A4C view.

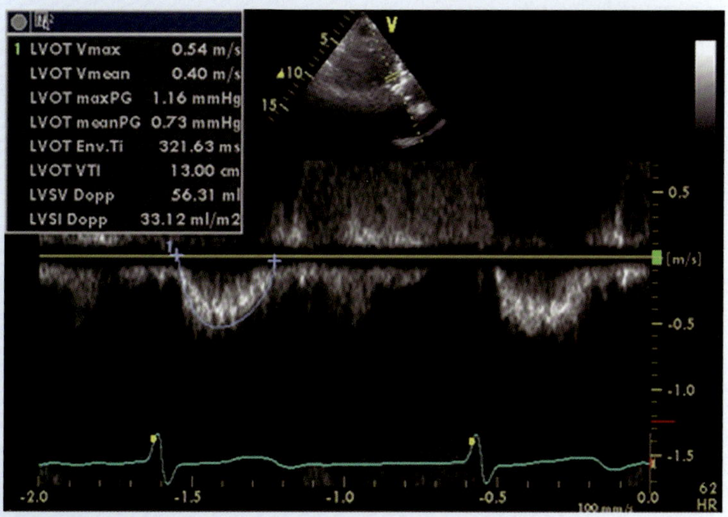

FIGURE 4.11 Apical long-axis view with CW demonstrates a peak gradient of 39.6 mm Hg and mean of 21.5 mm Hg and VTI of the velocity curve of 74.3 cm. TTE, CW Doppler from the AL axis view.

In this older woman, systolic function is preserved; however, the stroke volume is relatively low with a VTII of the LVOT of 13.0 cm and a VTI of the valve of 74.3 cm.

$$\text{Ao valve area} = 0.785 \times (2)^2 \times 13.0/74.3 = 0.55\ \text{cm}^2$$

This situation is in the category of severe AS, low flow, low gradient, and preserved LV systolic function. It has been shown that longitudinal function of the LV is abnormal by means of global systolic longitudinal strain.

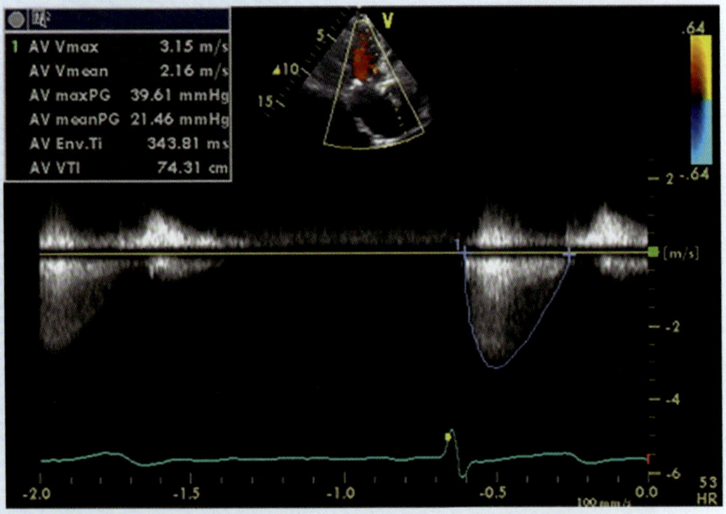

FIGURE 4.12 Pulsed wave Doppler interrogation of the LVOT velocity reveals that this value is low at 13.0 cm. TTE, PW Doppler, AL axis view.

ACC/AHA Guidelines for Aortic Valve Replacement

The ACC/AHA guidelines are available for application to individuals who have aortic valve stenosis and provide recommendations along with the level of evidence for the recommendation. In addition, information is given concerning the risk/benefit of the indication in various categories. The pathways that lead to the recommendations are in the following figure.

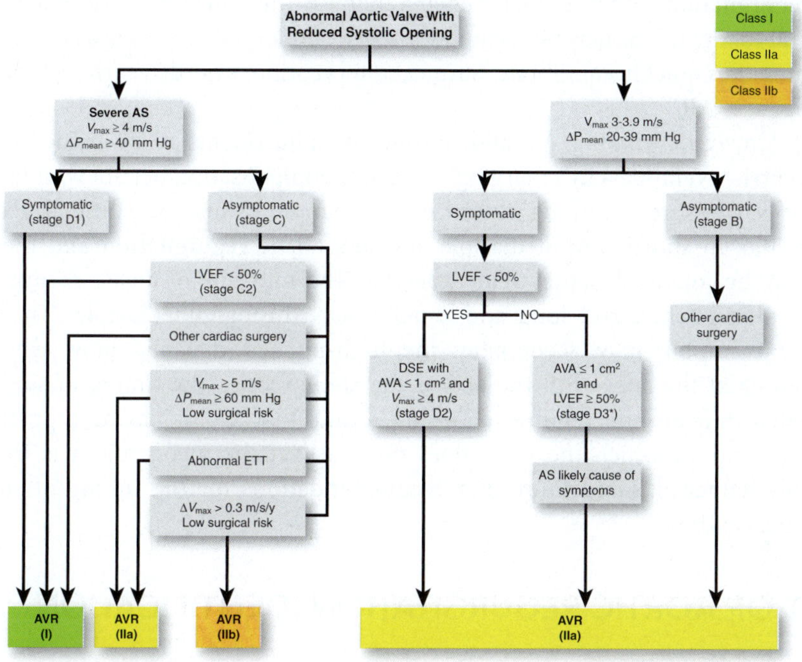

Arrows show the decision pathways that result in a recommendation for AVR. Periodic monitoring is indicated for all patients in whom AVR is not yet indicated, including those with asymptomatic AS (stage D or C) and those with low-gradient AS (stage D2 or D3) who do not meet criteria for intervention.

*AVR should be considered with stage D3 AS only if valve obstruction is the most likely cause of symptoms, stroke volume index is <35 mL/m², indexed AVA is ≤0.6 cm²/m², and data are recorded when the patient is normotensive (systolic BP <140 mm Hg).

AS indicates aortic stenosis; AVA, aortic valve area; AVR, aortic valve replacement by either surgical or transcatheter approach; BP, blood pressure; DSE, dobutamine stress echocardiography; ETT, exercise treadmill test; LVEF, left ventricular ejection fraction; ΔP_{mean}, mean pressure gradient; and V_{max}, maximum velocity.

FIGURE 4.13 Currently in the United States, TAVR is approved for use in individuals with high and intermediate risk, and low-risk individuals are under investigation in clinical trial. (Source: Nishimura RA, Otto CM, Bonow RO, et al. 2014 ACC/AHA Guideline for management of patients with valvular heart disease. A report of the ACC/AHA association task force on practice guidelines. *J Am Coll Cardiol.* 2014;63(22):e57-e185.)

SECTION 3

AORTIC REGURGITATION

Aortic regurgitation (AR) has a number of etiologies. In contrast to aortic stenosis, the etiologies are not as easily determined. They may be congenital or from other processes such as degeneration from aging, myxomatous changes, infection, trauma, or toxicity from drugs. In addition, they may be associated with abnormalities of the aortic root as seen with Marfan syndrome, aortic dissection, and infectious and inflammatory changes.[9,16]

AR may be acute or chronic. Acute AR is not tolerated well and might be seen in the setting of dissection, endocarditis, and trauma. In this setting, the left ventricle does not have time to compensate, end-diastolic pressures are high, early mitral valve closure is present sometimes with late diastolic mitral regurgitation, and pulmonary edema follows. The murmur of AR may be difficult to identify or may be early, low pitched, and rapidly tapering as the diastolic pressures quickly equilibrate. Surgical intervention is needed early in the course of acute AR.

Slowly developing AR allows time for adjustments to be made. The left ventricle remodels by enlarging, a state of compensation occurs with low diastolic pressures and long murmurs, and symptoms may be minimal. Exercise results in shortening of diastole and less aortic regurgitation and therefore may be tolerated better than expected. The murmur of aortic regurgitation is high pitched and long and usually lasts throughout diastole. An Austin Flint rumble may accompany the high-pitched diastolic blow when listening at the apex with the bell of the stethoscope. The timing of surgery is often difficult and requires choosing a time that avoids having a postoperative state in which the valve does not leak yet the myocardium is irreversibly damaged. Guidelines offer recommendations for the timing of surgical intervention.

JET OF AORTIC REGURGITATION IDENTIFICATION

When the jet of aortic regurgitation is identified, thoughts about etiology should be considered. A quick survey of the adjacent areas should be undertaken. The subvalvular area should be inspected for size and the presence of a membrane or a hypertrophic septum. The aortic annulus should be assessed looking for calcium that might extend up upon the leaflets. The thickness of the leaflets and their mobility should be noted. The size of the sinuses of Valsalva and how they relate to the sinotubular junction have important information as does the size of the ascending aorta above the sinotubular junction. Effacement of the sinotubular junction usually means that it is dilated. In the case of dissecting aortic aneurysm, a dilated ascending aorta is a clue, and searching for extra echoes in the lumen of the aorta that might be oscillating makes the diagnosis of dissection. Focusing on this area when seeing a jet of aortic regurgitation on 2D echocardiography usually makes the correct diagnosis as to etiology. Determination of severity of the aortic regurgitation follows.

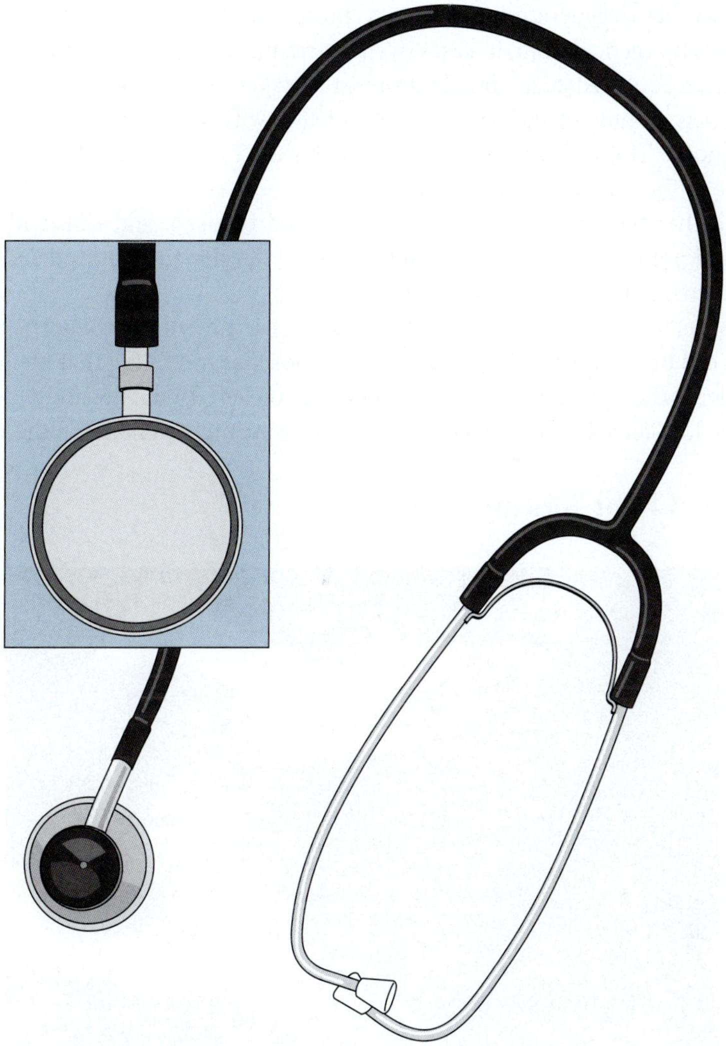

FIGURE 4.14

THE STETHOSCOPE

The murmur of aortic regurgitation may be soft and difficult to hear. It may be audible only in the sitting position with the individual leaning forward. In a noisy room with competing sounds from a ventilator in place and an overhead fan operating, auscultation is not ideal. At the present time, this is often the case.

On the other hand, if an individual presents to the emergency room with tearing back pain and a low diastolic pressure, identification of the murmur of aortic regurgitation is key to the next steps, which might be echocardiogram and CTA of the aorta. In a patient being treated for endocarditis, the sudden appearance of a prominent murmur of aortic regurgitation detected with the use of a stethoscope at the bedside means trouble and in itself suggests that surgical intervention may be needed and soon. In individuals with prosthetic tissue valves that have in place for a number of years, the detection of a murmur of aortic regurgitation often signals that degenerative changes are present and intervention may be needed. In the emergency room, in cases of chest trauma, murmur of aortic regurgitation means a ruptured cusp and action must be taken. When the murmur is so loud that it is audible to the patient, a brief listen with the stethoscope can give the diagnosis. The vibration frequencies of the valves on echocardiography are the same as those on the Doppler tracings.

So the stethoscope is in hand and should be used, and skill with this tool should not be lost and should continue to be developed in our nurses, students, residents, physicians, and cardiologists.[17]

Clues to the presence of aortic root disease as an etiology of aortic regurgitation can be identified by the use of the stethoscope, revealing that the murmur is louder at the right sternal border rather than the left. When the murmur is louder at the left sternal border, it suggests that the murmur originates in the valve.

The Austin Flint Murmur[9]

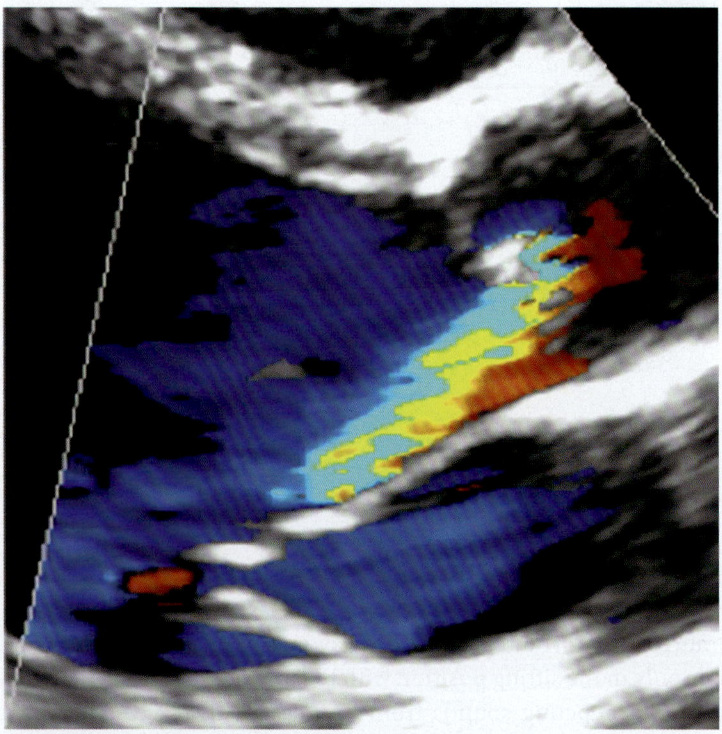

FIGURE 4.15 Still frame of the jet of aortic regurgitation blasting the AMVL.

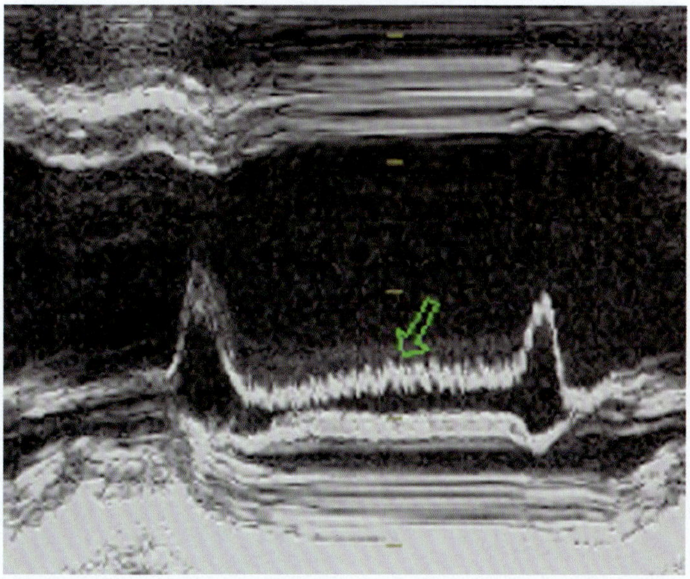

FIGURE 4.16 Fine flutter (*green open arrow*) of the AMVL caused by the jet of aortic regurgitation. M-mode echo.

Several possible mechanisms for production of the Austin Flint murmur have been put forth. These include sounds from blood flowing the partially closed mitral valve, vibrating of the anterior mitral leaflet, convergence jets from the aortic regurgitation, and the mitral inflow and the aortic regurgitation jet itself.

ASSESSMENT OF THE DEGREE OF AORTIC REGURGITATION (AR)

- The dimensions of the left ventricle
- Doppler parameters for assessment of AR
- Jet width and area relative to the LVOT
- Width of the vena contract
- PISA determinations
- Volumetric methods
- Pressure half time

CALCULATION OF THE EFFECTIVE REGURGITANT ORIFICE USING THE PISA METHOD

$$\text{ERO} = 2\pi r^2 \times \frac{\text{Aliasing Velocity}}{\text{Peak AR Velocity}}$$

$$\text{RV} = \text{ERO} \times \text{VTI}_{\text{AR Jet}}$$

$$\text{SV} = \frac{\pi}{4} \times D_{\text{LVOT}^2} \times \text{VTI}_{\text{LVOT}}$$

$$\text{RF} = \frac{\text{RV}}{\text{SV}}$$

CALCULATION OF THE EFFECTIVE REGURGITANT ORIFICE FROM THE PISA INFORMATION

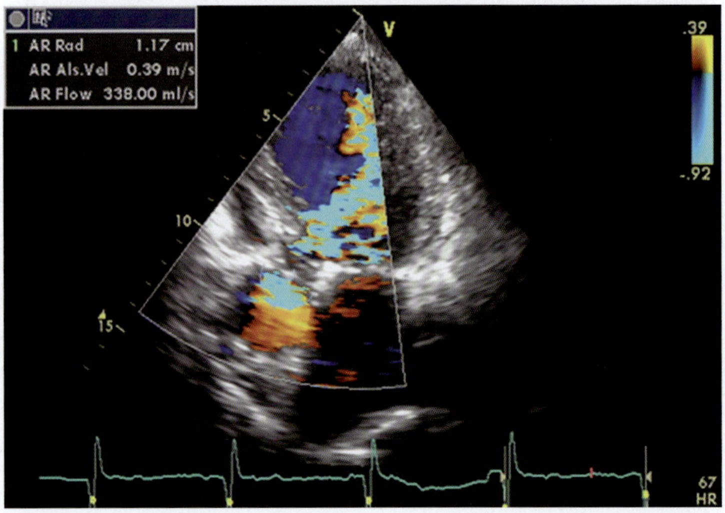

FIGURE 4.17 Aliasing velocity = 39 cm/s. PISA radius = 1.17 cm.

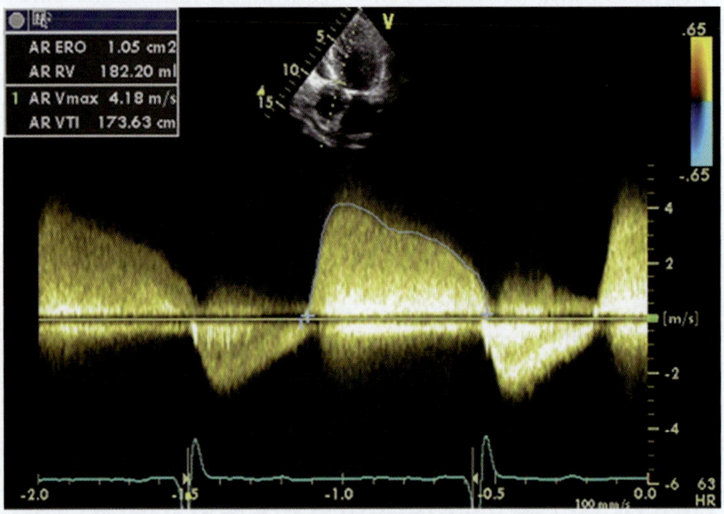

FIGURE 4.18 AR VTI = 174 cm. AR *V*max = 418 cm/s.

$$\text{ERO} = 2\pi r^2 \times \frac{\text{Aliasing Velocity}}{\text{Peak AR Velocity}}$$

$$\text{ERO} = 6.28 \times \left(1.17^2\right) \times \frac{39}{418} = 0.80 \ \text{cm}^2$$

$$\text{RV} = 0.80 \times 174 = 140 \ \text{mL}$$

An ERO of >0.3 cm^2 is consistent with severe AR as is a regurgitant volume of >60 mL (our example had 140 mL).

DOPPLER PARAMETERS OF SEVERE AORTIC REGURGITATION[9]

See Table 4.1.

TABLE 4.1 DOPPLER PARAMETERS

Vena contracta width	>0.6 cm
Jet width/LVOT width	>65%
Jet CAS/LVOT CSA	<60%
Regurgitant volume	>60 mL/beat
Regurgitant fraction	>50%
EROA	>30 cm^2

Chronic Aortic Regurgitation

Information Gathering in the Individual With Chronic Aortic Regurgitation

When assessing the status of an individual with any valve abnormality for intervention, one has to first ask the question about symptoms. In the case of aortic regurgitation or stenosis, one has to question the individual about exertion fatigue, light-headedness, or chest tightness. At first, the answer may be that the individual does anything that is desired and that there are none of the above symptoms. It may take more than one office visit and interrogation to determine that exercise tolerance has changed and that certain activities are avoided because of intolerance. It may even take a walk on the treadmill to determine that, instead of 9 minutes being tolerated only 3 minutes are tolerated. When this is determined, then the threshold from "no symptoms" to "symptoms" is crossed, and considerations for intervention are at hand (see below). A sentinel bout of pulmonary congestion during an upper respiratory illness might precipitate crossing this line, or a hike in a region that once was tolerated is not tolerated. Results of interrogations at the time of interview with the patient identify that action should be taken toward intervention and valve replacement. Identification of symptoms applies not only to those with aortic regurgitation but also to those with any valve abnormality. See below.

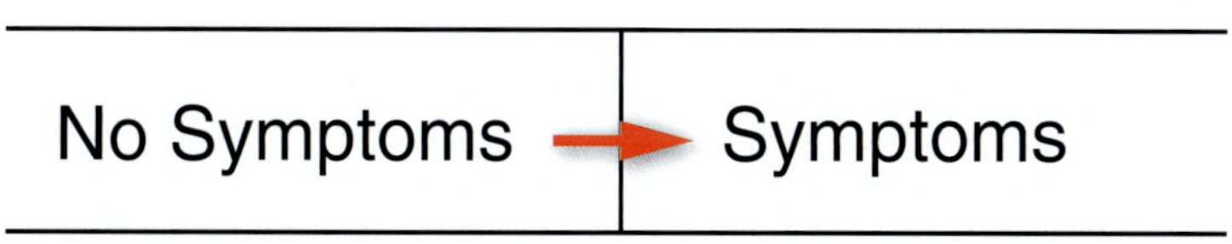

FIGURE 4.19

In the absence of symptoms after a thorough interrogation, it becomes more difficult in determining the timing of intervention for any valve abnormality. The guidelines offer various classes of recommendations and levels of evidence in these situations, but they are not absolute and require thought and discussion and assessment of overall risk. Parameters obtained from left ventricular dimensions, left ventricular systolic function, and Doppler parameters of severity must be integrated into the overall situation of decision-making. Classes of recommendation and levels of evidence in these situations of the asymptomatic individual change from this point. Careful assessment of echocardiographic information is needed and occasionally stress testing for assessment of ejection fraction and functional capacity can be helpful. Magnetic resonance imaging can also offer more information.

The following illustrations illustrate acquisition of some of the key information gathered in individuals with aortic regurgitation that allow decision-making and recommendations to take place. Knowledge of the current guideline and class of recommendations and level of evidence is important for the clinician in making recommendations to individual patients.

The Timing of Surgery for Chronic Aortic Regurgitation

The timing of surgical intervention for individuals with aortic regurgitation (AR) has always been difficult. On the one hand, in those with acute AR, surgery is needed immediately, and on the other hand, those with chronic AR may present with good exercise tolerance and wonder why someone wants to open their chest. Chronic AR requires thought processes about preservation of reasonably normal left ventricular function, both systolic and diastolic, and the overall state of health of the individual. If symptoms are present such as the development of fatigue with exertion, then, if risks are acceptable, replacement should be done. It is those individuals with asymptomatic AR that require discussion and explanation.

The guidelines from the ACC/AHA for chronic aortic regurgitation offer recommendations for intervention that have been well thought out and offer the latest thoughts concerning the timing of surgical intervention in these individuals.[9,10]

2014 ACC/AHA Guidelines for Chronic Aortic Regurgitation

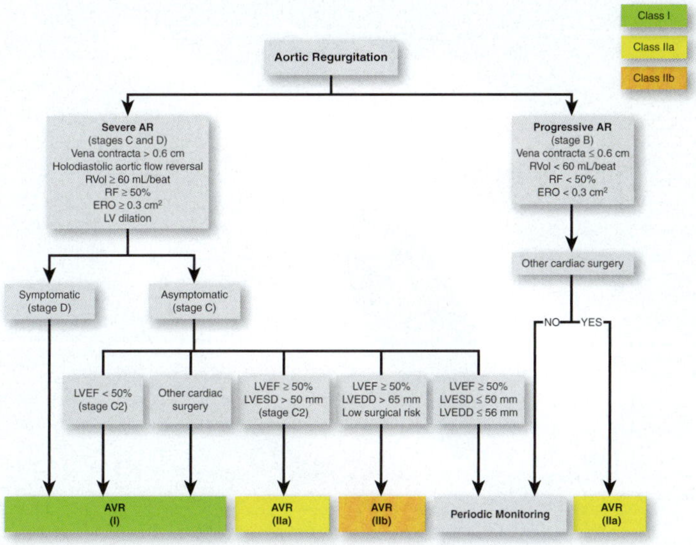

FIGURE 4.20 Source: Nishimura RA, Otto CM, Bonow RO, et al. 2014 ACC/AHA Guideline for management of patients with valvular heart disease. A report of the ACC/AHA association task force on practice guidelines. *J Am Coll Cardiol.* 2014;63(22):e57-e185.

SECTION 4

CONGENITAL ABNORMALITIES OF THE AORTIC VALVE

UNICUSPID AORTIC VALVE

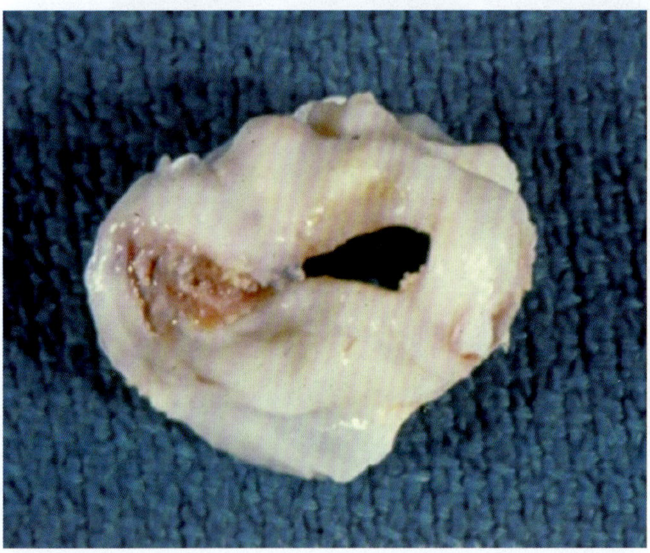

FIGURE 4.21

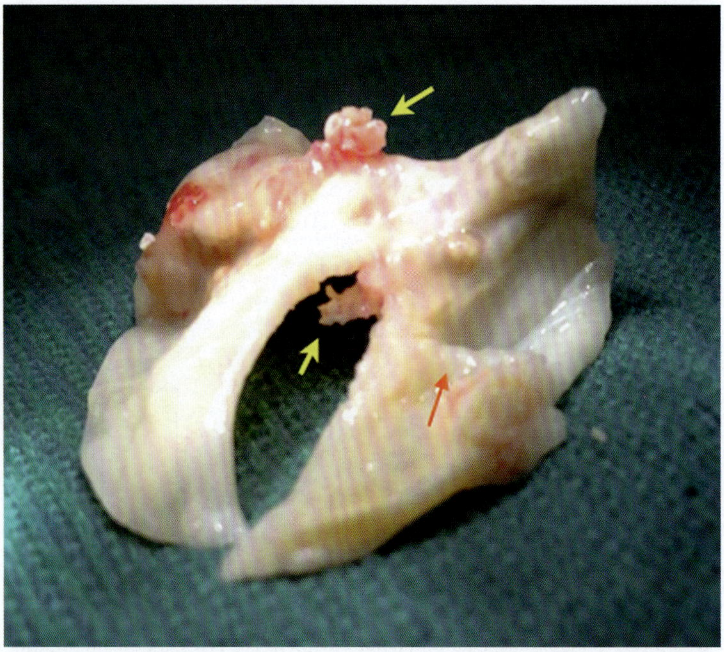

FIGURE 4.22

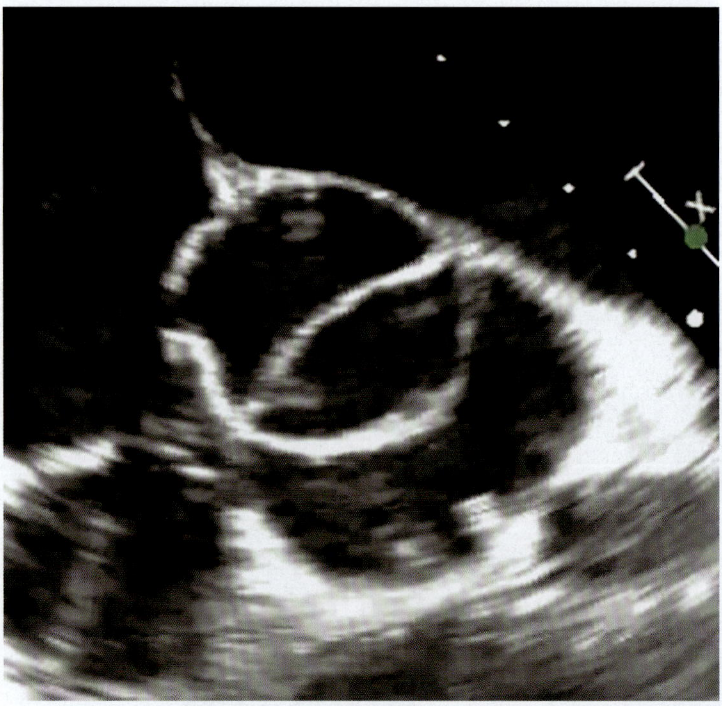

FIGURE 4.23

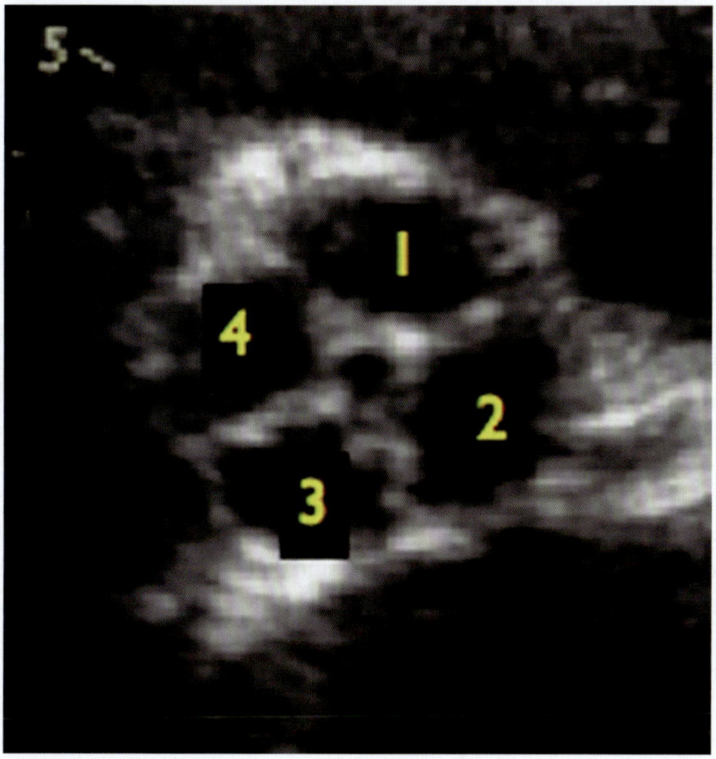

FIGURE 4.24

Individuals with a unicuspid aortic valve present earlier in life. These valves can be thicker at an earlier point in life and present more of a hemodynamic burden (A). Often, despite being classified as a unicuspid valve, there are remnants of a commissure (B). Individuals with bicuspid valve present with various manifestations from ejections sounds or clicks to aortic regurgitation and stenosis to an ascending aortic aneurysm. Other congenital abnormalities such as coarctation of the aorta have a high association with a bicuspid aortic valve. The most common type of bicuspid aortic valve is that of fusion of the right and left cusps, and it has the highest association with ectasia of the ascending aorta. Commonly, aortopathy is the term used to describe this ascending aortic abnormality. The rare quadracuspid aortic valve (D) is illustrated above and may be associating with a variable degree of functional abnormality, usually aortic regurgitation.[18,19]

BICUSPID AORTIC VALVE

- Fusion of the right and left coronary cusps is the most common.
- Fusion of the right and noncoronary cusps is the second most common.
- Fusion of the noncoronary cusp and the left coronary cusps is rare.
- Ascending aneurysm and coarctation are most commonly found with fusion of the right and left cusps.

SECTION 5

SURGICAL CHOICES FOR AORTIC VALVE REPLACEMENT

When symptoms develop in the presence of severe aortic valve disease, then consideration of intervention is at hand. Many factors enter into this decision-making. The age and expected longevity of the patient are important. Tissue valves may last 10 to 20 years and do not require anticoagulation but later may require another procedure. Overall state of health and potential for taking anticoagulants must be considered. Once committed to a mechanical valve, it is a long-term commitment. Considerations for potential noncardiac surgical procedures and bridging techniques must be considered.

Recently, the development of transcatheter techniques has offered treatment of those individuals with severe aortic stenosis who otherwise might not have had that opportunity. High-risk surgical situations and older individuals fall into this category. Furthermore, the "valve-in-valve" technique has become useful when tissue valves begin to deteriorate and offers these individuals relief when otherwise a "redo" surgical procedure would be needed. We are still learning about the durability of these valves.

The development of a team approach to transcatheter techniques has coupled the interventional cardiologist with the surgeon as a team, and the imaging specialist have been added to the equation. This approach has given options to the high-risk patient with severe aortic stenosis. This team approach has led to the success of the programs throughout the country and world.

In this chapter, various types of mechanical and tissue valves and their complications are illustrated.

TRANSCUTANEOUS AORTIC VALVE REPLACEMENT (TAVR)

View From the Control Room in the Cath Lab During Transcatheter Aortic Valve Replacement

Cardiologists are involved with TAVR in the cath lab and in the operating room. Not only do they need to know what to expect from the echo images and Doppler information, but knowledge about the happenings on the cath table and on the fluoroscopic screen is important. Positioning of the valve before deployment is monitored by fluoroscopy, valve calcifications and angiography. Pigtail catheters placed at the bottom of the cusps offer additional information. A careful assessment of the position of the take off of the coronary arteries is also important. These are complemented by echocardiographic images. Each modality should be familiar to each team member present at the table.

The following pages illustrate fluoroscopic images and hemodynamic information obtained from hemodynamic tracings. The hemodynamic effects of rapid pacing are also illustrated. Without this effect, the valve and balloon would be ejected into the aorta.

TAVR FROM THE CONTROL ROOM—THE HEMODYNAMIC TRACINGS

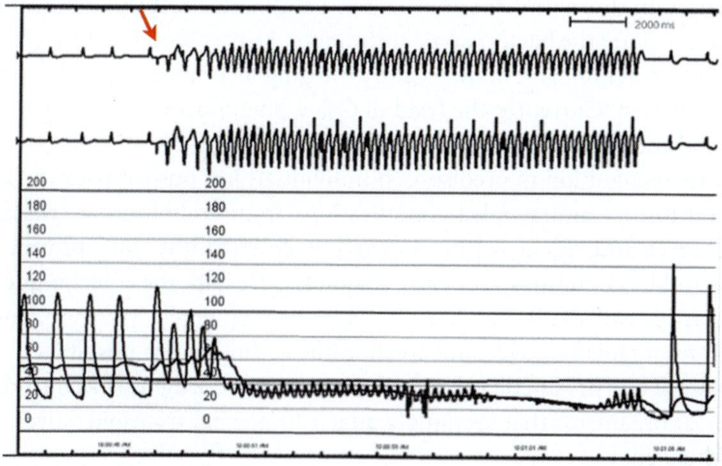

FIGURE 4.25 Rapid pacing (*red arrow*) and deployment of the valve as seen on the fluoroscopic monitoring screen.

PROSTHETIC VALVES

The choice of a prosthetic valve currently has to take into consideration several factors. If surgery is medium or high risk, then a TAVR can be considered. If anticoagulation is an issue or will be an issue in the future, then mechanical valve is not a choice. Tissue valves eliminate the need for anticoagulation unless atrial fibrillation is present. Durability of tissue valves comes into play since they last ~15 years, but currently, valve-in-valve techniques have taken on a new prospective from the standpoint of durability.

Monitoring of prosthetic valves of any type is required from the clinical standpoint, and imaging techniques include echocardiography and fluoroscopy. Illustrations of these techniques follow.

SECTION 6

ENDOCARDITIS OF THE AORTIC VALVE

CLASSIFICATION

- Infective endocarditis
  - Acute bacterial endocarditis
  - Subacute bacterial endocarditis
- Nonbacterial thrombotic endocarditis

Endocarditis as a disease entity has deep roots in medicine. The clinical syndrome has been described in detail by Sir William Osler in the late 1800s. Initially, it was termed malignant endocarditis since there was no specific treatment and individuals with this entity did not survive. Landmarks in the understanding of this disease include the bacteriologic techniques such as blood cultures, the development of penicillin, and more recently imaging techniques with ultrasound at the top of this list. Currently, the triad of Osler, pneumococcal meningitis, pneumonia, and endocarditis, is not often seen.

Early recognition in predisposed individuals has pushed back the syndrome's natural history and avoided complications from embolization. The axiom that fever in an individual with a murmur is endocarditis until proven otherwise leads to blood cultures and early diagnosis. Despite these techniques, the disease process still exists, but different forms have emerged. More virulent relatively resistant organisms have come forth in the setting of our hospital environments and attack our prosthetic valves and devices. Illicit drug use has introduced large doses of organisms that seemingly attach to normal tricuspid valves. The scene has changed.

The following sections illustrate some of the pathologic findings and images when endocarditis is present.

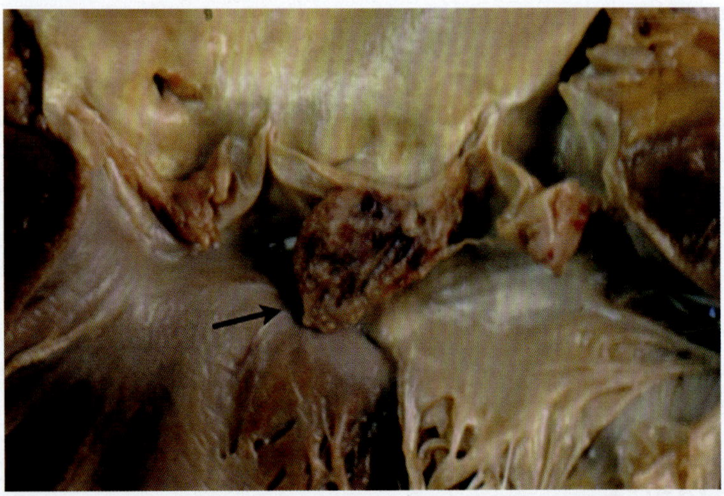

FIGURE 4.26 Large vegetation attached to the ventricular surface of the noncoronary cusp of the aortic valve (*black arrow*).

Bacteria attach to the endocardium that has been disturbed by flow disturbances such as the Venturi effect and already deposited platelets and fibrin. From there, they proliferate, invade, and destroy tissue. Multiple local factors are operative at these sites. Regurgitant lesions develop vegetations on the downstream side of the valve leaflets, or as in the above example, aortic regurgitation results in lesions on the ventricular side of the valve surface. Downstream lesions may be preset where jets have exerted their forces against surfaces such as on chordal structures or the walls of the left atrium. In the end, the valve tissue gets destroyed or becomes disrupted in one form or another, or perforations occur.[20]

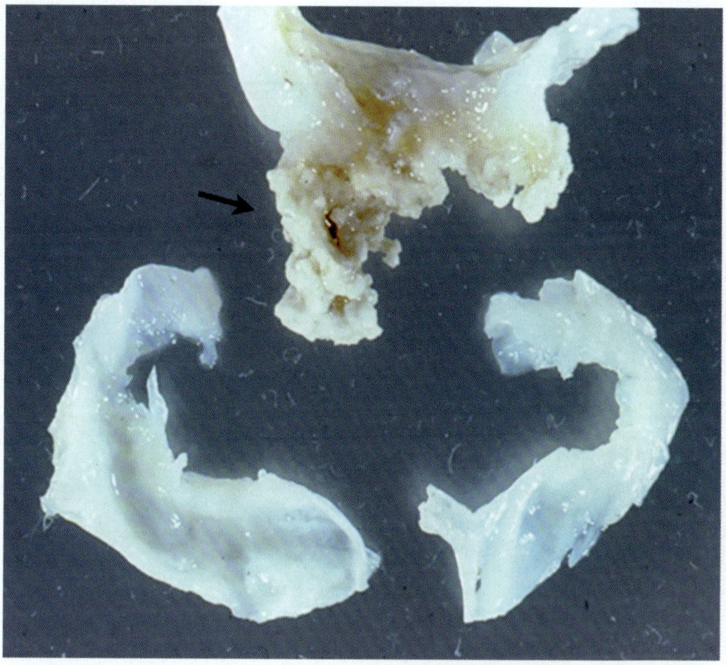

FIGURE 4.27 A large vegetation attached to the cusp of a surgically removed aortic valve with destruction of the valve leaflets. (*black arrow*).

SEVERE AORTIC REGURGITATION AND ENDOCARDITIS

In the setting of acute endocarditis involving the aortic valve, aortic regurgitation often becomes severe. If a virulent organism such as methicillin-resistant staphylococcus is the offender, the aortic valve can be destroyed quickly. A normal left ventricle does not handle the hemodynamic load of acute regurgitation, and after a brief course of antibiotics, intervention is needed. Once the blood cultures are positive, and antibiotics are made appropriate, careful observation at the bedside and with echocardiography is needed. Any change in the status of the patient requires intervention. A mobile vegetation >10 mm in length in itself suggests that the valve should be replaced on the basis of the embolic potential. Often, microemboli are occurring that are not noticed and are revealed by an MRI study. A visual field defect or a visual disturbance in one eye can herald an embolus. A blue toe or finger; classic splinter hemorrhage on the fingernails; a nodular, painful area at the tip of a finger (Osler node); and a painful erythematous areas of the soles of the hands or toes (Janeway lesion) can be clues to the presence of emboli from an infected valve. At the present time it is the job of clinicians to push this disease process back in its natural history such that in an individual with known murmur and fever has bacterial endocarditis until proven otherwise. Before antibiotics are given blood cultures should be drawn. These efforts have in recent years along with transesophageal echo in individuals with bacteremia of any type promoted discovery of early valve lesions and allow the process to be treated before the valve is destroyed.[9]

THE ECHOCARDIOGRAM AND AORTIC ENDOCARDITIS

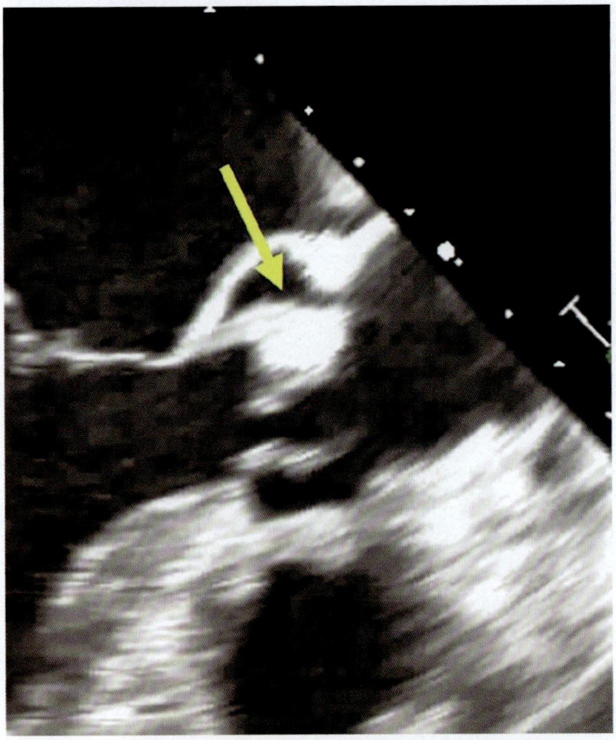

FIGURE 4.28 A large vegetation involves the LCC and moves with the aortic leaflet (*yellow arrow*). The LV is very hyperdynamic, a clue to the presence of severe AR. TEE, 120°.

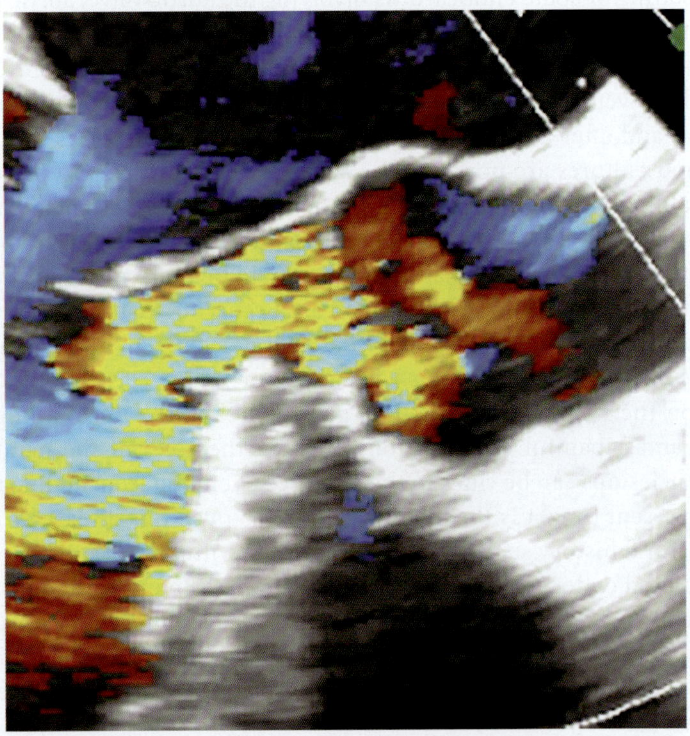

FIGURE 4.29 Color Doppler that demonstrates the severe AR and also the MR. The jet of AR fills most of the LVOT. TEE, 135° view.

MARANTIC ENDOCARDITIS

Marantic endocarditis is a noninfectious form of vegetation on cardiac endocardial surfaces. It is termed nonbacterial thrombotic endocarditis. It occurs in hypercoagulable states as seen in lupus erythematosus and the presence of antiphospholipid antibodies. The antiphospholipid syndrome has been described as an individual with an episode of thrombosis or two miscarriages plus very high anticardiolipid levels and a positive test for lupus anticoagulants more than 8 weeks apart. In this syndrome, thrombotic lesions develop on injured endocardial surfaces. Most commonly, it involves the coapting surfaces of the mitral valve and less often the aortic valve. Marantic endocarditis is also associated with underlying malignancies such as Hodgkin disease and adenocarcinoma of the lung, pancreas, stomach, and colon. The lesions seen on echocardiography often involve the mitral valve and less commonly the aortic valve and less often the right-sided valves. These verrucous lesions are usually but not always on the coapting surfaces of the valves on the upstream side. Often, multiple embolic phenomena occur. Anticoagulant therapy with warfarin is indicated if possible.[21-23]

Whereas usually the mitral valve is involved with these verrucous lesions, our examples involve the aortic valves and both presented with stroke.

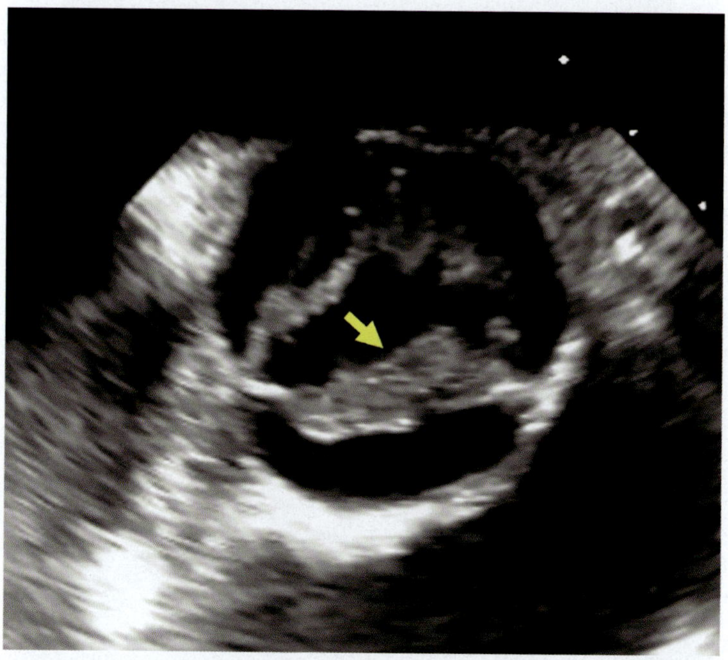

FIGURE 4.30 Freeze frame of the aortic leaflets demonstrates masses on the ventricular surface of all three leaflets (*yellow arrow*) at the coapting edges. TEE, cross-sectional view.

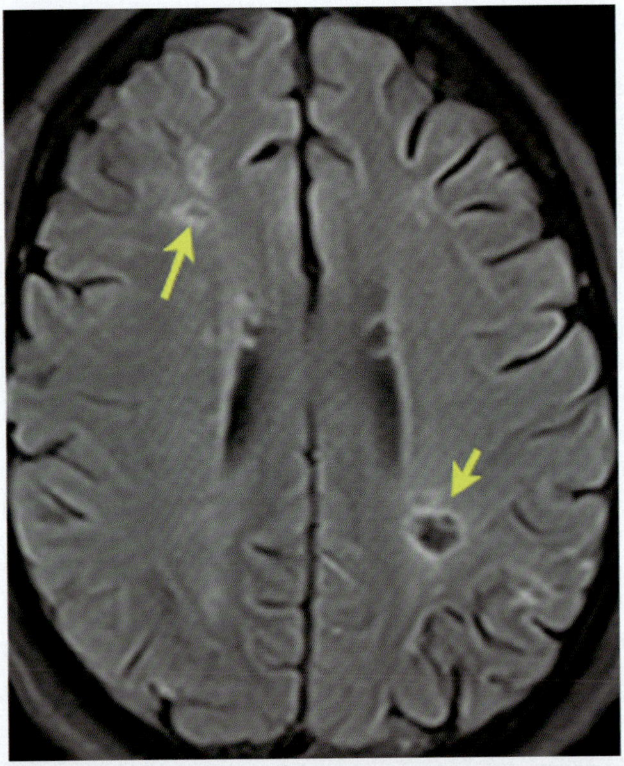

FIGURE 4.31 The MRI showing the results of multiple cerebral emboli (*yellow arrows*).

NORMAL BIOPROSTHETIC AORTIC VALVE

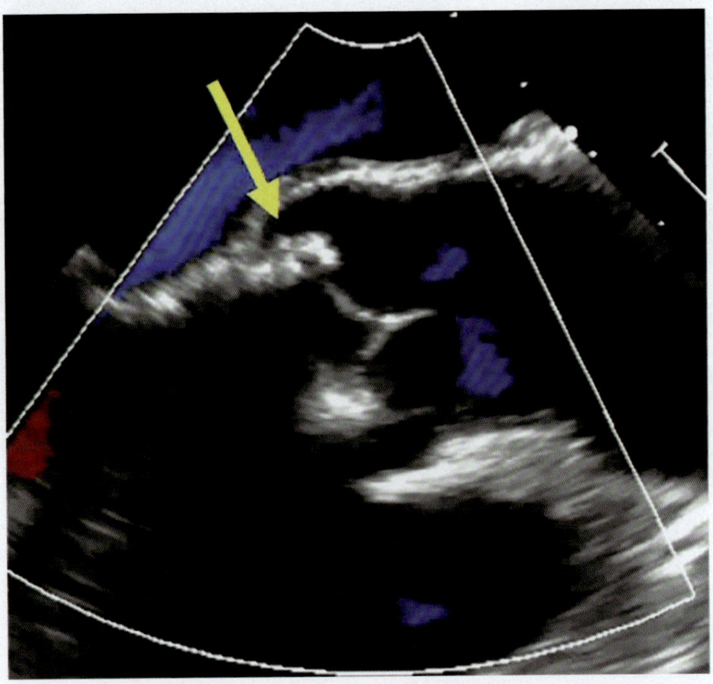

FIGURE 4.32 Normally functioning Carpentier-Edwards Magna bovine pericardial bioprosthetic valve. Note the struts (*yellow arrow*), the thin leaflets, and no aortic regurgitation.

VALVE RING ABSCESS AND PSEUDOANEURYSM OF THE MITRAL AORTIC INTERVALVULAR FIBROSA

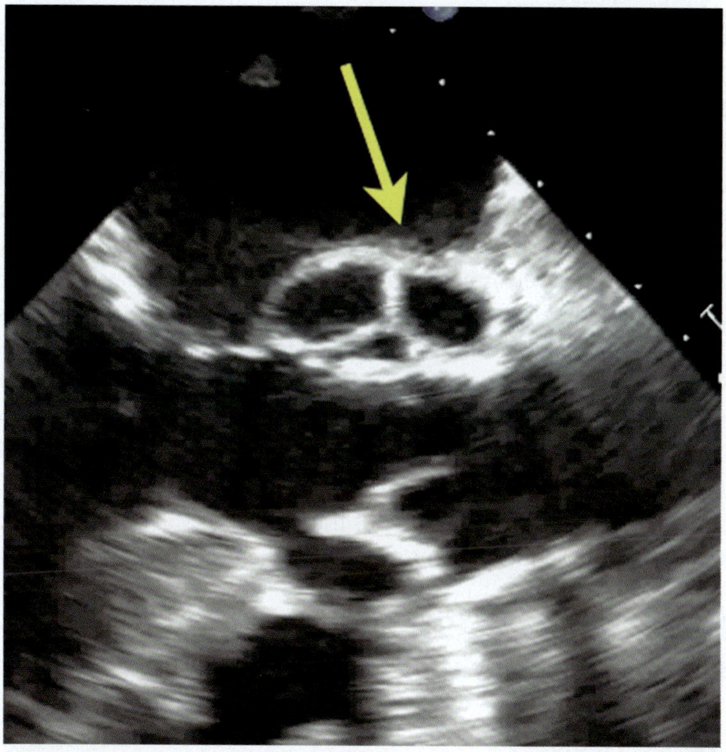

FIGURE 4.33 Expanding area posterior to the aorta is shown in this long-axis view TEE from 132° (*yellow arrow*).

Mechanical Prosthetic Valves

Mechanical aortic valves are usually bileaflet valves, but on occasion, a ball-in-cage valve is used. Echocardiography allows viewing of the motion of the leaflets or the ball in cage and surrounding tissues. Mobile vegetations and valve ring abscesses can be visualized. In addition, Doppler information can assess the presence of a valvular regurgitation and the gradient across the valve. Acceptable gradients are available for each valve and each size of the valve.

Fluoroscopy is always an excellent way to assess mechanical valves and motion of their components. Gradients can be influenced by the presence of anemia and other factors, and fluoroscopy is an additional modality that can offer information about valve function.[24]

SECTION 7

OTHER ABNORMALITIES OF THE AORTIC VALVE

PAPILLARY FIBROELASTOMA ON THE AORTIC VALVE

These benign tumors are small and usually attached to the aortic valve most commonly but sometimes attached to the mitral valve and rarely in other areas of the heart. They usually have a stalk and therefore have some mobility. Most commonly, they are single; however, as in the following example, they may be multiple. Under the microscope, they have a characteristic appearance described as a "sea anemone" in that they have hyaline material lined with endothelium. These do have embolic potential, which comes to mind when these small tumors are visualized on echocardiography and have been removed surgically when this has occurred.

The following illustrations demonstrate one of these tumors at postmortem examination and one that was discovered as part of an evaluation for hypertrophic cardiomyopathy. The example of the on mitral valve had embolized to the retina and was subsequently removed.[25]

PAPILLARY FIBROELASTOMA AORTIC VALVE PATHOLOGY SPECIMEN

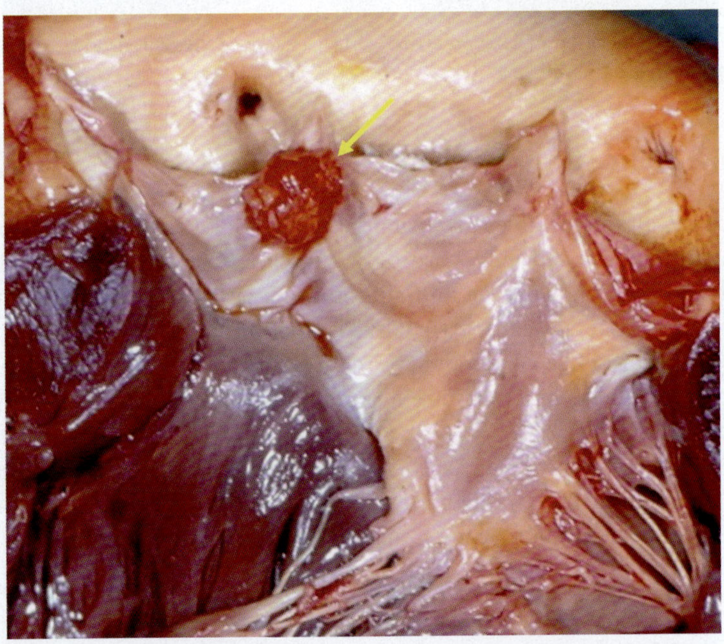

FIGURE 4.34 An autopsy specimen that shows an incidentally found papillary fibroelastoma. It appears as a small rounded multilobulated mass attached to the edge of the aortic valve cusp on the ventricular side of the valve (*yellow arrow*).

Lambl Excrescences

Lambl described in 1856 these small filiform lesions that occur on the ventricular surface of the aortic valve in normal and abnormal valves. On mitral valves, they appear on the atrial surface and rarely are they seen in right-sided valves. They consist of collagen tissue and have an endothelial lining. They are linear and vary from 5 to 10 mm in length and ~1 mm in diameter. They are filiform or threadlike and oscillate back and forth with the cardiac cycle. Their etiology is uncertain and thoughts about a thrombotic etiology have been entertained as seen with Libman-Sacks endocarditis; however, they have more structure than the lesions seen in lupus erythematosus or other states that have hypercoagulability. In a personal communication, the late Dr. Michael Gravanis did some work with electron microscopy and thought that they were extruded collagen fibrils from the valve. Uncommonly, individuals who have these have cerebral embolic ischemia.[26-28]

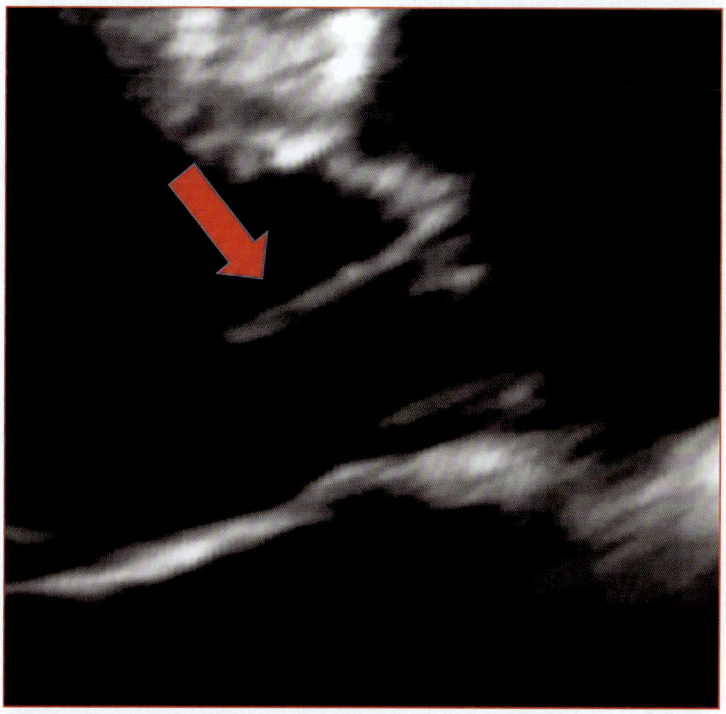

FIGURE 4.35 Freeze frame of aortic valve Lambl prolapsing as a linear structure into the LVOT in diastole (*red arrow*)—transthoracic echo. TTE, PLA view.

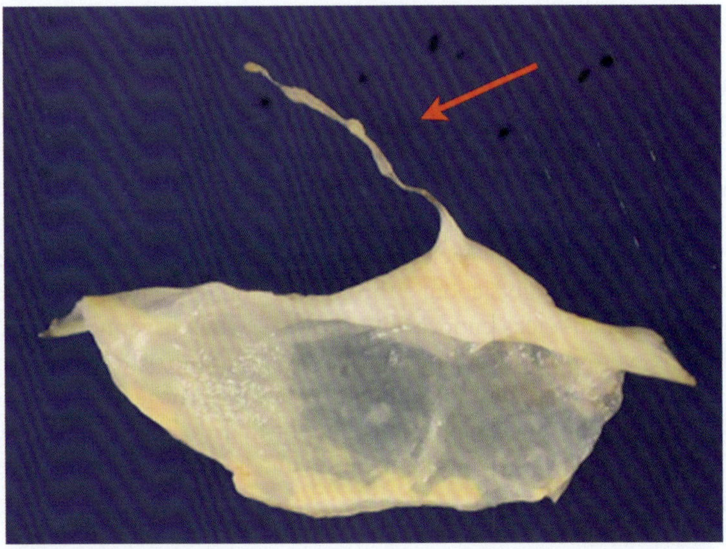

FIGURE 4.36 Specimen from the above patient above after surgical resection for aortic valve replacement—note that the Lambl has its origin from the ventricular surface of the aortic valve (*red arrow*).

SECTION 8

DISCRETE MEMBRANOUS SUBAORTIC STENOSIS

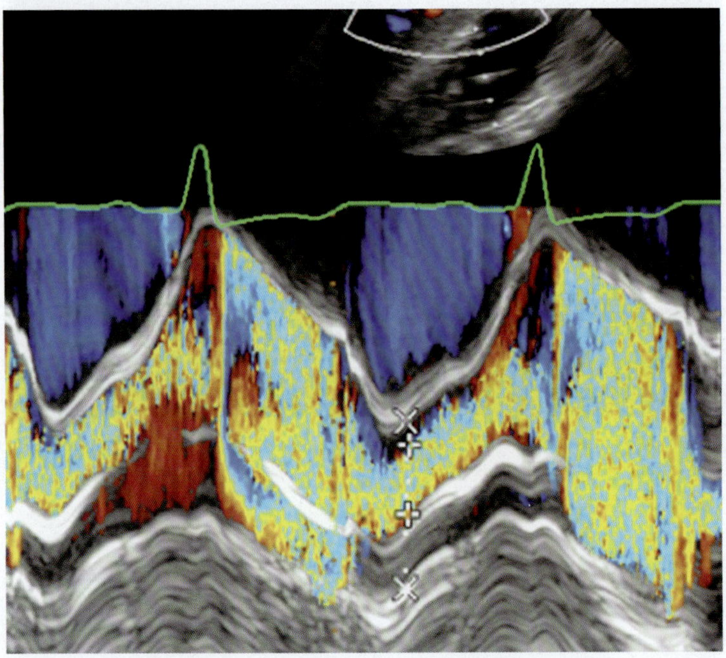

FIGURE 4.37 Color M-mode sampling through the aortic valve leaflets.

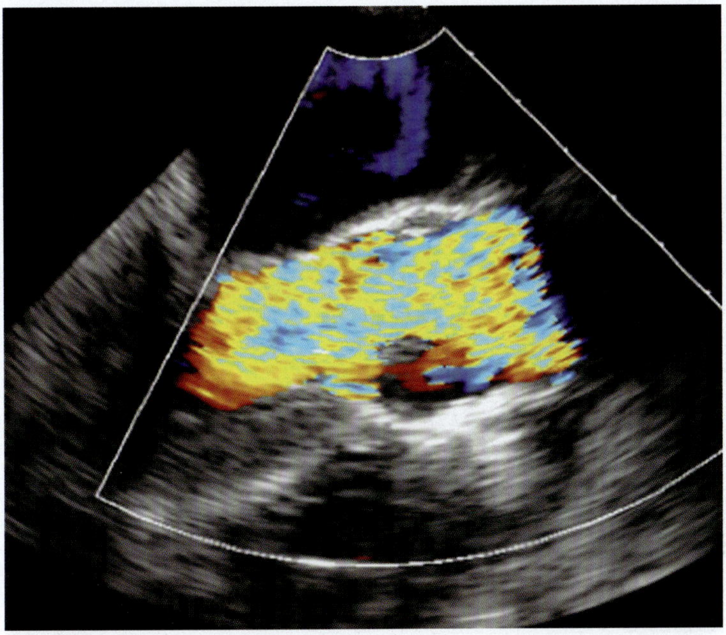

FIGURE 4.38 Intense turbulence arriving below the aortic valve and blasting through the aortic leaflets and aortic root.

In discrete membranous subvalvular aortic stenosis, the membrane is circumferential and creates a chamber between the membrane and the aortic valve. Within this chamber, there is severe turbulence as this is the first chamber to receive the jet created by the stenosis. The membrane is usually thin and fibrous and results in a jet that hits the aortic valve leaflets. Over time, the endothelium is damaged, platelets and fibrin get deposited, the valve thickens, and function abnormalities follow. Valve stenosis can be of variable degree but is usually not severe and neither is the regurgitation. Surgical resection of this membrane is done through the aortic valve, and often, removal of a surprisingly small amount of tissue results in significant hemodynamic improvement.[29,30]

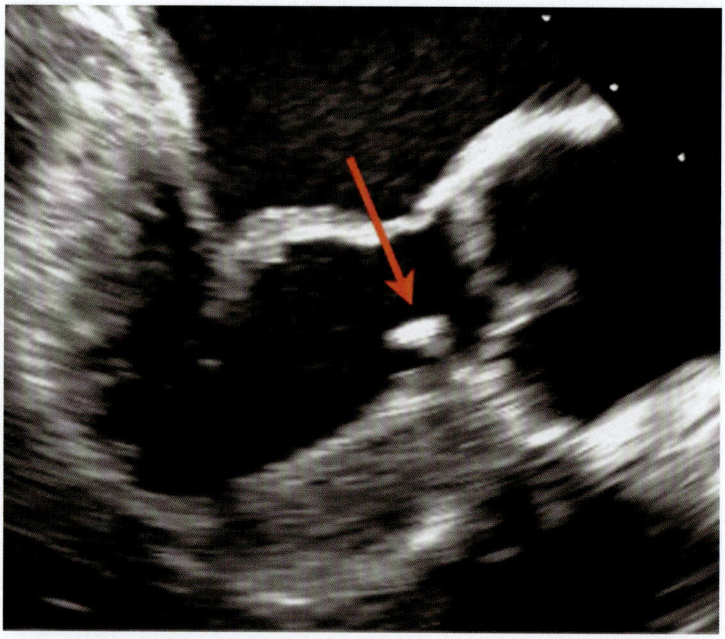

FIGURE 4.39 The discrete subvalvular membrane most prominent on the septal side of the LVOT but also associated with thickening on the anterior mitral leaflet—*red arrow* points to the septal side of the membrane.

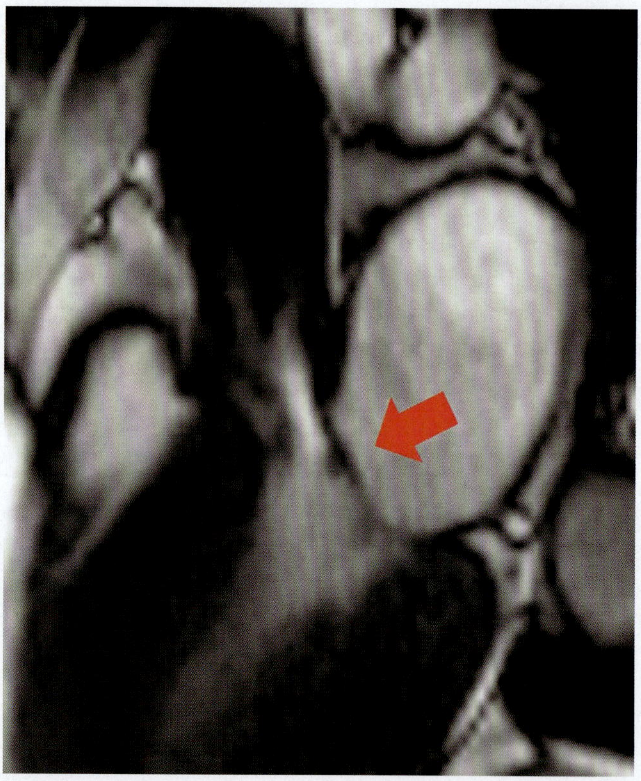

FIGURE 4.40 Long-axis systolic freeze frame view of a T2 image of the left ventricle showing the subaortic membrane (*red arrow*). Note that there is a portion of this membrane located on the anterior leaflet of the mitral valve and also the interventricular septum. The jet produced by the subaortic membrane blasts toward the aortic valve leaflets and in the long term causes thickening and insufficiency of this valve.

SECTION 9

AORTIC ANEURYSMS, AORTIC DISSECTION, AND OTHER AORTIC ABNORMALITIES

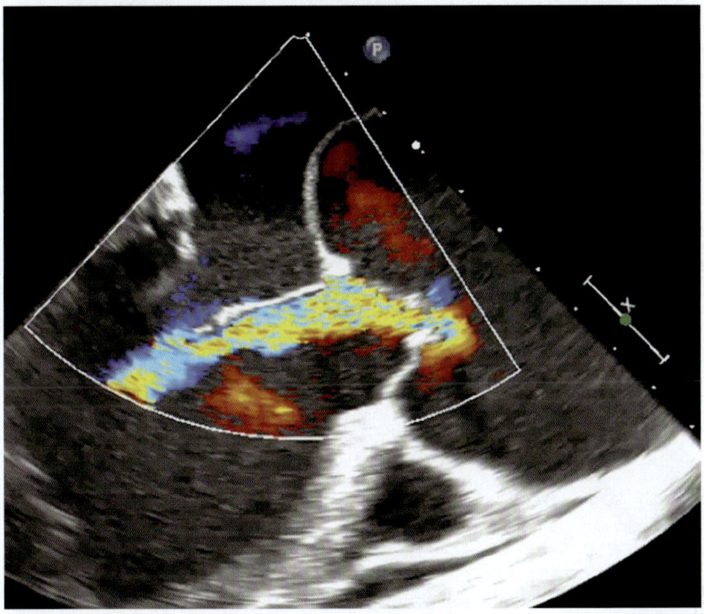

FIGURE 4.41 Marfan syndrome with a very dilated aorta in the sinus of Valsalva area and aortic regurgitation. TEE, 138° view.

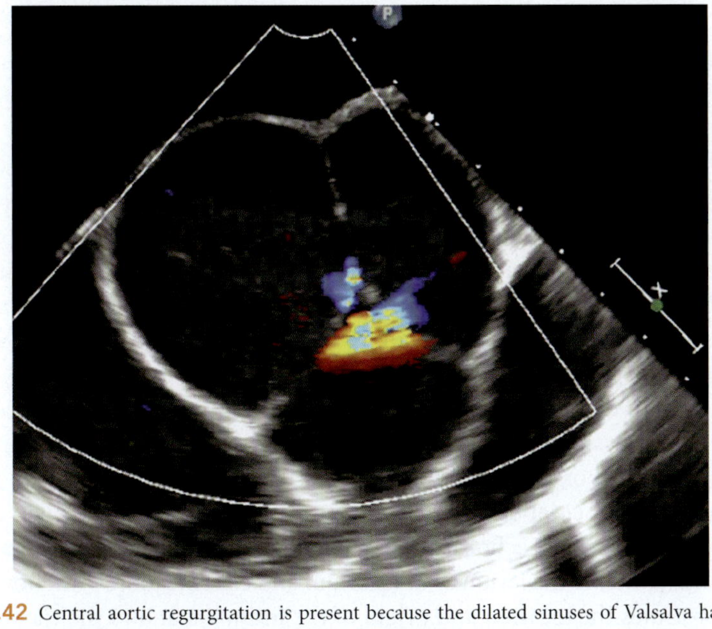

FIGURE 4.42 Central aortic regurgitation is present because the dilated sinuses of Valsalva have pulled the central portions of the valve apart. Freeze framed, TEE, 50° view at the coaptation area.

DISSECTING ANEURYSM OF THE AORTA

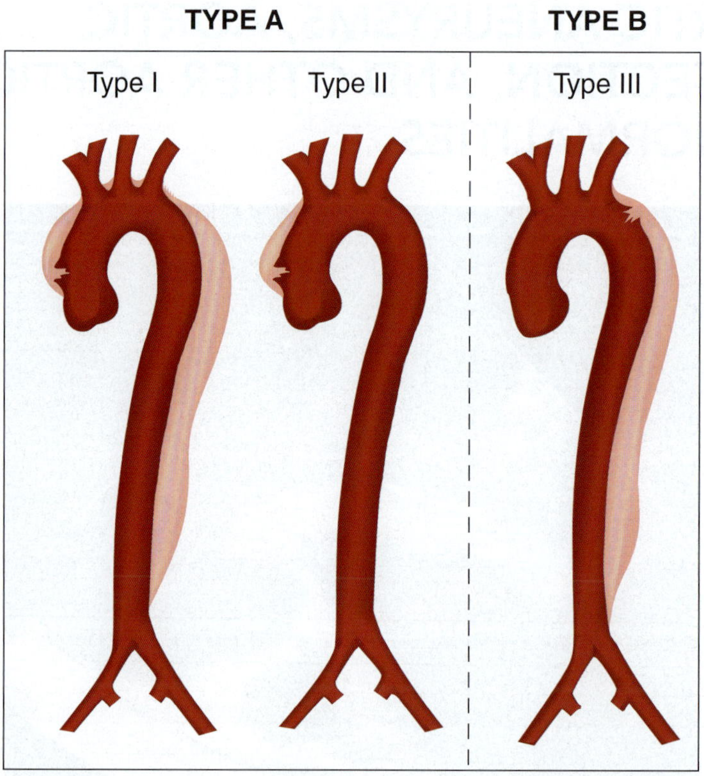

FIGURE 4.43 In these drawings, the calcification of aortic dissection according to the DeBakey and the Stanford is illustrated. In the DeBakey type I, the intimal tear is in the ascending sort, and the dissection extends at least into the arch and often further. In the DeBakey type II, the intimal tear is in the ascending aorta, and the dissection extends superior but is confined to the aorta proximal to the innominate artery. The Stanford calcification includes both of these two in the type A classification since they both require emergency surgery using the same type of median sternotomy approach. DeBakey type III or Stanford type B begins in the descending aorta and extends distally to a variable degree and usually is treated medically. (Source: Figure taken from Braverman A. Acute aortic dissection. *Circulation.* 2010;122:184-188.)

Individuals presenting to the emergency room with chest pain with a component of back pain provoke thinking immediately about the possibility of aortic dissection. This syndrome coupled with the absence of a peripheral pulse, discrepant blood pressures in the arms, stroke, or even myocardial infarction brings this to the top of this list of the differential diagnosis. A history of Marfan's syndrome, Loeys-Dietz syndrome, Ehlers-Danlos syndrome and bicuspid aortic valve all are strong predisposing factors.[31,32]

A prompt diagnosis is needed as is classification of the defect since Stanford type A aneurysms or DeBakey types I and II require immediate surgery and Stanford type B or DeBakey type III are usually treated medically. In the emergency setting, a computerized tomographic x-ray with contrast will define the lesion. Transthoracic echocardiography and transesophageal echocardiography can further define the lesion as to its origin and classification. The above diagram demonstrates the location and origin of the intimal tear and the classification of dissecting aneurysms.

STANFORD TYPE A DISSECTING ANEURYSM OF THE AORTA AS VIEWED ON TRANSTHORACIC ECHO

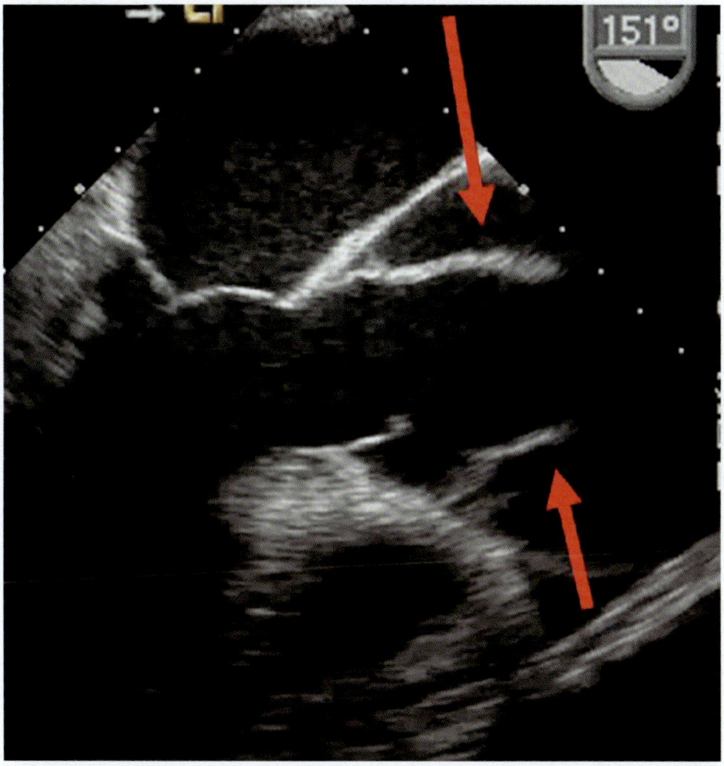

FIGURE 4.44 Stanford type A aortic dissection with intimal flap moving with the aortic leaflets (*red arrows*). The ascending aorta is very ectatic. TEE, 153°.

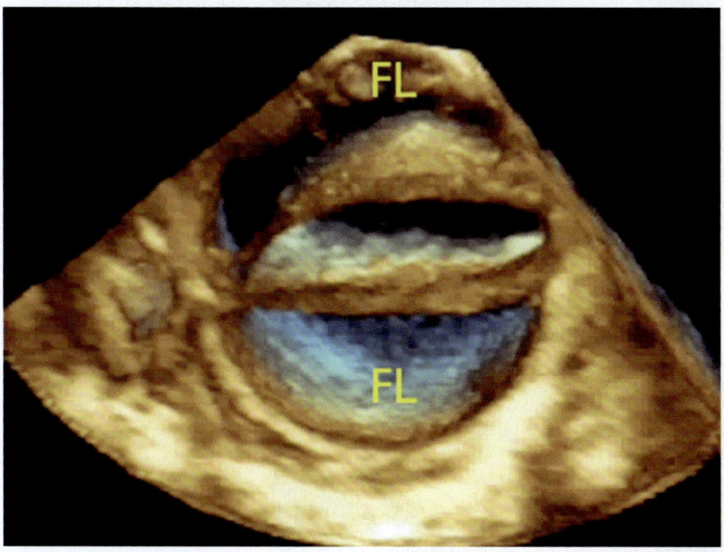

FIGURE 4.45 The three-dimensional views of the dissected descending thoracic aorta showing a near circumferential dissection. The true lumen is in the central location, and the false (*FL*) is surrounding. TEE, 3D views.

STANFORD TYPE B OR DEBAKEY TYPE III AORTIC DISSECTION

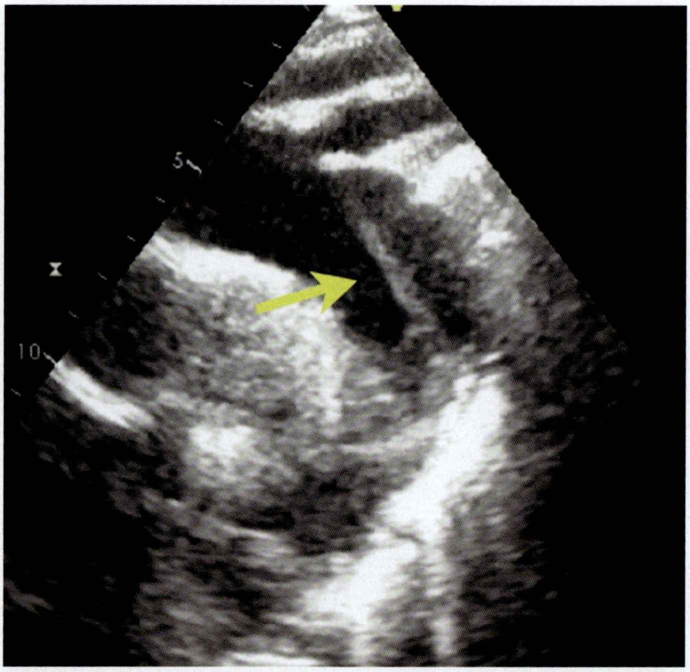

FIGURE 4.46 The first clues from the suprasternal notch show an intimal flap (*yellow arrow*) originating from just below the left subclavian artery.

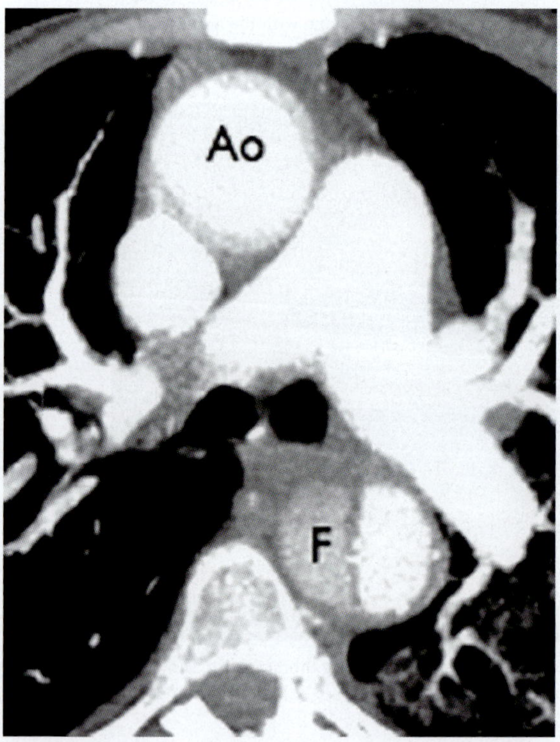

FIGURE 4.47 Cross-sectional view on CT showing the dissected descending aorta (*F*, false lumen) and not the ascending aorta (*Ao*).

SECTION 10

ATHEROSCLEROSIS OF THE AORTA

ATHEROSCLEROSIS OF THE AORTIC ARCH AND THE DESCENDING AORTA AS A SOURCE OF EMBOLUS TO THE BRAIN OR STRUCTURES DISTAL

As plaques progress in size and atherosclerotic activity, they can rupture and leave small cavities in the aorta at various locations. The endothelium becomes disrupted, and portions loosen and become mobile and oscillate back and forth from systole to diastole. Sometimes these pieces of endothelium develop into a linear configuration and appear whiplike as they move with the cardiac cycle. The plaques empty their contents, and loose endothelium is noted to a variable degree depending on shape. All of this leads to small and larger degrees of embolization.

CASE PRESENTATION

A 53-year-old man presented to the emergency room with right-sided weakness and dysphagia. Transesophageal echo was done as part of a "stroke evaluation."

Mobile atherosclerotic plaque noted in the proximal descending thoracic aorta in the individual presenting with a stroke. Atherosclerotic plaque can become ulcerated and various types and sizes of thrombi can form and embolize distally. When the plaque initially ruptures, small particles of its contents can go distally and cause small-vessel occlusion. This phenomenon is seen in aortic aneurysms and results in the so-called blue toe syndrome. The

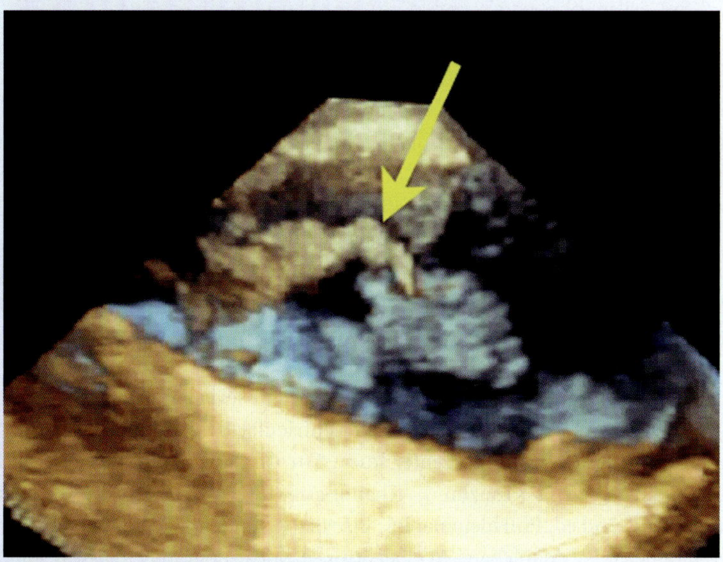

FIGURE 4.48 Another view of the proximal descending aorta demonstrating the mobile disrupted plaque (*yellow arrow*). Still frame, TEE, 3D.

endothelial lining of the aorta can be left dangling after the contents are spilled and result in mobile areas as seen in this individual. The mobile area probably has complex components of endothelial wall and thrombus. In this individual, the mobile areas appear like tentacles and potential for more embolization is present. When these are present in the arch or proximal distal portion of the aorta, they have the capability of embolizing into the cerebral circulation and causing stroke. It is true that during the course of pulsatile flow, there is a forward surge of flow but also a small degree of flow reversal that can result in embolization to the cerebral vessels.

REFERENCES

1. Weyman AE. *Principles and Practice of Echocardiography.* 2nd ed. Philadelphia, PA: Lea & Febiger; 1994:499.
2. Ross J, Braunwald E. Aortic stenosis. *Circulation.* 1968;38(suppl 5):V61-V67.
3. Distinguishing severe from nonsevere aortic stenosis in patients with depressed left ventricular function and low transvalvular gradients. *J Am Cardiol.* 1995;75:191-194.
4. deFilipppi CR, Willett DL, Bricker E, et al. Usefulness of dobutamine echocardiography in distinguishing severe from nonsevere aortic stenosis in patients with depressed left ventricular function and low transvalvular gradients. *J Am Cardiol.* 1995;75:191-194.
5. Lang RM, Goldstein SA, Kronzon I, Khandheria BK, Mor-Avi V. *ASE's Comprehensive Echocardiography.* 2nd ed. Philadelphia, PA: Elsevier (Saunders); 2016:417-421.
6. Oh JK, Seward JB, Tajik AJ. *The Echo Manual.* 3rd ed. Philadelphia, PA: Wolters Kluwer/ Lippincott Williams & Wilkins; 2007:192-199.
7. Pibarot P, Dumesnil JG. Low-slow, low gradient aortic stenosis with normal and depressed left ventricular ejection fraction. *J Am Coll Cardiol.* 2012;60(19):1845-1843.
8. Pireira JJ, Lauer MS, Bashir M, et al. Survival after aortic valve replacement for severe aortic stenosis with low transvalvular gradients and severe left ventricular dysfunction. *J Am Coll Cardiol.* 2002;39:1356-1363.
9. Nishimura RA, Otto CM, Bonow RO, et al. 2014 AHA/ACC Guideline for management of patients with valvular heart disease. A report of the ACC/AHA association task force on practice guidelines. *J Am Coll Cardiol.* 2014;63(22):e57-e185.
10. Vahanian A, Alfieri O, Andreotti F. Guidelines on the management of valvular heart disease (version 2012): the Joint Task Force on the Management of Valvular Heart Disease of the European Society of Cardiology (ESC) and the European Association for Cardio-Thoracic Surgery (EACTS). *Our Heart J.* 2012;33:2451-2496.
11. Pibarot P, Dumesnil JG. Low-flow, low-gradient aortic stenosis with normal and depressed left ventricular ejection fraction. *J Am Coll Cardiol.* 2012;60:1845-1853.
12. Mehrotra P, Jansen K, Flynn AW, et al. Differential left ventricular remodeling and longitudinal function distinguishes low flow from normal-flow preserved ejection fraction, low gradient severe aortic stenosis. *Our Heart J.* 2013;34:1906-1914.
13. Adda J, Mielot C, Giorgi R, et al. Low-flow, low gradient severe aortic stenosis despite normal ejection fraction is associated with severe left ventricular dysfunction as assessed by speckle tracking echocardiography: a multi-center study. *Circ Cardiovasc Imaging.* 2012;5:27-35.
14. Lang RM, Goldstein SA, Kronzon I, Khandheria BK, Mor-Avi V. *ASE's Comprehensive Echocardiography.* 2nd ed. Philadelphia, PA: Elsevier (Saunders); 2016:422-426.
15. Clavel MA, Ennezat PV, Marechaux A, et al. Stress echocardiography to assess stenosis severity and predict outcome in patients with paradoxical low-flow, low-gradient aortic stenosis and preserved LVEF. *J Am Coll Cardiol.* 2013;6:175-183.

16. Lang RM, Goldstein SA, Kronzon I, Khandheria BK, Mor-Avi V. *ASE's Comprehensive Echocardiography*. 2nd ed. Philadelphia, PA: Elsevier (Saunders); 2016:438-446.
17. Vukanovic-Criley JM, Criley S, Warde CM, et al. Competency in physical examination skills in medical students, trainees, physicians and faculty: a multi-center study. *Arch Intern Med.* 2006;166:601-616.
18. Fedak PW, Verma S, Davie TE, Leask RL, Weisel RD, Butty J. Clinical and pathophysiological implications of a bicuspid aortic valve. *Circulation.* 2002;106:900-904.
19. Michelena HI, Desjardins VA, Avierinos JR, et al. Natural history of asymptomatic patients with normally functioning or minimally dysfunctional bicuspid aortic valve in the community. *Circulation.* 2008;117(21):2776-2778.
20. Robard S. Blood velocity and endocarditis. *Circulation.* 1963;27:18-28.
21. Libman E, Sacks B. A hitherto undescribed form of valvular and mural endocarditis. *Arch Intern Med.* 1924;33:701-737.
22. Hojnik M, George J, Ziporen L, Shoenfeld Y. Heart Valve Involvement (Libman-Sacks Endocarditis) in the antiphospholipid syndrome. *Circulation.* 1996;93(8):1579-1587.
23. Oh JK, Seward JB, Takik AJ. *The Eho Manual.* 3rd ed. Philadelphia, PA: Wolters Kluwer/ Lippincott Williams & Wilkins; 2007:249-250.
24. Lancellotti P, Pibarot P, Chambers J, et al. Recommendations for the imaging assessment of prosthetic heart valves: a report from the European Association of Cardiovascular Imaging endorsed by the Chinese Society of Echocardiography, the Inter-American Society of Echocardiography, and the Brazilian Department of Cardiovascular Imaging. *Eur Heart J Cardiovasc Imaging.* 2016;17(6):589-590.
25. Kalarich KW, Wnriquez-Sarano M, Gura GM, et al. Papillary fibroelastoma: echocardiographic characteristics for diagnosis and pathologic correlation. *J Am Coll Cardiol.* 1997;30:784-790.
26. Lambl VA. Papillare escrescenze und der semilunar-klapple der aorta. *Wein Med Wochenschr.* 1856;16:244-250.
27. Roldan CA, Shirley BK, Crawford MH. Valve excrescences: prevalence, evolution and risk for cardioembolism. *J Am Coll Cardiol.* 1997;30(5):1308-1315.
28. Gravanis M. Personal communication.
29. Choi JY, Sullivan ID. Fixed subaortic stenosis: anatomical spectrum and nature of progression. *Br Heart J.* 1991;65:280-286.
30. Katz NM, Buckley MJ, Liberthson RR. Discrete membranous sub aortic stenosis. Report of 31 patients, review of the literature, and delineation of management. *Circulation.* 1977;56:1034-1038.
31. Braverman A. Acute aortic dissection. *Circulation.* 2010;122:184-188.
32. Loeys BL, Schwarze U, Holm T, et al. Aneurysm syndromes caused by mutations in the TGF-beta receptor. *N Engl J Med.* 2006;355(8):788-798.

5

The Right Atrium

SECTION 1

ANATOMY OF THE RIGHT ATRIUM

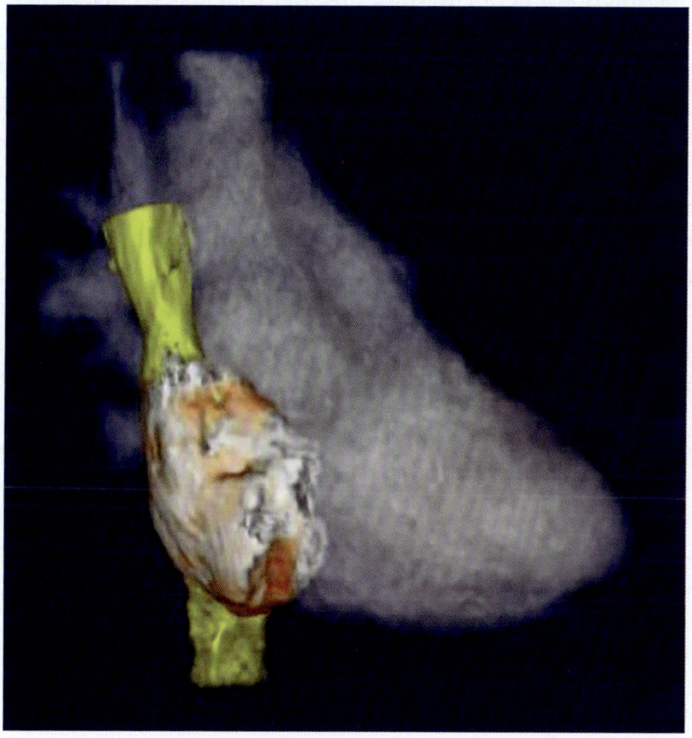

FIGURE 5.1 3D image of the right atrium processed from a computerized tomographic image.

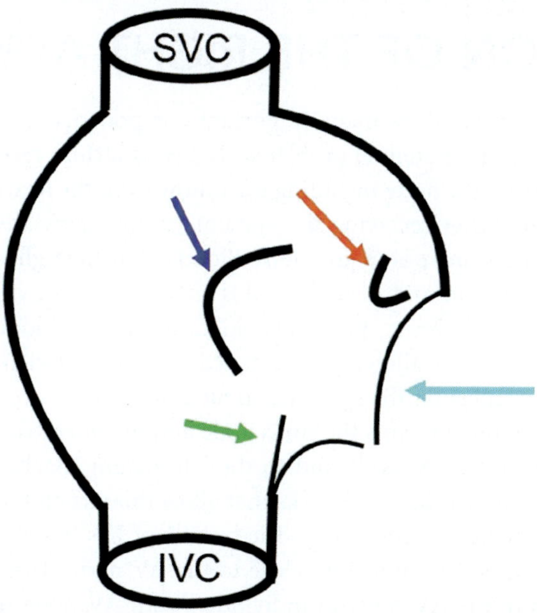

FIGURE 5.2 Stick diagram of the RA and important structures within. *Blue arrow*, fossa ovalis; *red arrow*, coronary sinus and thebesian valve; aqua arrow, tricuspid valve; *green arrow*, eustachian valve; SVC, superior vena cava; IVC, inferior vena cava.

The right atrium (RA) is the entranceway to the heart, receiving blood from the inferior and superior vena cava (SVC) and the coronary sinus. Embryologically, it is generally divided in two morphologically distinct parts. The superior-posterior portion or the sinus venous portion is relatively smooth and nontrabeculated, while the inferior-anterior portion or atrial appendage portion is trabeculated. The two areas are separated by the crista terminalis, which begins at the SVC and extends to the inferior vena cava (IVC) in a crescent-shaped fashion. The right atrial appendage is located in the trabeculated region. The sinus venous portion includes the SVC and IVC, the entrance to the RA or vestibule, and the interatrial septum. As placental blood enters the RA from the IVC, it is baffled by the eustachian valve (named after Bartolomeo Eustachi or Eustachius) toward the foramen ovale and into the systemic circulation. The eustachian valve is a residual of the right valve of the sinus venous and usually involutes during childhood. The eustachian valve sometimes persists to a variable degree in adulthood and can create confusion for imaging. After birth, the foramen generally closes, and systemic venous blood is collected in the RA and pumped toward the right ventricle in late diastole.

Sometimes, there is a prominent veil-like filamentous network in the lower aspects of the right atrium known as the Chiari network (named after Hans Chiari). It has variable attachments (in contrast to the eustachian valve) including the crista terminalis, the upper regions of the RA, the interatrial septum, the floor of the RA, and the opening of the coronary sinus. The exit of the coronary sinus is guarded by the thebesian valve (named after Adam Christian Thebesius). This thebesian valve is sometimes present and other times completely absent.[1-4]

SECTION 2

FUNCTION OF THE RIGHT ATRIUM

The right atrium contains many important components, and each has its own set of functions and potential problems. The right atrium receives all of the systemic blood from the body including the inflow from the heart itself through the coronary sinus. After receiving the systemic venous flow, the right atrium has reservoir, conduit, and pump functions. Blood enters the right atrium passively, is stored there briefly in mid-diastole, and is pumped into the right ventricle in late diastole. In the embryonic stage, IVC blood or placenta blood is baffled by way of the eustachian valve allowing oxygenated and nutrient-rich blood to cross the foramen ovale and enter the systemic circulation.

The right atrium contains the sinus node and the interatrial conduction pathways leading to the AV node and to the left atrium (Bachmann bundle). The AV node has endocardial landmarks that allow this structure to be avoided during electrophysiologic procedures. The bundle of His has characteristic electrical potentials in the right atrium close to the AV node. These landmarks allow identification of the AV node in individuals with AV node reentry tachycardia and subsequent ablation if needed. Ablation of the AV node and pacemaker is sometimes needed in individuals with uncontrolled ventricular responses to atrial fibrillation. The counterclockwise pathways of atrial flutter are located in the right atrium. Pacemakers usually have atrial attachments in the right atrial appendage. Theos of the coronary sinus is located on the floor of the right atrium. Electrophysiologists place pacemaker leads in this vessel as a portal to the lateral wall of the left ventricle that allows for bi-ventricular pacing. Accessory bundles course from the sinus node around the AV node by way of the right atrium and lead to conduction tissue beyond the AV node creating ventricular preexcitation.

In open heart procedures, the right atrium is the first area that is cannulated to withdraw venous blood for the pump oxygenator. The os of the coronary sinus offers an avenue for retrograde cardioplegia. The fossa ovalis is the portal to the left atrium for electrophysiologic and structural heart procedures via transseptal puncture. In congenital heart disease, the atrium can be used as a pathway to the pulmonary circulation when tricuspid or pulmonary atresia is present.

Inflow of blood can deliver undesirable objects, abnormal cells, tumors, or thrombi to the right atrium and subsequently to the right ventricle and the lungs. Tumors growing in the vena cava may appear in the right atrium. Primary cardiac tumors or tumors of adjacent tissues may be visible in the atrial wall. The right atrium is generally the cardiac chamber with the lowest mean pressure; therefore, internal and external pressure changes readily alter its shape and hemodynamics.[4] The abnormalities below illustrate some of these occurrences. The right atrium contains many important components, and each has its own set of functions and potential problems. The right atrium receives all of the systemic blood from the body including the inflow from the heart itself through the coronary sinus. After receiving the systemic venous flow, the right atrium has reservoir, conduit, and pump functions. Blood enters the right atrium passively, is stored there briefly in middiastole, and is pumped into the right ventricle in late diastole. In the embryonic stage, IVC blood or placenta blood is baffled by way of the eustachian valve allowing oxygenated and nutrient-rich blood to cross the foramen ovale and enter the systemic circulation.

SECTION 3

THE NORMAL RIGHT ATRIUM

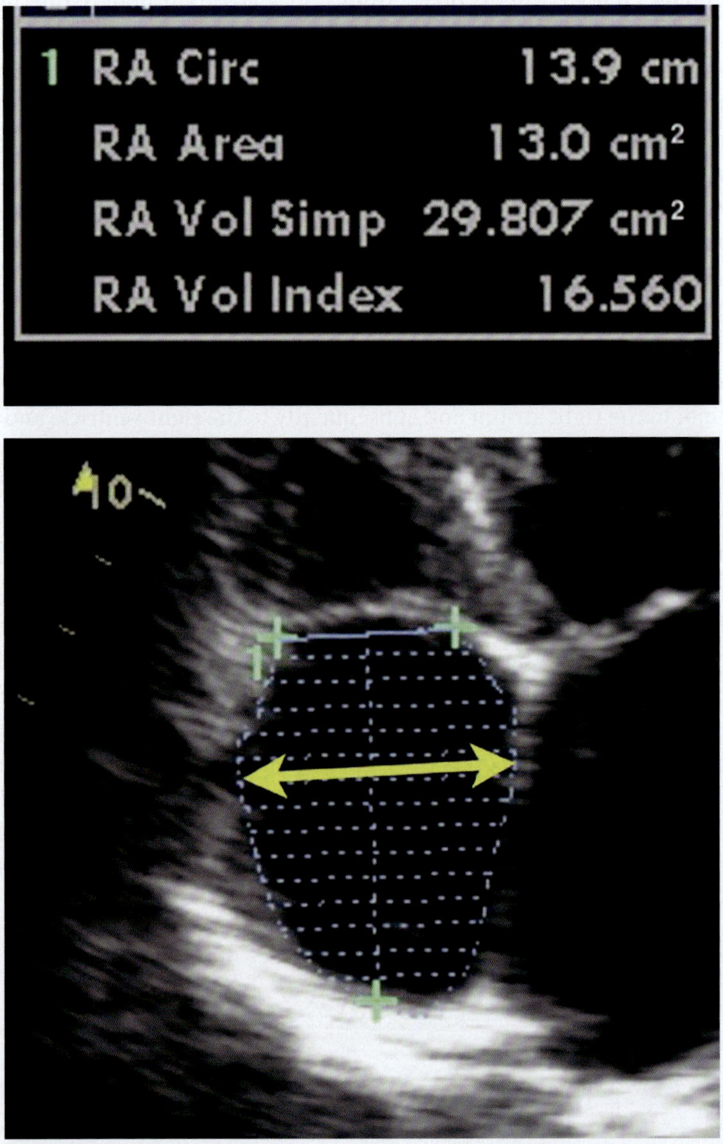

FIGURE 5.3 The normal right atrium should be measured from the apical four chamber view. The minor axis of the right atrium is measured from the interatrial sepal to lateral wall from a line that is perpendicular to the long axis of the right atrium (*yellow double headed arrow*). This dimension is parallel to the plane of the tricuspid valve annulus. The volume of the right atrium is measured by tracing the blood to atrial wall border with the base being a line across the tricuspid annulus. The disk summation technique will result in a volume. These volumes are calculated from a single plane in contrast to those calculated from the biplane left atrial calculations. Normal is different for males and females in contrast to the left atrial dimensions. Normal values for the right atrial minor axis is 1.9 ± 0.3 cm/m^2 for women and 1.9 ± 0.3 cm/m^2 for men. For the major axis normal is 2.5 ± 0.3 cm/m^2 and for women and 2.4 ± 0.3 cm/m^2 for men. Normal volume indices for males is 25 ± 7 mL/m^2 and for females is 21 ± 6 mL/m^2. Note that these values are indexed for body surface area. The above example is from a female. (From Lang RM, Badano LP, Mor-Avi V, et al. Recommendations for chamber quantification by echocardiography in adults: an update from the American Society of Echocardiography and the European Association of Cardiovascular Imaging. *J Am Soc Echocardiogr*. 2015;28:1-39.)

The normal right atrium should be measured from the apical four-chamber view. The minor axis of the right atrium is measured from the interatrial septal to lateral wall from a line that is perpendicular to the long axis of the right atrium (yellow double-headed arrow). This dimension is parallel to the plane of the tricuspid valve annulus. The volume of the right atrium is measured by tracing blood to the atrial wall border with the base being a line across the tricuspid annulus.

The disk summation technique will result in a volume. These volumes are calculated from a single plane in contrast to those calculated from the biplane left atrial calculations. Normal values are different for males and females. Normal values for the right atrial minor axis is 1.9 ± 0.3 cm/m^2 for women and 1.9 ± 0.3 cm/m^2 for men. For the major axis, normal values are 2.5 ± 0.3 cm/m^2 for women and 2.4 ± 0.3 cm/m^2 for men. Normal volume indices are 25 ± 7 mL/m^2 for males and 21 ± 6 mL/m^2 for females. Note that these values are indexed for body surface area. The above example is from a female.[5]

SECTION 4

ABNORMALITIES OF THE RIGHT ATRIUM

PATENT FORAMEN OVALE

The incidence of patent foramen ovale (PFO) in the general population has been well studied. In 1984, Hagan found in 1000 normal hearts at autopsy that the incidence was ~27%. Various estimates have been made in various settings, but they all are more or less in this range. Large defects have different implications than small defects.[6]

Embryologically, PFO occurs when the left-sided septum primum and the right-sided septum secundum do not fuse. In the region of the fossa ovalis, this leaves overlapping membranes that in certain circumstances allow venous blood, clots, air, and other right atrial contents to cross from right to left. This overlapping occurs to varying degrees resulting in a variety of anatomic configurations. If they do not completely overlap, a secundum atrial septal defect occurs. When a PFO is present, these overlapping membranes can best be visualized by transesophageal echocardiography in the ~70° view. In ordinary circumstances, this communication remains closed under the influence of slightly higher pressures on the left side. These membranes respond to competing pressures. When the right-sided pressures are elevated, the septum primum component of the PFO bulges to the left and uncouples the relationship between the membranes opening the pathway between the two chambers. The length of the pathway appears as a tunnel of variable lengths. Microbubbles injected into a peripheral vein ordinarily do not cross to the left-sided circulation. If a PFO is present, microbubbles will cross to the left side under certain circumstances. Maneuvers that transiently increase right atrial volume and pressure, such as coughing, laughing, sneezing, and deep breathing or releasing a Valsalva maneuver, increase the right atrial volume and pressure and facilitate crossing of the microbubbles from right to left. The most dreaded consequence of this physiology is the paradoxical embolism whereby an embolus in transit in the right atrium can cross the PFO in the setting of transient elevated right atrial pressure and enter the left-sided circulation. Paradoxical embolism can have various consequences in the left circulation including stroke.[7-10] Sometimes the foramen may be open from left to right when the atrium is dilated and the left atrial pressure is very high.

PFO may be an etiologic factor in the syndrome of platypnea-orthodeoxia syndrome (platypnea, shortness of breath when sitting or standing, and orthodeoxia, deoxygenation when sitting or standing) in which cyanosis may be present when assuming the upright position. The position of the heart in the chest, the diaphragm, gravity, and the state of respiration facilitate right-to-left shunting in some individuals with PFO, and closure of this defect can improve this situation.[11] Closure of PFO in the setting of cryptogenic stroke still remains a difficult issue despite a number of studies.[12-14]

In the following examples, these issues are illustrated.

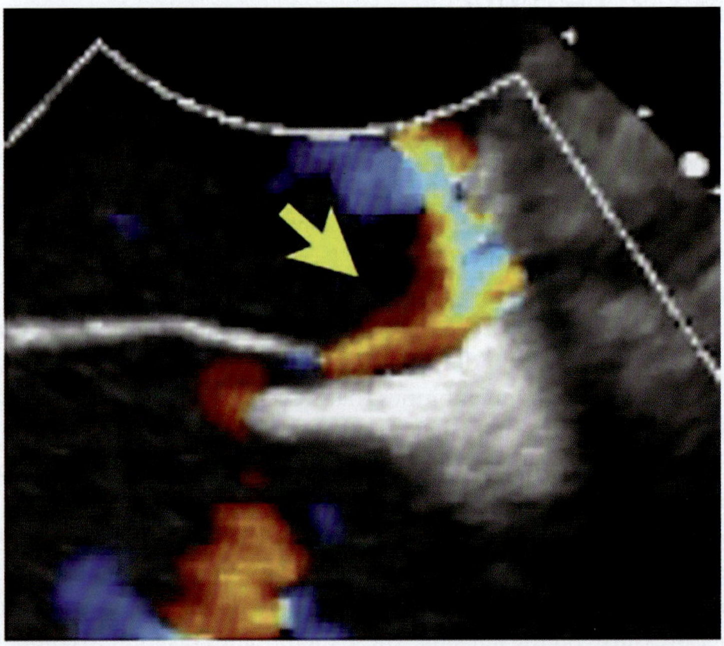

FIGURE 5.4 In this freeze frame, flow is noted as it courses from right to left (*yellow arrow*). Taken from the TEE image on the right.

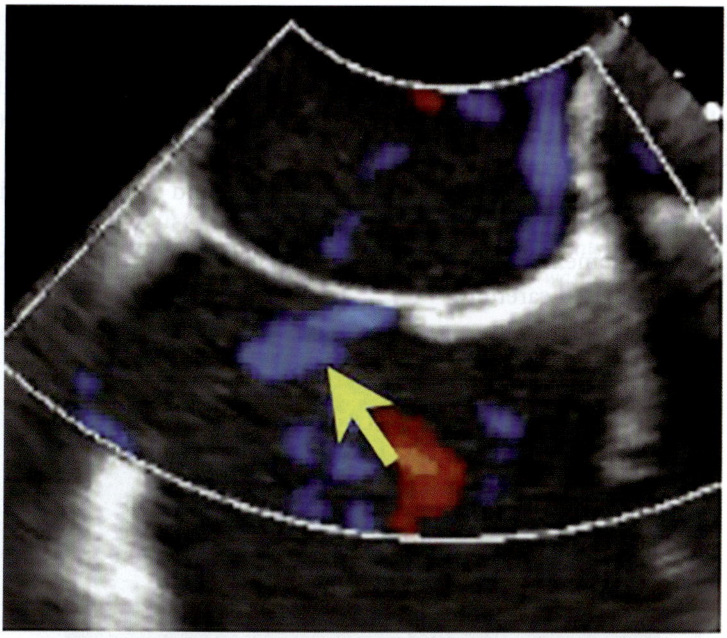

FIGURE 5.5 Another freeze frame of the TEE image on the right demonstrating flow from left to right—blue flame (*yellow arrow*).

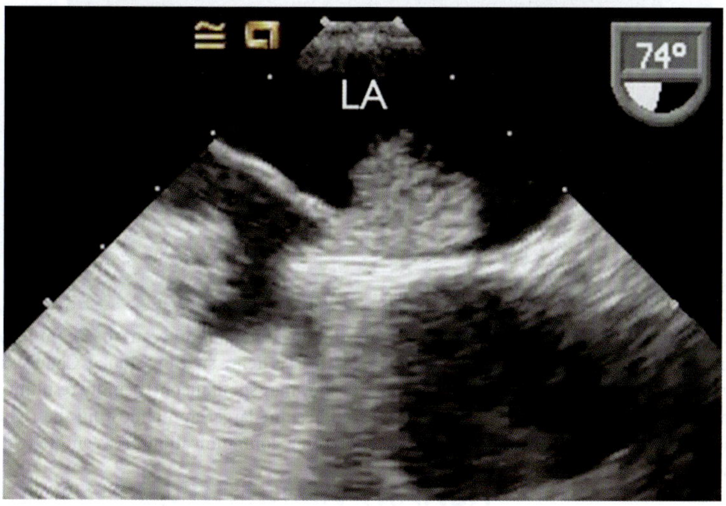

FIGURE 5.6 A larger patent foramen ovale that demonstrated more left-to-right shunting on deep inspiration. The thin interatrial septum shifts to the left and allows a bolus of microbubbles to enter the left atrium. This individual has experienced a transient ischemic attack, and this defect was closed with a percutaneous device. LA, left atrium. TEE, 74° view.

INTERATRIAL SEPTAL ANEURYSM[8]

When the interatrial septum is very thin (septum primum) it is subject to oacillation from side to side especially when left and right atrial pressures are similar. The reciprocal relationship between these two pressures facilitates this phenomenon.

right atrial pressure is high, then there is an opportunity for the thrombus to course through the PFO to the left circulation.[15,16] Examples of these problems are shown in the pages that follow.

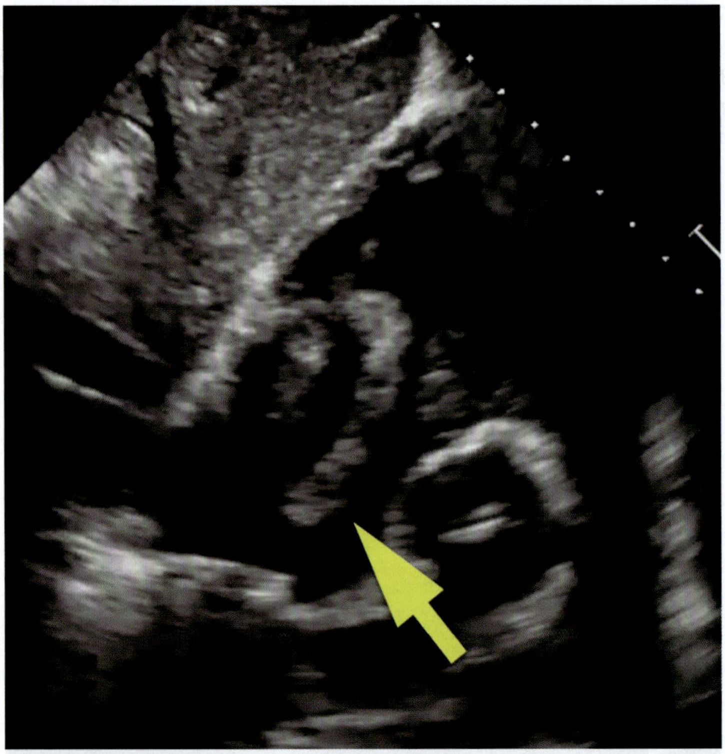

FIGURE 5.9 Serpentinelike mass in the right atrium (*yellow arrow*) associated with a dilated vena cava. Subcostal short-axis view on TEE.

RENAL CELL CARCINOMA

Tumors have various methods of metastasizing to the heart. These include lymphatic, hematogenous, contiguous, and direct extension through vessels. Renal cell carcinoma is the most noted tumor to extend directly by way of the IVC to the right atrium. A second tumor that has this capability is hepatic carcinoma. Echocardiography plays a role in making this diagnosis, but other modalities such as cardiac magnetic resonance imaging define these abnormalities in great detail.[17]

The sections that follow illustrate some of these abnormalities.

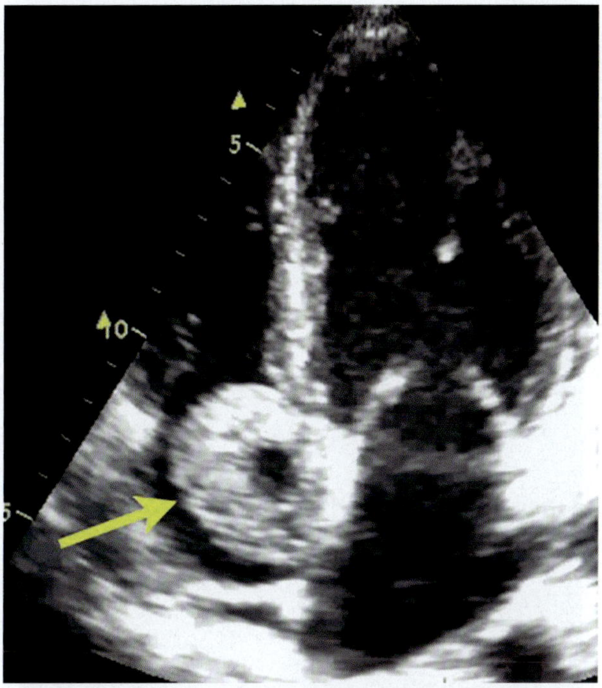

FIGURE 5.10 Right atrium filled with a rounded mass (*yellow arrow*) without a well-defined attachment. The central hypoechoic area could be vascularity or a large area of necrosis. A4C view.

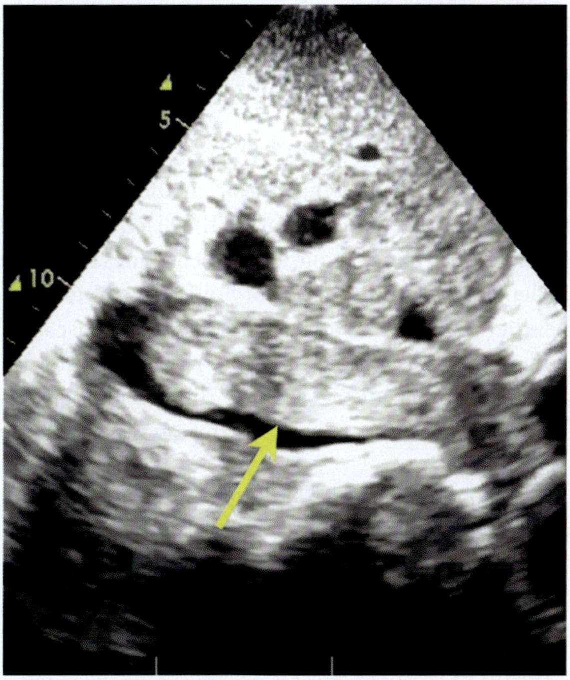

FIGURE 5.11 An important part of evaluation of a right atrial mass is to view the inferior vena cava as shown here in this patient. The cava is filled with tumor coming from below and extending into the right atrium (*yellow arrow*). This information now suggests that this is a tumor extending from below. If originating from the renal vein, it is most often renal cell carcinoma. TTE, subcostal view.

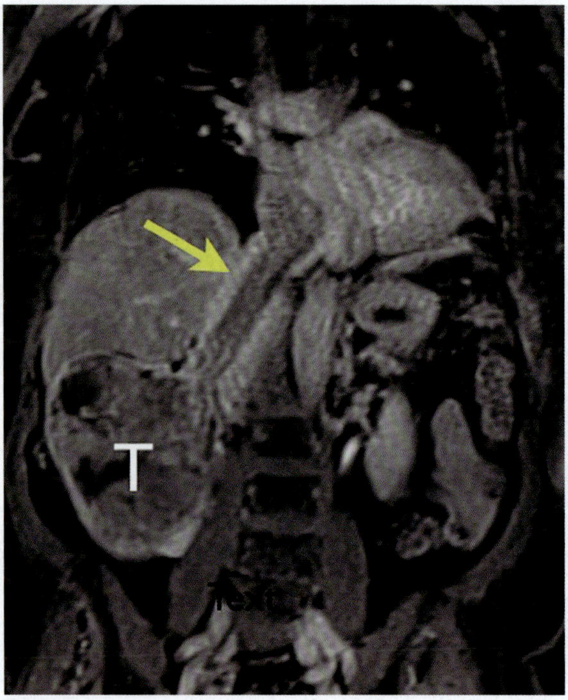

FIGURE 5.12 Right lower pole renal tumor (*T*) extending up the inferior vena cava (*yellow arrow*) to the right atrium.

MRI and Renal Cell Tumors

RIGHT ATRIAL MYXOMA

Echocardiography has played a major role in the diagnosis of atrial myxoma. From defining large symptomatic tumors to the discovery of incidental myxomas, all are much related to echocardiographic techniques. In earlier days, the clinical diagnosis depended on obstructive or embolic symptoms. Echocardiography has allowed earlier diagnosis at an earlier stage of the disease. Other techniques such as cardiac magnetic resonance and computerized tomographic imaging also take credit for discovery of these tumors incidentally. On occasion, a “tumor blush” will appear on a coronary arteriogram that is a clue to a myxoma being present.[18,19]

Myxomas not only obstruct and embolize but also can be associated with systemic symptoms such as fever and serologic abnormalities that offer clues to the underlying diagnosis of myxoma.[20,21]

CASE PRESENTATION

A 45-year-old gentleman who had a cough, had dyspnea on exertion, and had been treated with antibiotics several times in the past few weeks. In the emergency room, he was screened with a chest CT with contrast that showed a right atrial mass.

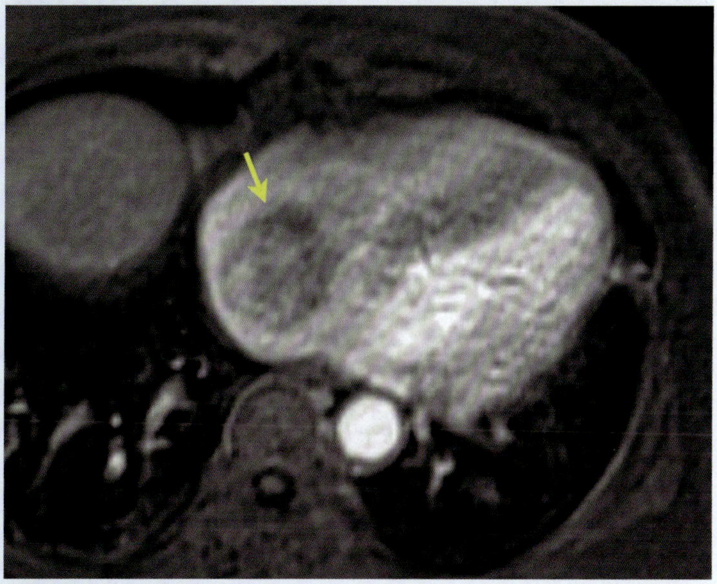

FIGURE 5.13 This individual had presented to the emergency room with generalized weakness, fever, and cough. This illness has been present for a few weeks. In addition, he was discovered to have mild anemia. A CT scan was ordered to evaluate for pulmonary emboli since he had just been on a long airplane ride. The images revealed a rounded mass in the right atrium (*yellow arrow*), and right atrial myxoma was suspected. The echo on the next panel belongs to this individual. Intracardiac masses are now discovered on CT scans with contrast ordered for various reasons such as pulmonary emboli and pulmonary infiltrates and even occasionally for spine or abdominal abnormalities. The surgical specimen from this patient is shown on the right.

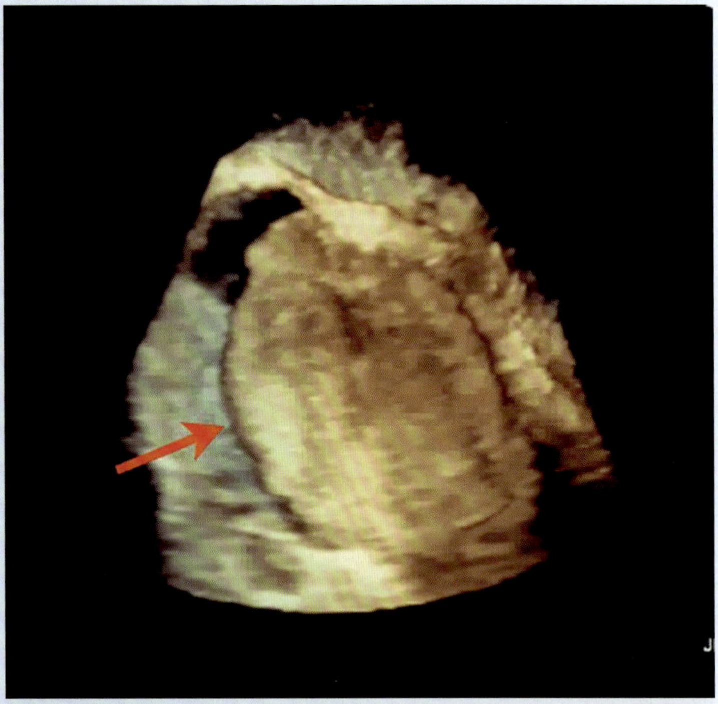

FIGURE 5.14 Three-dimensional views showing the myxoma (*red arrow*) pulling at the interatrial septum. The typical origin of a myxoma on the inferior limbus of the fossa ovalis. 3D live, 0°.

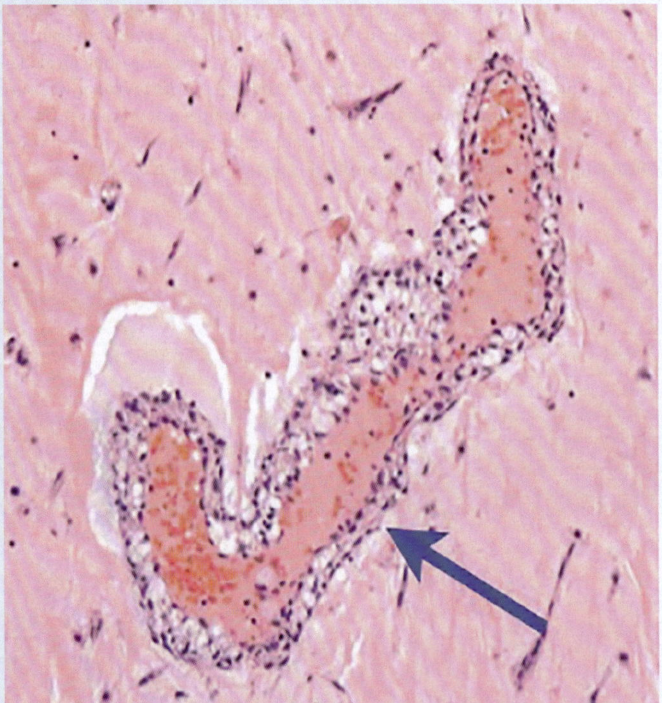

FIGURE 5.15 Myxoma cells (*blue arrow*) gathered about a vessel in a typical perivascular location.

EXTRINSIC COMPRESSION OF THE RIGHT ATRIUM

The right atrium is the chamber with the lowest pressure and therefore is the most vulnerable to compression by extrinsic forces. This can range from pericardial fluid under pressure to tumors in the adjacent areas or even a large hiatal hernia. The right atrium is one of the sentinel areas when cardiac tamponade is being considered. Pericardial pressure can increase to the point of compressing the right atrium, a sign of early tamponade. Extrinsic organs to masses can compress the right atrium and be confused for an intracardiac mass or clot. An example of this is discussed below in a postoperative individual who has a large pericardial clot. Blood accumulates in the pathway of least resistance, which can be the space surrounding the right atrium. A hiatal hernia may mimic an intracardiac mass by compression in the area of the right atrium. This can be clarified by a sip of soda or observation of peristalsis of boluses of air. Solid tumors in the area can also compress the right atrium.

Illustrations of those issues follow.

Hiatal Hernia Compressing the Right Atrium

Historically, this individual has a history of a large hiatal hernia, which is demonstrated on the left on plain chest x-ray and on the MRI noted above. At the time of the reading of the echocardiogram, this was not known, and in an individual with a history of ovarian cancer who was undergoing chemotherapy, this report caused alarm. Further investigation into the history revealed the history of the hiatal hernia, and the correct diagnosis was made. Sometimes, when reading echoes, one has to pursue history that is not given on the request in order to give an accurate diagnosis. Additionally, during echo, if such a finding is encountered, a carbonated drink can be given and will cause this area to become very echogenic and thus identifies this structure as esophagus.

6

The Tricuspid Valve

SECTION 1

THE TRICUSPID VALVE AT THE BEDSIDE AND THE ECHOCARDIOGRAPHY AND CARDIAC CATHETERIZATION LABS

Of the four valves, the tricuspid valve may produce the most visible signs of dysfunction. Manifestations of dysfunction of the tricuspid are visible from the head to the ankles. Individuals with severe tricuspid regurgitation sometimes have visible pulsatile veins on their forehead, systolic propulsion of the eyeballs, moving earlobes, distended external jugular veins, pulsating internal jugular veins, ascites, and peripheral edema.

A careful look at the patient at 30° elevation is revealing and can suggest the presence of severe tricuspid regurgitation. A search for the other signs follow, and the echocardiogram then can be used to define, quantitate, and explore etiologies.

In the cardiac cath laboratory, transducers from femoral sheaths demonstrate large systolic valves, and the pulse wave tracings in the right atrium show similar configurations as are found in the right ventricle.

In the echocardiography laboratory, the right atrium is filled with color on Doppler tracings, the inferior vena cava and hepatic veins are full and have flow reversal, and various abnormalities of the valve are visualized. The right ventricle dilates and takes away the interventricular septum from the left and has a configurational change from triangular to rounded. As the right ventricle dilates, the tricuspid annulus dilates in a direction opposite to the interventricular septum, and the tricuspid valve line of coaptation is pulled apart and tricuspid regurgitation of various degrees follows.

SECTION 2

ANATOMY OF THE TRICUSPID VALVE

The tricuspid valve consists of anterior, posterior, septal leaflets and the tricuspid annulus. The right ventricle supports the papillary muscles and the chordal structures. The atrium also supports the annulus. The annulus of the tricuspid valve is nonplanar with two high points: one in the anterior septal region and the other on the opposite side of the annulus. Viewed from above the plane of the annulus, it is elliptical in shape. It is subject to being dilated by various conditions. The interventricular component does not dilate since it abuts the ventricular septum, so the remainder of the circumference of the annulus dilates in response to such conditions as volume and pressure overload of the right ventricle.

The anterior and posterior leaflets of the tricuspid valve are opposed, and the septal leaflet coapts with a portion of each of them creating three commissures. The anterior leaflet is the largest of the three, the posterior leaflet the smallest, and the septal leaflet in between in size. The posterior leaflet sometimes has scallops. The septal leaflet is the most variable in size. There are generally three papillary muscle groups with the anterior that is the largest. The anterior papillary muscle has its origin in the region of the moderator band. The anterior papillary muscle sends chords to the anterior and posterior leaflets and the posterior papillary muscle sends chords to the posterior and septal leaflets. The septal papillary muscles may be just chordae that course from the interventricular septum to the septal leaflet, and sometimes a few of these connect to the anterior leaflet.[1-3]

Abnormal function of the tricuspid valve results from various conditions such as the annulus becoming dilated (the most common cause), inflammatory and infectious processes, mechanical influences by pacer and defibrillator leads, and congenital abnormalities.

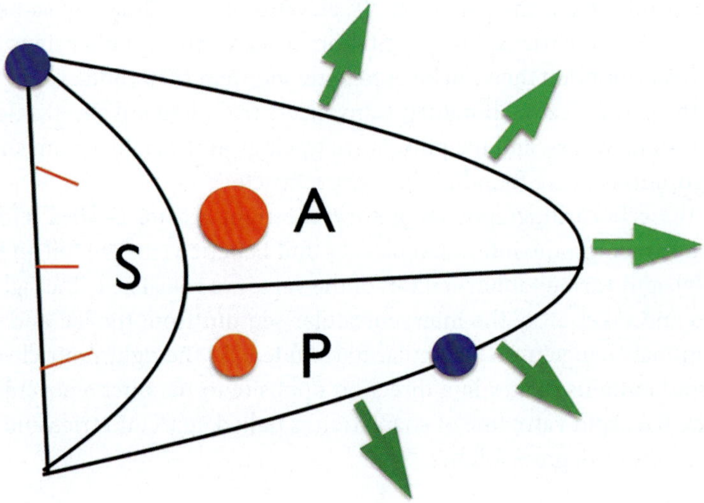

FIGURE 6.1 Stick diagram of the tricuspid valve. A, anterior; P, posterior; S, septal.

The tricuspid valve is depicted in Figure 6.1. The anterior leaflet is quite variable. Papillary muscles to the anterior leaflet (larger red circle) arise from the moderator band, and their chordal structures extend to the anterior leaflet and septal leaflet (large red circle). The smaller posterior papillary muscle (smaller red circle) sends chordal structures to the posterior leaflet and the septal leaflet. The septal leaflet has chords (red lines) that arise from the septum itself and usually do not have muscle attached.

Usually on 2D echocardiography, all three leaflets cannot be visualized simultaneously because of the nonplanar configuration. The anterior leaflet is the most obvious from the mitral inflow view and the apical four-chamber view. Next, the septal leaflet can be visualized with the anterior leaflet in the easily obtained RV inflow view. The posterior leaflet is the most elusive but can be visualized from the RV inflow view with a more posterior angulation. On live 3D echocardiography all three of the tricuspid leaflets can frequently be visualized simultaneously. As with the mitral valve annulus, there is a saddle shape to the tricuspid annulus with high points at the aorta and an opposite position on the other side of the annulus (blue circles). Low points are on the opposite poles. When the tricuspid annulus dilates, it can only do so laterally (green arrows). The septal region does not expand.

In the apical four-chamber view the tricuspid annulus measures 28 ± 5 mm in diastole and a significantly dilated tricuspid annulus is >35 mm. A systolic diameter of >3.2 cm and a diastolic annular diameter of >3.4 cm are markers of significant TR. Physiologically, the tricuspid annulus may decrease its annular area by 25%, so this is a dynamic structure. Surgeons take into account the size of the tricuspid annulus when performing mitral surgery and in deciding which type of surgical procedure might be most appropriate.[4]

SECTION 3

THE NORMAL TRICUSPID VALVE

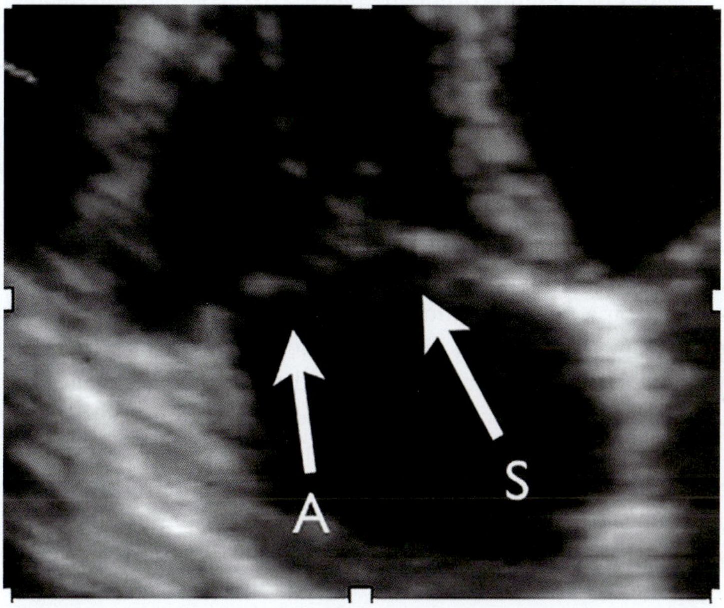

FIGURE 6.2 Freeze frame of the image on the left. A, anterior; S, septal.

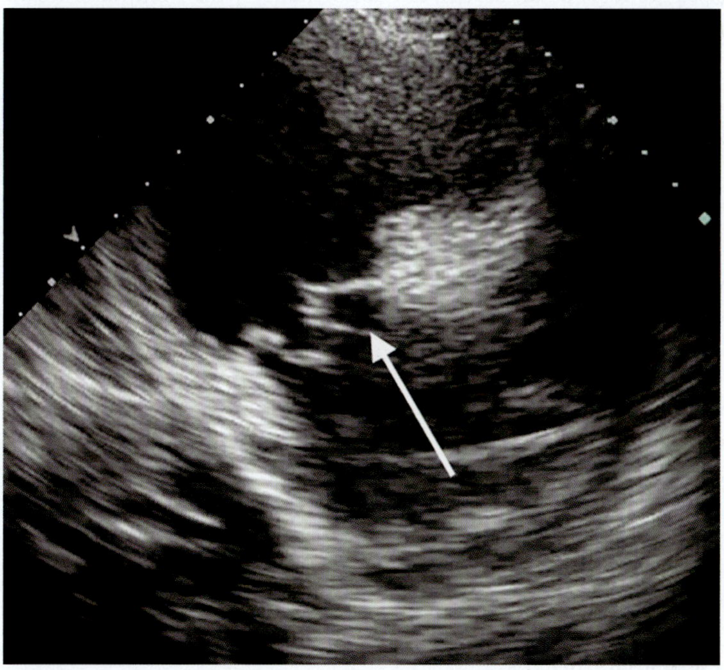

FIGURE 6.3 Freeze frame of the image on the left.

ABNORMALITIES OF THE TRICUSPID VALVE

The most common etiology of tricuspid valve abnormalities that result in tricuspid regurgitation is a secondary cause. When the right ventricle dilates in response to a pressure and/or a volume overload, then the tricuspid annulus dilates in a lateral fashion (see stick diagram) since the septal portion of the annulus cannot dilate. This may be in response to abnormalities in the pulmonary vasculature from pulmonary vascular disease or something else such as pulmonary embolus. In addition, as the left-sided structures develop abnormalities, they reflect back to the right side. For example as mitral stenosis worsens the right sided pressures elevate and the right ventricle dilates resulting in the tricuspid valve failing. Infective endocarditis is always a threat to the tricuspid valve especially in the setting of IV drug use or in the presence of foreign bodies such as central lines and pacemaker leads. The list is long of conditions that can result in tricuspid regurgitation.

The tricuspid valve leaflets are vulnerable to various abnormalities that range from rheumatic inflammatory changes and myxomatous changes to trauma or even compromise from a cardiac tumor. Humoral substances that arise from the GI tract may result in scarred, retracted leaflets as seen in the carcinoid syndrome or from systemic-taken diet drugs. Pacemaker leads can prop the valve leaflets open, or adhesions may develop that scar the leaflets to the point of causing functional abnormality. Trauma can rupture a leaflet or chord and result in severe regurgitation.

There is a long list of abnormalities that cause tricuspid regurgitation and a shorter list that cause tricuspid valve stenosis. Rheumatic disease can produce tricuspid stenosis as an associated abnormality with rheumatic mitral stenosis. See Table 6.1.

TABLE 6.1 ABNORMALITIES OF THE TRICUSPID VALVE

Tricuspid Regurgitation

- Enlarged right ventricle
- Infective endocarditis
- Myxomatous degeneration
- Marfan syndrome
- Carcinoid syndrome
- Pacemaker leads and adhesions
- Myocardial biopsy
- Trauma
- Radiation
- Diet drugs
- Congenital
  - Ebstein anomaly
  - Tricuspid atresia
  - A-V canal abnormalities

(Continued)

TABLE 6.1 ABNORMALITIES OF THE TRICUSPID VALVE (*Continued*)

Tricuspid Stenosis

- Rheumatic disease
- Carcinoid syndrome
- Infective endocarditis
- Valvulitis (lupus)
- Benign and malignant tumors
- Pacemaker leads and adhesions
- Congenital

SECTION 4

FLAIL ANTERIOR LEAFLET OF THE TRICUSPID VALVE DUE TO TRAUMA

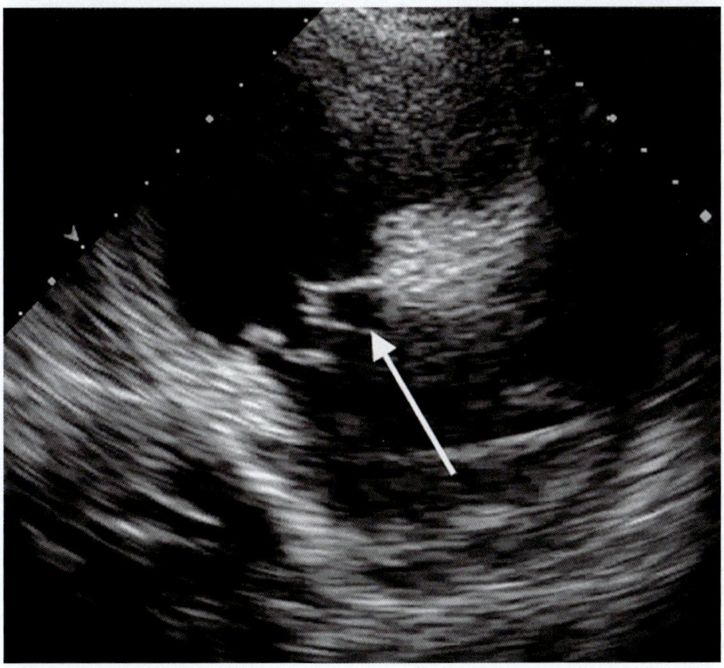

FIGURE 6.4 Two leaflets of the tricuspid valve are visible in this RV inflow view. The anterior leaflet and the septal leaflet. The anterior leaflet is flail as is the septal leaflet (*white arrow*). Identificaton of these leaflets can be difficult since slight variation in transducer position can identify either the anterior or posterior leaflet. Neither leaflet coapts properly and prolapses into the right atrium in systole. TTE RV inflow view.

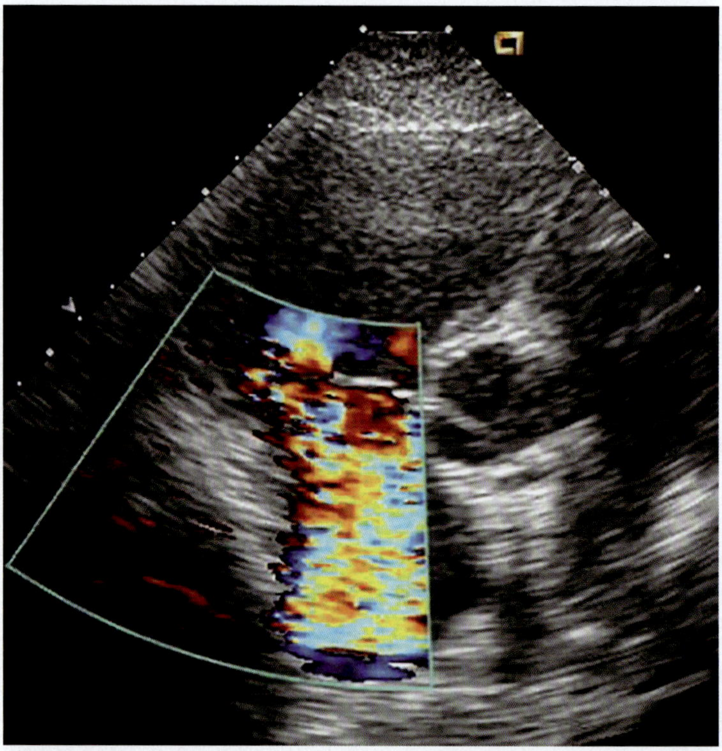

FIGURE 6.5 High cross-sectional view of the RA and RV with color Doppler showing severe tricuspid regurgitation.

The tricuspid valve unlike the mitral valve does not lend itself to repair. The lines of coaptation are complex, and each leaflet has more complex papillary muscle relationships, or in the case of the septal leaflet, there are often no papillary muscle attachments. The chords of the septal leaflet often connect directly to the interventricular septum. In this individual with flail anterior and septal leaflets, the valve was replaced.

SECTION 5

CARCINOID SYNDROME AND CARCINOID HEART DISEASE

Carcinoid syndrome is a rare syndrome produced by a neuroendocrine tumor usually located in the small intestine or colon. Embryologically, these tumors can have their origin in other areas; however, the lower intestine is the most common location. They have endocrine activity in that they secrete substances that are vasoactive, the most common one being serotonin. In individuals with this syndrome, symptoms include sensations of flushing, diarrhea, and bronchospasm. Plasma levels of serotonin are high, and the metabolic end product 5-hydroxyeidoleacteic acid (5-HIAA) is high in the urine, a marker of the disease.

High levels of serotonin are associated with carcinoid heart disease and usually mean that hepatic metastasis is present, releasing the vasoactive substances into the systemic circulation. Exposure of the heart to these substances results in plaquelike areas of endocardial thickening on the tricuspid and pulmonic valve surfaces resulting in scarring, retraction, function regurgitation, and stenosis. Left-to-right shunting or pulmonary metastasis can result in left-sided lesions in the heart.[5,6]

Currently, improvements in treatment modalities have allowed improved survival, and on occasion, the tricuspid and pulmonic valves have been replaced.

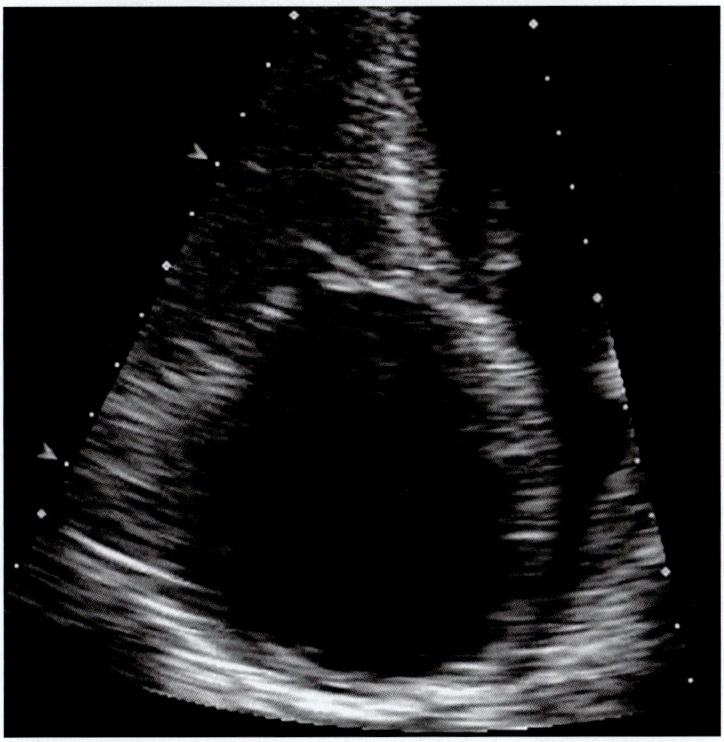

FIGURE 6.6 Relatively fixed tricuspid leaflets, a characteristic finding in carcinoid involvement of the tricuspid valve. The septal and anterior leaflets are visualized. TTE, A4C view.

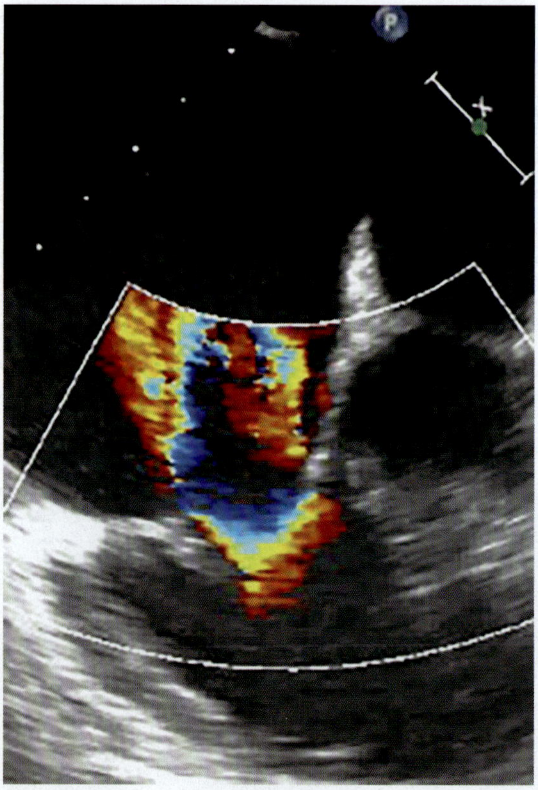

FIGURE 6.7 A very dilated right atrium and severe tricuspid regurgitation. PISA appearing with diastolic flow across the valve and with the tricuspid regurgitation. TEE, 32° view.

SECTION 6

CONTINUOUS WAVE DOPPLER AND SEVERE TRICUSPID REGURGITATION

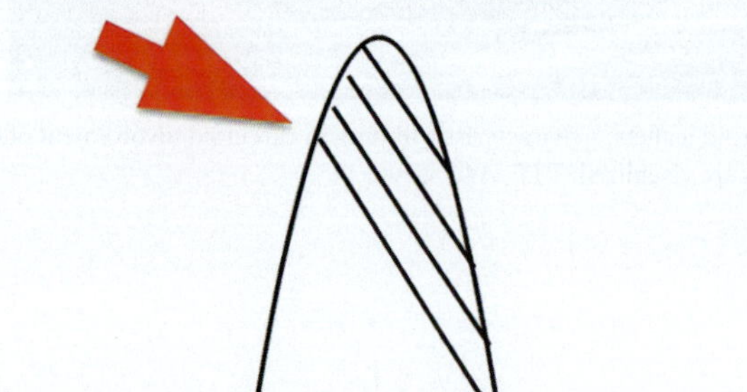

FIGURE 6.8 In the setting of severe tricuspid regurgitation, the velocity profile reaches a peak quickly and falls precipitously as if it has been cutoff (*red arrow*).[7,8]

SECTION 7

THE "CUTOFF SIGN" OF SEVERE TRICUSPID REGURGITATION

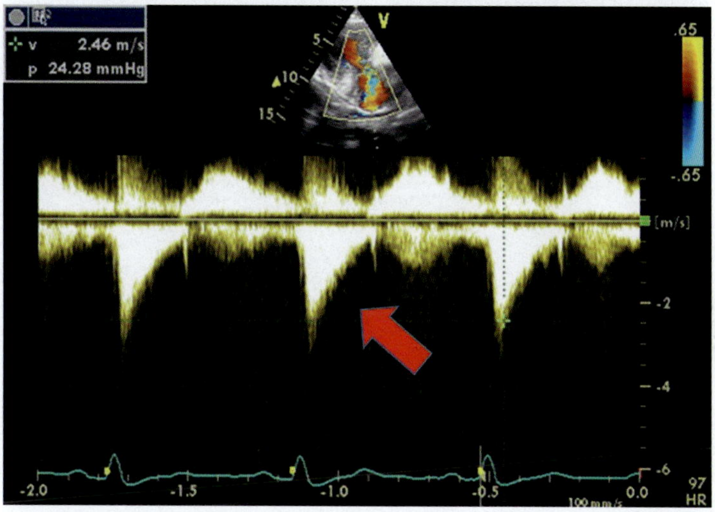

FIGURE 6.9 Continuous wave Doppler showing a relatively low peak velocity of tricuspid regurgitation and more importantly a rapidly decreasing velocity profile consistent with severe regurgitation. The velocity profile of the CW tracing appears to have been "cut off" after reaching a peak (*red arrow*). This is a sign of severe regurgitation of velocity profiles in general. Sometimes this gives one the false impression of right ventricular pressures being lower than they are in reality. The right atrial pressure is often higher than 15 mm Hg in these cases.

SECTION 8

MYXOMATOUS DEGENERATION OF THE TRICUSPID VALVE WITH TRICUSPID VALVE PROLAPSE

In the setting of severe myxomatous changes of the mitral valve, one should investigate for similar changes in the tricuspid valve. This is the case in the following example. Both valves have severe myxomatous change with billowing and prolapse of the leaflets and various degrees of regurgitation.

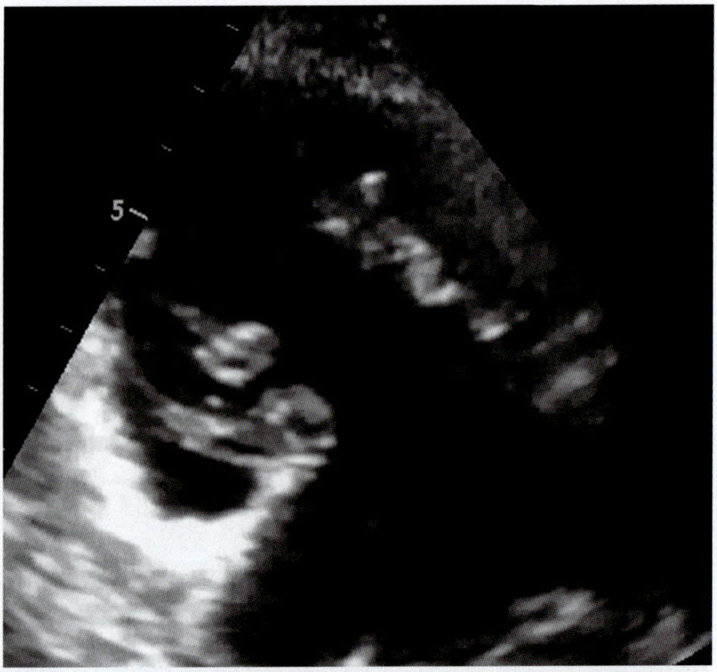

FIGURE 6.10 In this RV inflow view of the tricuspid valve, the anterior and septal leaflets open in diastole before prolapsing in systole well into the right atrium. TTE, RV inflow view.

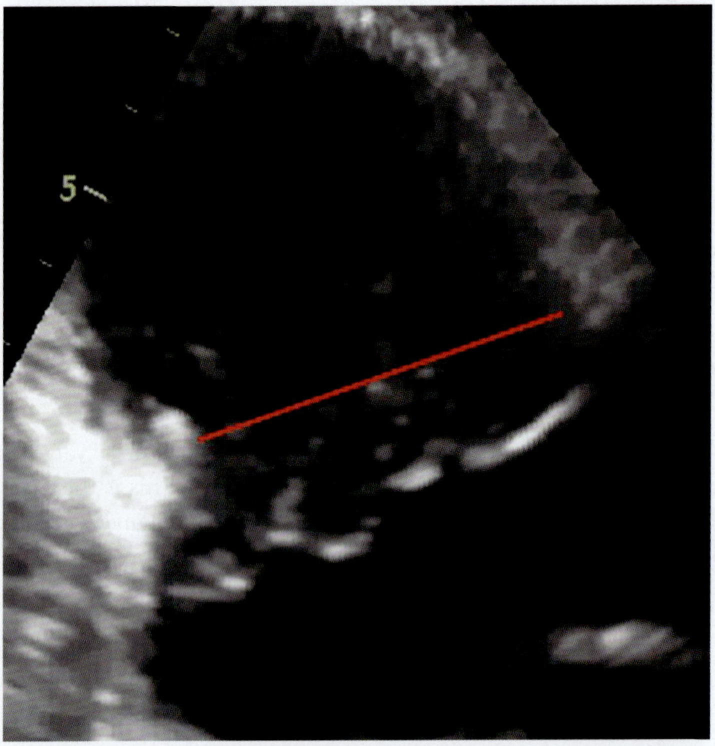

FIGURE 6.11 RV inflow view in systole demonstrating myxomatous leaflets prolapsing well above the plane of the tricuspid annulus (*red line*). TTE, RV inflow view.

SECTION 9

TRICUSPID VALVE/PACEMAKER LEAD ENDOCARDITIS

Tricuspid valve endocarditis is a severe complication in the setting of intravenous drug use. The tricuspid valve is the first to be exposed to bacteria from unsterile techniques and needles. Once this valve becomes infected, destruction follows with rupture of the valve apparatus, perforation, and embolization to the lungs. Valve replacement is often needed only to be followed on occasion by infection of the prosthetic valve.[9]

When pacemaker leads become infected, they may be associated with infection of the tricuspid valve since they are in contact with the valve. Removal of the pacemaker lead can be challenging since vegetations and thrombi are stripped from the lead as it is withdrawn. In addition, the lead may have become attached to the tricuspid apparatus, and it can be damaged also as the lead is withdrawn.

Examples of these infections are illustrated in the following pages.

PACEMAKER LEAD ENDOCARDITIS ADJACENT TO THE TRICUSPID VALVE

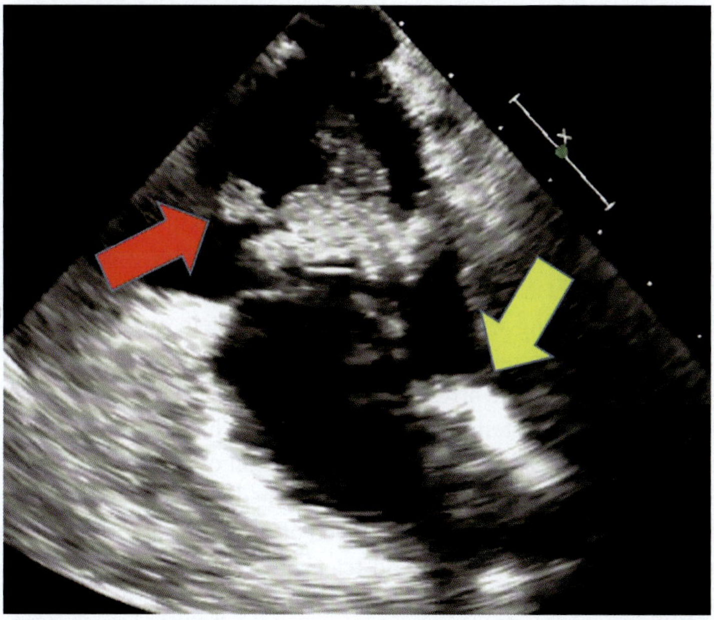

FIGURE 6.12 Very large vegetations (*red arrow*) as seen in fungal endocarditis that are associated with the defibrillator lead (*yellow arrow*); from this view, one has to assume that the tricuspid valve leaflets are also involved. As it turned out, this was not the case. TEE, 0° view.

SECTION 10

EBSTEIN ANOMALY OF THE TRICUSPID VALVE

In 1866, Wilhelm Ebstein described this anomaly of the tricuspid valve. It is currently one of the most well-known congenital heart abnormalities and bears the name of Wilhelm Epstein. In this abnormality the anterior tricuspid leaflet is very large, downwardly displaced and tethered by chordal structures to the wall of the right ventricle. In addition, the valve has a much lower origin in the ventricle and not the tricuspid annulus itself. Normally, the tricuspid valve has a slightly lower origin relative to that of the mitral valve. In Ebstein's, the attachment is much lower within the right ventricle—an index value of 8 mm/m^2 below the annulus of the mitral valve as measured in the apical four-chamber view allows one to make the diagnosis of Ebstein anomaly.

Not only does this abnormality result in hemodynamic abnormality, but arrhythmias are always a consideration. Various supraventricular tachycardias can be present along with accessory pathways. Atrial fibrillation is always a threat in the setting or ventricular preexcitation. Very rapid ventricular rates can result in collapse. This is a prime indication for electrophysiologic intervention. In addition, various other congenital abnormalities are associated with Ebstein's such as atrial septal defect.

Abnormal tethering of the anterior tricuspid valve leaflet does not allow coaptation, and varying degrees of tricuspid regurgitation follow. A lower attachment of the leaflets makes for a region of the ventricle that becomes atrialized and has electrical characteristics of the ventricle yet is part of the atrium. This arrangement allowed for the diagnosis of Ebsten's to be made by comparing hemodynamic tracings to electrical signals. An electrical signal that had the characteristics of a ventricular tracing and a hemodynamic tracing that appeared to come from the atrium made the diagnosis of a displaced tricuspid valve.

The dilated right atrium and large right ventricle result in a characteristic electrocardiogram. Along with tricuspid atresia, Ebstein anomaly has the tallest P waves of all. Those found in Ebstein anomaly are only equaled by the Himalayan P waves seen in tricuspid atresia.

Additionally in Ebstein's, the QRS complexes have a peculiar RBBB pattern, described as being "splintered." The combination of very large P waves plus low-voltage "splintered" QRS complexes makes the diagnosis.

Echocardiography eliminated the need of such efforts, and simply imaging the relative positions of the mitral and tricuspid valves makes the diagnosis at the present time along with assessment of RV function and the degree of associated tricuspid regurgitation.[10]

Examples of Ebstein anomaly of the tricuspid valve follow.

EBSTEIN ANOMALY OF THE TRICUSPID VALVE (ELECTROCARDIOGRAM)

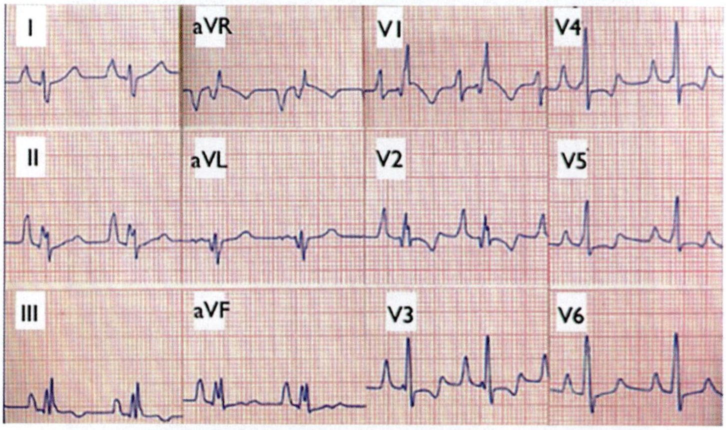

FIGURE 6.13 Large P waves especially in lead II and unusual right bundle-branch block exhibiting a bizarre "splintered" configuration in the precordial leads.

Ebstein anomaly of the tricuspid valve consists of a downward displacement and hypoplasia of the septal leaflet of the tricuspid valve, hypoplasia of the posterior leaflet, and a very large prominent fenestrated anterior leaflet that has various degrees of tethering. This large leaflet may be very mobile and flail open and closed. Sometimes, when it closes, it causes a loud sound that is called a "sail" sound. The degree of downward displacement, the fenestrations, and the degree of tethering of the large leaflet are related to its insufficiency and the degree of tricuspid regurgitation. Downward displacement into the right ventricle of the septal leaflet of the tricuspid valve relative to the mitral annulus of 8 mm/m^2 or greater defines this anomaly. A portion of the ventricle by virtue of the tricuspid valve being downwardly displaced becomes "atrialized." Often, the tricuspid regurgitation is severe and results in a very large right atrium and very large P waves on ECG.

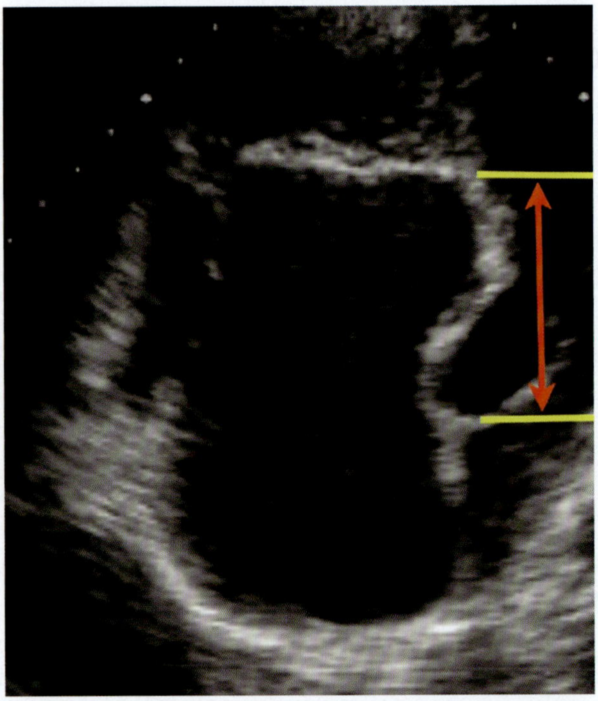

FIGURE 6.14 In Ebstein anomaly, one of the criteria for diagnosis especially in milder cases is that the distance from the mitral to the tricuspid valve insertions into the septum in the A4C view is 0.8 cm/m^2 or greater. In this example, the total distance is 4.8 cm, so those criteria are far exceeded. The *yellow lines* indicate the tricuspid leaflet insertion and the mitral leaflet insertion with the *red arrow* indicating the distance between.

REFERENCES

1. Rogers JH, Bolling SF. Contemporary reviews in cardiovascular medicine, the tricuspid valve. Current perspective and evolving management of tricuspid regurgitation. *Circulation.* 2009;119:2718-2725.
2. Fukuda S, Saracino G, Matsumura Y, et al. Three-dimensional geometry of the tricuspid annulus in healthy subjects and in patients with functional tricuspid regurgitation: a real-time, 3-dimensional echocardiographic study. *Circulation.* 2006;114(1 suppl):1492-1498.
3. Anwar AM, Gelijnde ML, Soliman OI, et al. Assessment of normal tricuspid valve anatomy in adults by real-time three-dimensional echocardiography. *Int J Cardiovasc Imaging.* 2007;23(6):717-724.
4. Lancellotti P, Moura L, Pierand LA, et al. European Association of Echocardiography recommendation for the assessment of valvular regurgitation. Part 2: mitral and tricuspid regurgitation (native valve disease). *Eur Heart J Cardiovasc Imaging.* 2010;11(4):307-332.
5. Kulke MH, Mayer RJ. Carcinoid tumors. *N Engl J Med.* 1999;340(11):858-868.
6. Anderson AS, Krauss D, Lang R. Cardiovascular complications of malignant carcinoid disease. *Am Heart J.* 1997;134(4):693-704.
7. Geode JB, Scantlebury DC, Thomas JD, Nishimura RA. Hemodynamic evaluation of severe tricuspid regurgitation. *J Am Coll Cardiol.* 2013;62(20):e441-e441.

8. Firstenberg MS, Vandervoort PM, Greenberg NL, et al. Noninvasive estimation of transmittal pressure drop across the normal mitral valve in humans: importance of convective and inertial forces during left ventricular filling. *J Am Coll Cardiol.* 2000;36:1942-1949.
9. Byrne JG, Rezia K, Sanchez JA, et al. Surgical management of endocarditis: the society of thoracic surgeons clinical practice guideline. *Ann Thorac Surg.* 2011;91:2012-2019.
10. Jost CHA, Connolly HM, Detrain JA, Edwards WD, Danielson GK. Ebstein's anomaly. *Circulation.* 2007;115:277-285.

7

The Right Ventricle

SECTION 1

ANATOMY OF THE RIGHT VENTRICLE

The right ventricle is located anterior to and wraps around the left ventricle. The entrance to the right ventricle is defined by the tricuspid annulus and the tricuspid valve leaflets. The exit is the right ventricular outflow tract and the pulmonary valve. In cross-sectional views, it has a crescent shape. In the apical four-chamber view of the echocardiogram, the right ventricle has a triangular shape. Anatomically from the anterior view with the free wall is removed, it resembles a check mark with the tricuspid valve at the entrance and the pulmonary valve at the exit. When the heart is viewed on chest x-ray, the right margin of the heart forms an acute angle with the diaphragm resulting in this region being called the acute margin of the heart. The acute marginal branches of the right coronary artery lie in this anatomic area. In contrast to the prolate ellipse shape of the left ventricle, the overall shape of the right ventricle defies traditional geometry.

In general, the right ventricle can be divided into three anatomic regions: the inlet, apical, and outlet regions. The inlet region consists of the tricuspid valve and its apparatus. The apical region of the right ventricle has several heavy trabeculations including the apically located moderator band and the septomarginal band. These prominent trabeculations are thick and distinguish the right ventricle from the less trabeculated left ventricle. The third region or outflow region is less trabeculated and leads to the pulmonary valve. From the frontal view, the outflow region of the right ventricle crosses the midline and situates itself to the left of the left ventricular outflow tract. This results in the left and right circulations crossing each other in the frontal plane—a feature that is not present in some congenital abnormalities such as transposition of the great arteries.

The interventricular septum is a part of all three regions of the right ventricle. It supports the apical region, the tricuspid valve apparatus, and the outlet region. It gives rise to papillary muscles and trabeculations and supports the outlet region. The interventricular septum is muscular except for the membranous portion of the septum. The membranous septum usually gives rise to the septal leaflet of the tricuspid valve. The upper regions of the interventricular septum support the pulmonary valve. The left side of the septum relates to the right cusp area of the aortic valve.

The right ventricle has two layers of myocardium in contrast to the left, which has three. The thin-walled right ventricle has an outer, subepicardial circumferential layer and an inner subendocardial longitudinal layer. The shape of the right ventricle and the muscle fiber arrangement make remodeling a challenge. These factors are especially important in clinical situations such as pulmonary hypertension and transposition of the great vessels in which the right ventricle faces pressures that can be in the systemic range.

The blood supply of the right ventricle consists of a conus branch, acute marginal branches, and, to a small degree, the posterior descending. The conus branch supplies the right ventricular outflow tract area and may continue and supply some of the interventricular septum. The acute marginal branches supply the free wall of the right ventricle. The posterior descending coronary artery supplies the surface of the right ventricle close to the interventricular groove. A proximal occlusion of the right coronary artery before the conus branch and the acute marginal branches can result in the serious right ventricular infarction syndrome in which there are high central venous pressures and low cardiac output.[1]

LINEAR MEASUREMENTS OF THE NORMAL RIGHT VENTRICLE

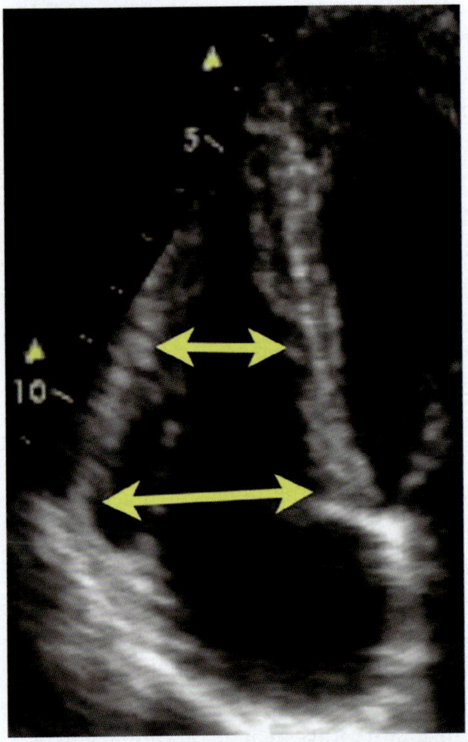

FIGURE 7.1 In general, the measurements for the right ventricular size are taken from the A4C view with the left ventricle at the center and the right ventricle imaged such that the transverse dimensions appear the largest. Diameters of >41 mm at the base and >35 mm at the midlevel suggest that the right ventricle is dilated.

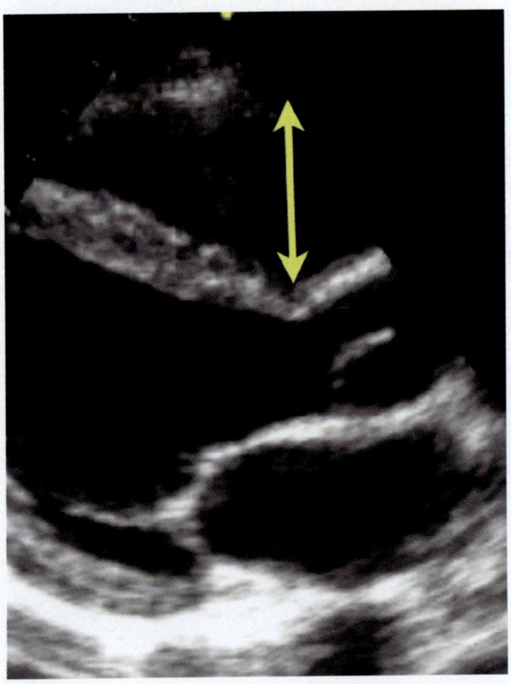

FIGURE 7.2 The parasternal long-axis view offers an opportunity to view the right ventricular outflow tract for the first time and gives clues to the size of the right-sided chambers. This is measured from the base at the junction of the interventricular septum and the free wall of the right ventricle and normally varies from 7 to 27 mm.

NORMAL VALVES FOR RV CHAMBER SIZE

Parameter	Mean ± SD	Normal Range
RV basal diameter (mm)	33 ± 4	25-41
RV mid diameter (mm)	27 ± 4	19-35
RV longitudinal diameter (mm)	71 ± 6	59-83
RVOT PLAX diameter (mm)	25 ± 2.5	20-30
RVOT proximal diameter (mm)	28 ± 3.5	21-35
RVOT distal diameter (mm)	22 ± 2.5	17-27
RV wall thickness (mm)	3 ± 1	1-5
RVOT EDA (cm^2)		
Men	17 ± 3.5	10-24
Women	14 ± 3	8-20
RV EDA indexed to BSA (cm^2/m^2)		
Men	8.8 ± 1.9	5-12.6
Women	8.0 ± 1.75	4.5-11.5
RV ESA (cm^2)		
Men	9 ± 3	3-15
Women	7 ± 2	3-11
RV ESA indexed to BSA (cm^2/m^2)		
Men	4.7 ± 1.35	2.0-7.4
Women	4.0 ± 1.2	1.6-6.4
RV EDV indexed to BSA (mL/m^2)		
Men	61 ± 13	35-87
Women	53 ± 10.5	32-74
RV ESV indexed to BSA (mL/m^2)		
Men	27 ± 8.5	10-44
Women	22 ± 7	8-36

EDA, end-diastolic area; ESA, end-systolic area; PLAX, parasternal long-axis view; RVOT, RV outflow tract.

FIGURE 7.3 The following recommendations for chamber quantification have been established by the ASE/EACI. From Lang RM, Badano LP, Mor-Avi V, et al. Recommendations for chamber quantification by echocardiography in adults: an update from the American Society of Echocardiography and the European Association of Cardiovascular Imaging. *J Am Soc Echocardiogr.* 2015;28:1-39.

STANDARD VIEWS OF THE RIGHT VENTRICLE, INFLOW, AND OUTFLOW

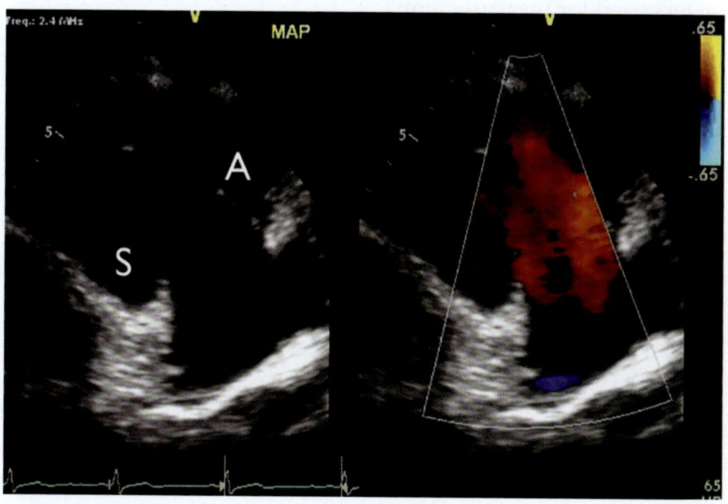

FIGURE 7.4 The RV inflow tract view is easily obtained by tilting the transducer under the sternum from the parasternal long-axis view. The inflow portion of the RV is visualized along with the anterior and septal leaflets of the tricuspid valve. S, septal; A, anterior.

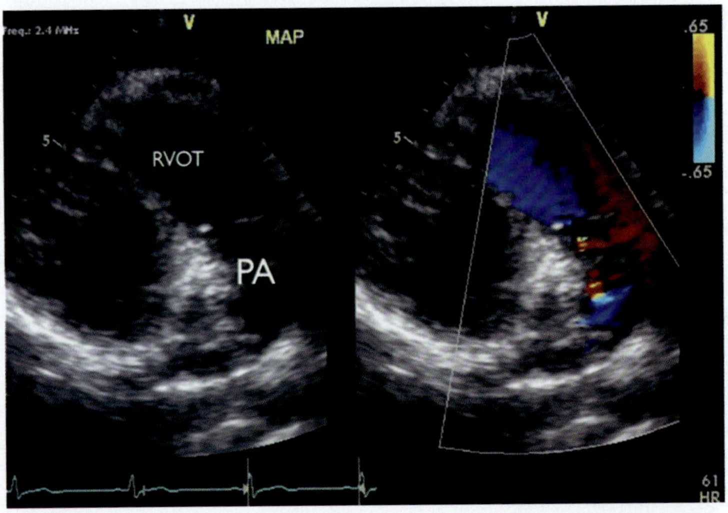

FIGURE 7.5 The RV outflow tract to include the pulmonary valve and proximal pulmonary arteries. RVOT, right ventricular outflow tract; PA, pulmonary artery.

SECTION 2

RIGHT VENTRICULAR SYSTOLIC FUNCTION

Parameters used for measurement:

- Visual examination of the size and contraction pattern of the right ventricle
- Fractional area change (FAC)
- Tricuspid annular plane excursion (TAPSE)
- Tricuspid annular systolic velocity (TASV)
- dP/dT of the tricuspid regurgitation velocity profile
- Longitudinal strain imaging using speckle tracking
- Velocity profiles of the free wall of the right ventricle using tissue Doppler
- Three-dimensional echo volume and ejection fraction
- Index of myocardial performance (RIMP)—global right ventricular function

SYSTOLIC FUNCTION OF THE RIGHT VENTRICLE[2,3]

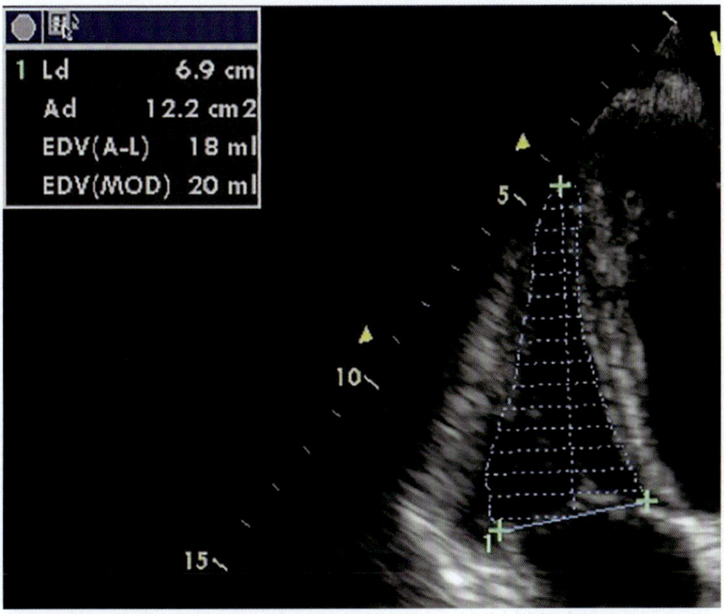

FIGURE 7.6 End-diastolic frame has been traced here to include the trabeculations of the right ventricle and the moderator band if visible. A focus view of the right ventricle is used from the apex. The tracing begins at the tricuspid annulus and extends around to the apex and back to the opposite annulus and a line is drawn across the tricuspid valve annulus.

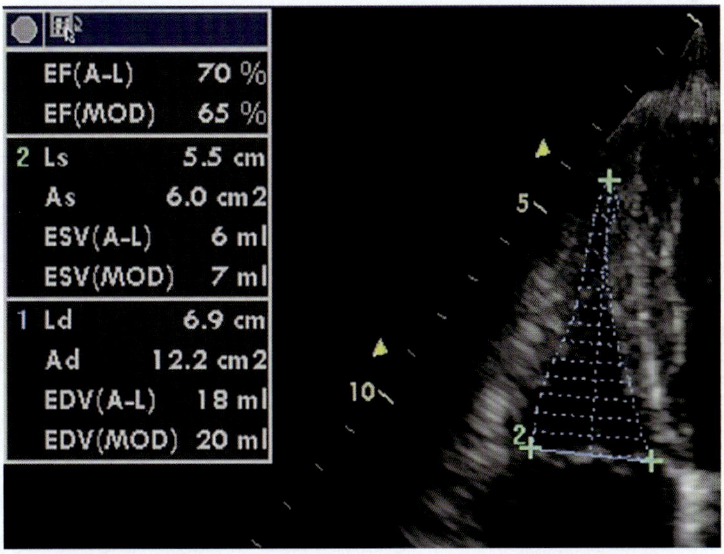

FIGURE 7.7 A similar line is drawn from a focused view in systole to include trabeculations and moderator band. The fractional area change is obtained by taking the systolic area divided by the diastolic area, which in this case is EDA – ESA/EDA = 6.2/12.2 = 51%. Normal is >35%. (The 2015 ASE guidelines suggest that 3D volumes be used when possible. The above program uses the method of disks and calculates a volume using the same software as for the left ventricle.)

FOUR ADDITIONAL METHODS FOR ASSESSMENT OF RIGHT VENTRICULAR SYSTOLIC FUNCTION

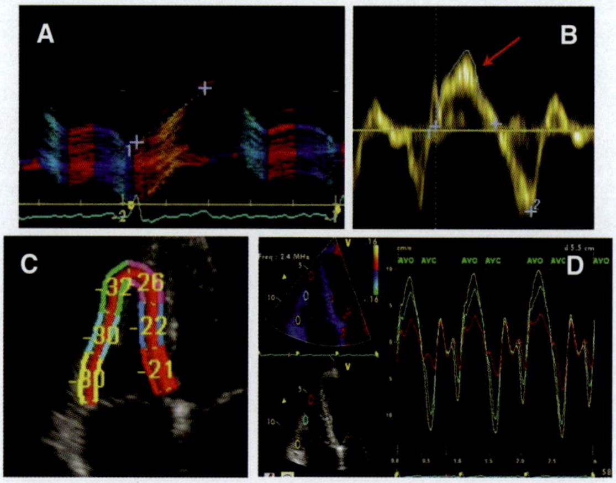

FIGURE 7.8 Each of the above displays illustrates techniques for evaluation of systolic function of the right ventricle (RV). The overall assessment of the right ventricle requires a coalition of multiple modalities. **A:** Tricuspid annular plane systolic excursion (TAPSE) is most commonly used to assess systolic function of the RV and has been studied extensively in the setting of pulmonary hypertension. **B:** Tricuspid annular systolic velocity (TASV) is a measure of the downward velocity of the lateral tricuspid annulus and offers another modality that gives information on systolic function of the RV. **C:** RV strain by speckle tracking is a third method for evaluation of systolic function of the RV. **D:** Tissue Doppler assessment of RV systolic function by analysis of velocities at selected points along the free wall of the RV. Each has something to offer, and overall assessment is enhanced by analysis of several modalities.

SECTION 3

RIGHT VENTRICULAR DIASTOLIC FUNCTION

Evaluation of diastolic function of the right ventricle is similar to that of the left ventricle. Pulse wave analysis of the tricuspid inflow velocity profile sampled at the tips of the tricuspid leaflets produces E and A waves. Tissue Doppler analysis of the lateral tricuspid annular velocities also offers analysis of e′ and a′ values. Similar patterns to those on the left allow for identification of abnormal relaxation, pseudonormal filling, and restrictive filling. Usually, abnormal findings of these patterns are associated with significant findings in functional class and other findings such as a dilated right atrium, dilated inferior vena cava, hepatic vein flow abnormalities, and elevated pressures on the right.

Parameters that indicate abnormal relaxation include E/A ratio of <0.8 or e′/a′ <0.5. E/A ratio of 0.8 to 2.1 or e′/a′ of 0.5 to 1.9 suggests high filling pressures. E/e′ < 6 or diastolic flow predominance in the hepatic veins suggests pseudonormal filling, and E/A > 2.1 and e′/a′ > 1.9 and an abbreviated deceleration time <120 ms along with diastolic integrate flow in the pulmonary artery suggests restrictive filling.[4]

SECTION 4

RIGHT VENTRICLE AND PULMONARY HYPERTENSION

The right ventricle is designed to function by generating volume and not pressure. Abnormalities that result in pressure overload result in remodeling of the right ventricle in response to the imposed load. As the right ventricle changes shape, distorts the interventricular septum, and dilates the tricuspid annulus, coaptation of the tricuspid valve is compromised and tricuspid regurgitation results.

Elevations of right ventricular systolic pressure can occur in several clinical settings. Individuals with chronic obstructive lung disease, idiopathic pulmonary hypertension, pulmonary embolism, and systemic diseases such as systemic sclerosis and many others can result in elevations in pressures in the right ventricle and the pulmonary artery. Much interest has been present in recent years in measuring and estimating these pressures associated especially since a host of novel drugs are available to alter pulmonary vascular resistance.

The importance of carefully separating out primary elevations of pulmonary artery pressure from secondary elevations has become important. Elevations in left ventricular filling pressure or pulmonary artery wedge pressure >15 mm Hg changes the target of treatment from the pulmonary circulation to the left ventricle and the systemic circulation. Once this issue has been eliminated, focus can be directed to the pulmonary vasculature at rest and sometimes with exercise.

Echocardiography and right heart catheterization have played a major role in the diagnosis of pulmonary hypertension and in the treatment and follow-up of interventions. Measurements of the tricuspid regurgitation jet velocity along with estimation of right atrial pressure offer a noninvasive approach for estimation of right ventricular systolic pressure. Direct measurement of these pressures with Swan-Ganz catheters offers objective information for diagnosis and treatment of these conditions. Many standards have been set, but currently mean pulmonary artery pressures at rest of >25 mm Hg and mean pulmonary artery pressures with exercise >30 mm Hg define pulmonary hypertension. This assumes pulmonary capillary wedge pressure is <15 mm Hg. Pulmonary arterial resistance as measured in Wood units normally should be <2 units. Generally when pulmonary hypertension is present, the pulmonary vascular resistance is >3 Wood units. These standards have been outlined in recent publications.[5,6]

Examples of alterations of the right ventricle and estimations of right ventricular systolic pressure as estimated by echocardiography and Doppler techniques are illustrated in the following pages. It should be noted that in the absence of right ventricular outflow obstruction, pulmonary valve stenosis or stenosis within the pulmonary arteries right ventricular systolic pressure is the same as pulmonary artery systolic pressure.[7]

CASE PRESENTATION

Chronic Obstructive Lung Disease

A 56-year-old woman with pulmonary hypertension associated with severe COPD and bullous emphysema (negative perfusion scans) and having symptoms of exertional shortness of breath.

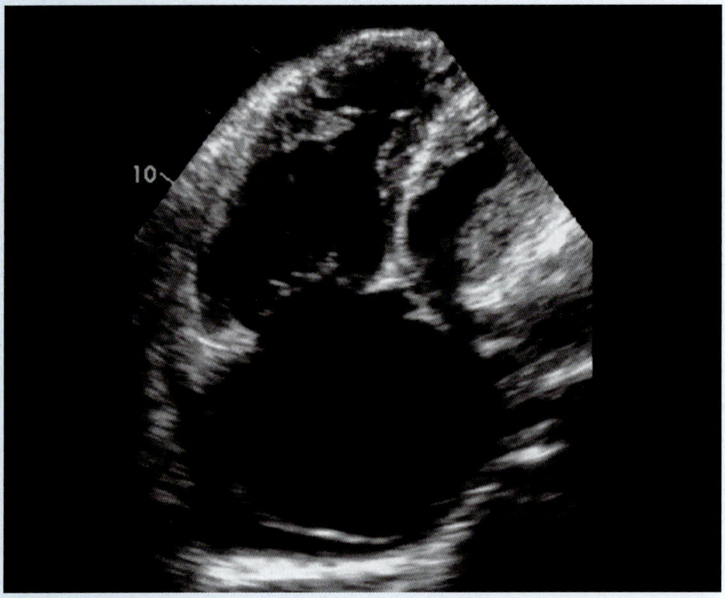

FIGURE 7.9 Dilated right ventricle and atrium. Both LV and RV are compressed by the large right-sided chambers. TTE, A4C view.

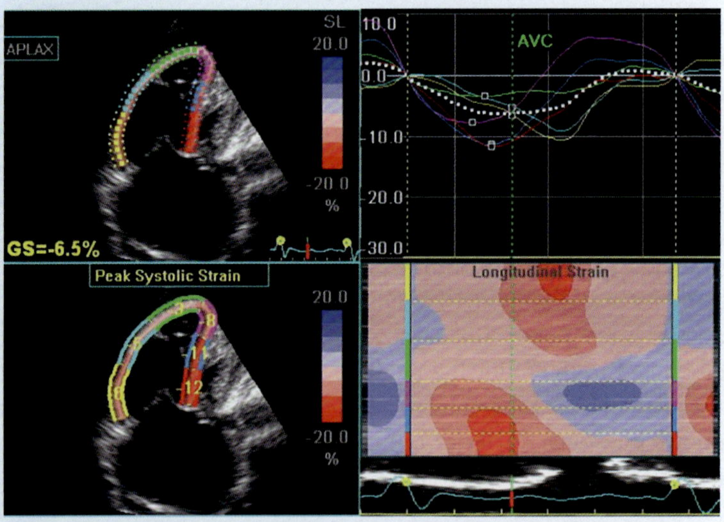

FIGURE 7.10 Global RV strain demonstrated to be very abnormal (normal > 20%).

CASE PRESENTATION

Sarcoidosis

A 48-year-old man with sarcoidosis with these images obtained on presentation. Calculation of right ventricular systolic pressure was in the 120-mm Hg range with similar findings on right heart catheterization. He was treated with sildenafil and warfarin for several years. Amiodarone was used when atrial fibrillation developed.

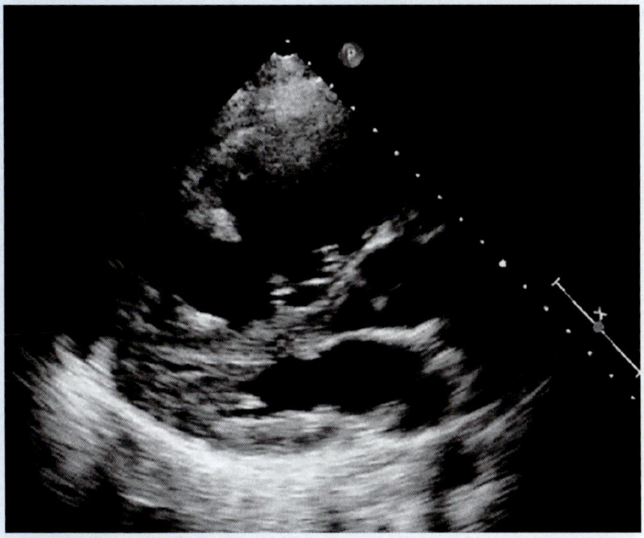

FIGURE 7.11 Very dilated right ventricle almost inverting the interventricular septum. Certainly this alters filling of the left ventricle. TTE, PLX view.

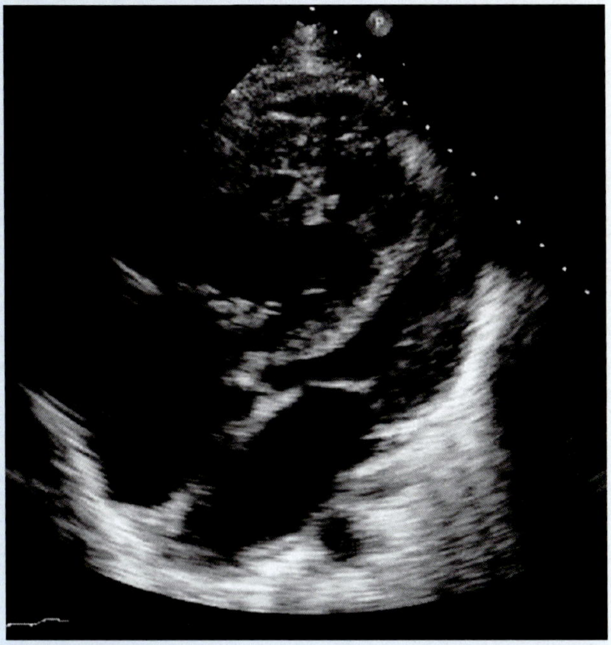

FIGURE 7.12 Apical four-chamber view showing the thickened right ventricular wall measuring >1 cm. with the normal being 0.5 cm or less.

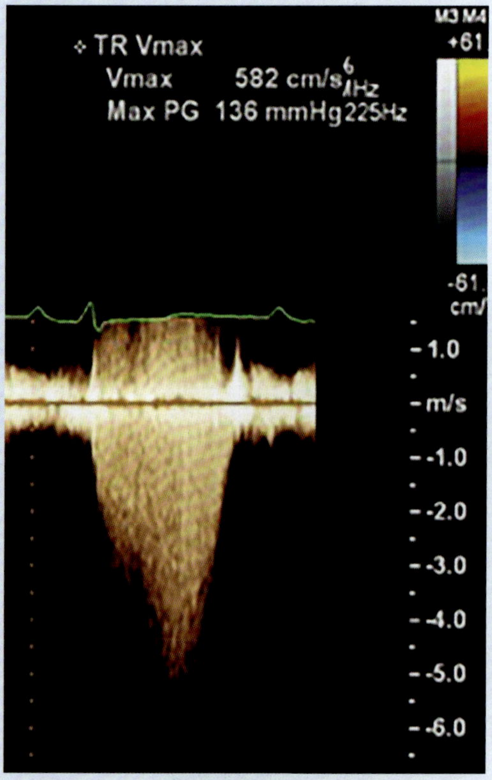

FIGURE 7.13 The jet of tricuspid regurgitation demonstrating spectral broadening and a very high velocity.

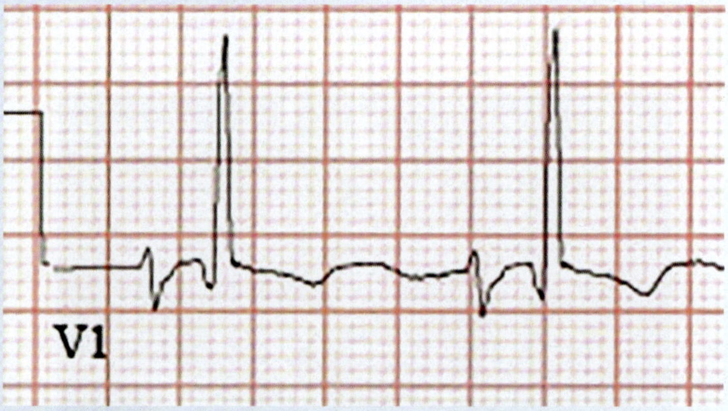

FIGURE 7.14 A portion of the EKG showing the type of P waves seen in other situations of a very large right atrium such as tricuspid atresia with the so-called Himalayan P waves and the changes of RVH to include right axis deviation and a qR in lead V1.

IDIOPATHIC PULMONARY HYPERTENSION

This disease process is probably more common than previously thought. Individuals often present with advanced disease and severe elevations in pulmonary artery pressures (>40 mm Hg mean) and have to be treated urgently with advanced measures even to include lung transplant. Most often, idiopathic pulmonary hypertension is seen in young women in the absence of other cardiac abnormalities such as valve disease or pulmonary emboli. They initially require a careful evaluation to separate out other abnormalities such as systemic diseases and left-sided valve disease or left ventricular dysfunction.

Echocardiography plays a major role in the initial diagnosis and follow-up of these individuals. Earlier recognition of this disease and the use of currently available medical treatments will hopefully in the future offer opportunities for reversal of the process and improved survival.[8,9]

CASE PRESENTATION

A 37-year-old woman with idiopathic pulmonary hypertension. She expired the day after this study.

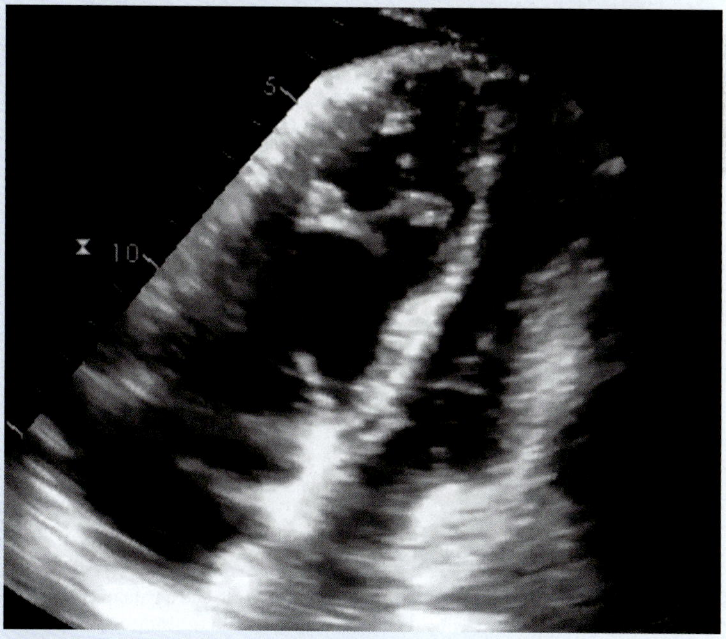

FIGURE 7.15 From the apex, the dilated trabeculated right ventricle stealing away the septum and compressing the left ventricle. TTE, A4C view.

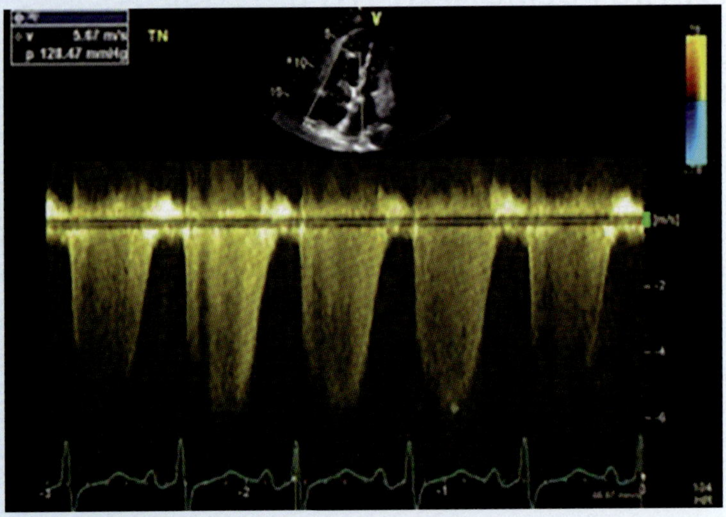

FIGURE 7.16 The TR jet measuring 5.67 m/s allowing calculation of the RVSP to be in the 140 mm Hg range. CW Doppler from the apex.

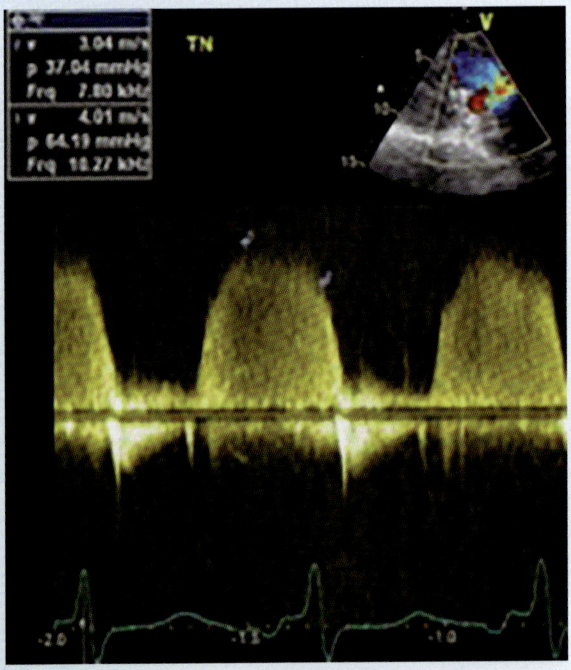

FIGURE 7.17 The PR jet showing a mean pressure of about 80 mm Hg and a pulmonary artery diastolic pressure of about 50 mm Hg. CW Doppler. Applying the Bernoulli equation to the early diastolic velocity and adding CVP estimates the mean pulmonary artery pressure, and in a similar fashion, the late diastolic velocity estimates the pulmonary diastolic pressure.

PULMONARY HYPERTENSION, "D"-SHAPED INTERVENTRICULAR SEPTUM, AND THE "FLYING W"

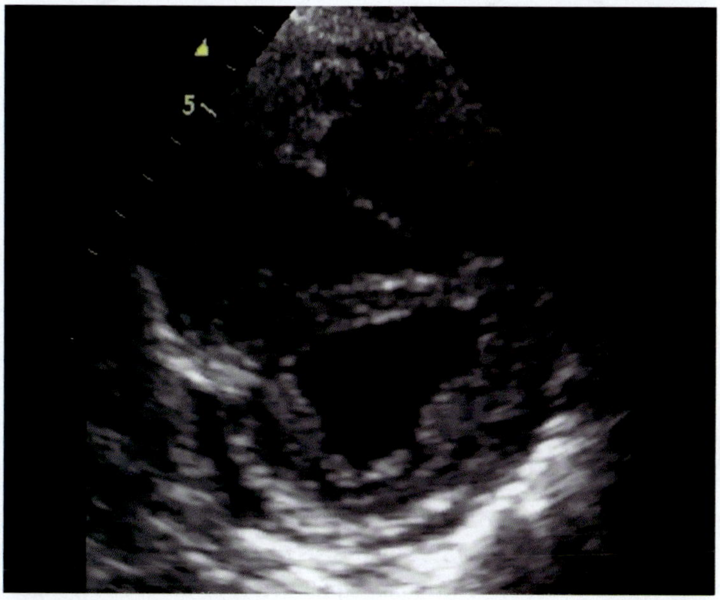

FIGURE 7.18 Cross-sectional view showing the dilated right ventricle and the "D"-shaped left ventricle. The normal crescent shape of the right ventricle is lost, and a more efficient and more spherical shape or prolate eclipse shape is assumed. The left and right ventricles exchange shapes in cross-sectional views. TTE, cross-sectional view.

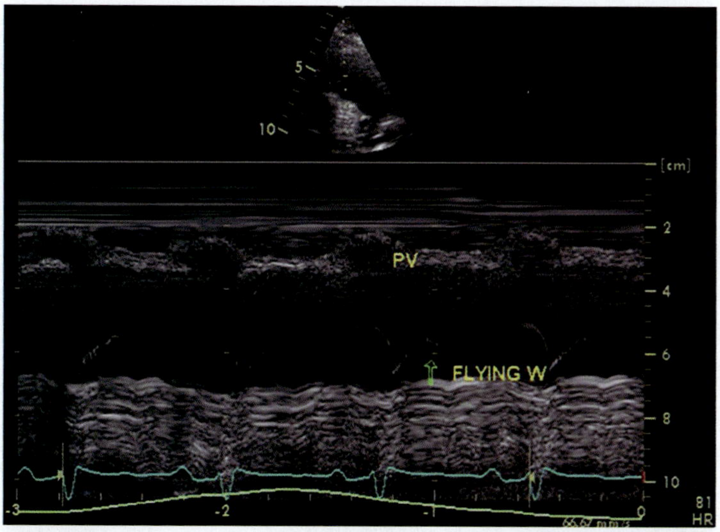

FIGURE 7.19 M-mode tracing through the pulmonary valve (*PV*) showing no "a" wave and midsystolic closure of the valve—this is consistent with elevated pressures in the pulmonary artery and is sometimes called the "flying W (*open arrow*)." The pressures in the pulmonary artery are so high that atrial systole cannot leave its imprint of the pulmonic valve and the compromised right ventricle cannot keep the pulmonic valve fully open in systole.[10]

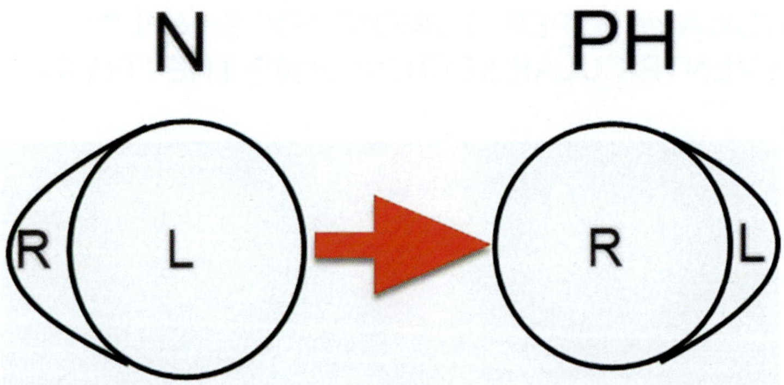

FIGURE 7.20 For the sake of mechanical advantage, the left and right ventricles exchange shapes at least in the cross-sectional views. Despite this, the right ventricle still has a geometric disadvantage in his overall shape and in the longer run does not handle pressure loads. R, right; L, left; N, normal; PH, pulmonary hypertension.

SECTION 5

EISENMENGER PHYSIOLOGY

This well-known condition was named by Dr. Paul Wood but first described by Dr. Victor Eisenmenger in 1897. It consists of an intracardiac shunt from usually an atrial septal defect or ventricular septal defect or other left to right shunt that in the course of the disease is associated with the development of elevated pulmonary vascular resistance and reversal of flow to right to left. The associated clinical findings of cyanosis, low oxygen saturations, and clubbing of the digits fulfill the criteria for the Eisenmenger syndrome. Currently, major efforts are made on the part of clinicians to correct shunts early and avoid these set of findings. Despite these efforts, individuals with these abnormalities still appear in our clinics.[11,12]

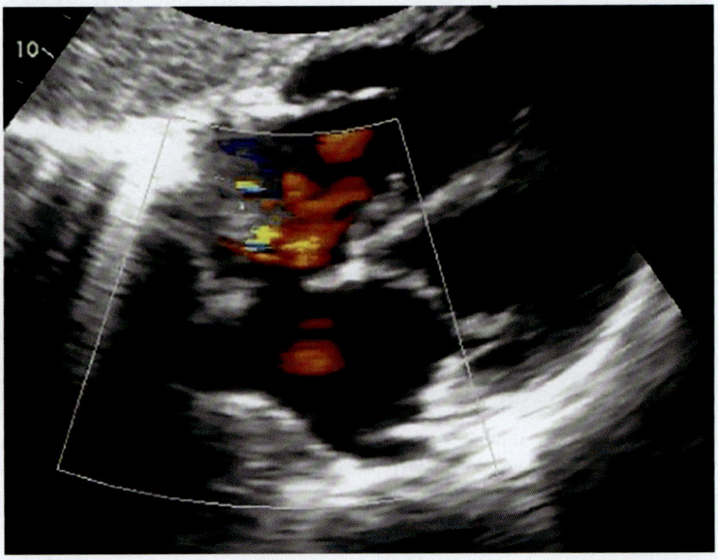

FIGURE 7.21 Color Doppler from the subcostal view showing flow across the secundum ASD. Despite the high pressures on the right, there is still some "red flow" across the IAS.

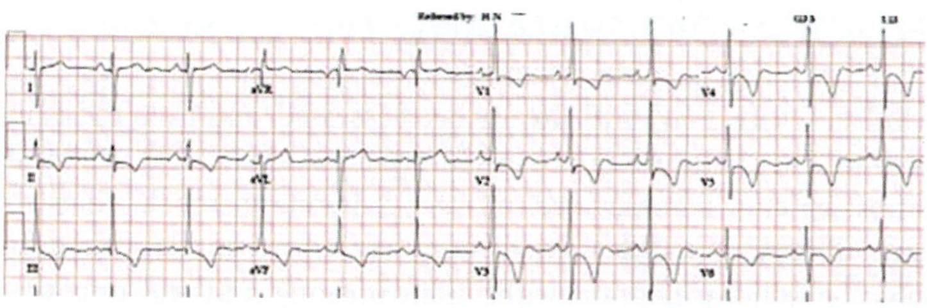

FIGURE 7.22 This individual's EKG has morphed into a pattern of RVH from what was once incomplete RBBB. Now, there is right axis deviation and very prominent initial anterior forces with a tall R wave in V1-V2. The T vector is turned away from the right ventricle as seen with RVH and "strain" pattern. The P wave is tall in V1 consistent with right atrial enlargement.

SECTION 6

PULMONARY EMBOLUS AND THE RIGHT VENTRICLE

The diagnosis of pulmonary embolism is often made in the emergency room or in hospitalized patients after a surgical procedure and many other situations. First, one has to be suspicious of the diagnosis, and that suspicion comes in the setting of any individual in respiratory distress. There may not be much to find on the physical examination but a faster than usual heart rate. Data need to be collected quickly including oxygen saturations and an electrocardiogram.

The electrocardiogram can be nearly normal, or it may show one of the characteristic changes (sinus tachycardia, S1, Q3, T3, or inverted T waves in the precordial leads).[13,14] Once the diagnosis of pulmonary embolus is at the top of the differential list, CT scan with contrast of the chest is needed (if renal function allows) to further diagnose the problem and define the clot burden. The echocardiogram is helpful to define hemodynamics on the right ventricle and calculate pressures in addition to clarify the presence or absence of additional clots that might be present in the right atrium (pulmonary embolus in transit) yet to course to the pulmonary circulation.[15] The presence or absence of right ventricular stain influences the choice of therapy between anticoagulation and thrombolytic therapy. Furthermore, the overall status of the heart needs definition.

Once as much of this information as possible is collected and the diagnosis is clear, therapy is needed as quickly as possible. Definition of the magnitude of the clot burden and the secondary effects on the right ventricle often define the course of therapy.[16-18] The electrocardiogram and the echocardiogram play a major role in this process.

Examples of abnormalities seen in pulmonary embolism will follow.

THE ECHOCARDIOGRAM AND THE CT SCAN

The clinical setting may have already been assessed, and from there, information is gathered. The echocardiogram has information about right ventricular systolic pressures, which will be elevated in larger pulmonary emboli. The right ventricle becomes dilated, and a McConnell sign may be present. Similar information is available on echocardiogram with strain imaging and will uncover abnormal global longitudinal strain. The CT scan may reveal a saddle embolus, and at times, the RV/LV ratio from the 4C view on CT scan is available. Values >1.0 suggests increased mortality and morbidity. This information can be collated to aid decision-making about the mode of intervention that is needed for therapy with systemic anticoagulation, intravenous or regional thrombolysis, or even catheter thrombectomy or surgical thrombectomy.

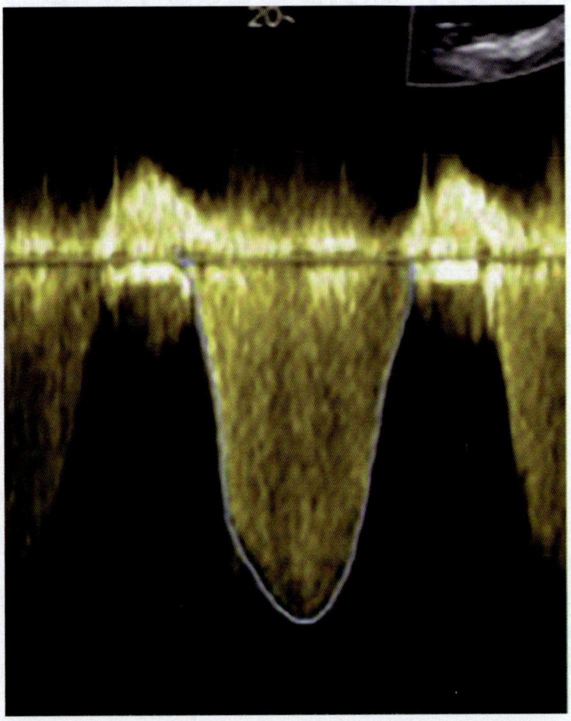

FIGURE 7.23 TR jet of 3.92 m/s and mean of 2.65 m/s indicate a calculated right ventricular systolic pressure of 72 mm Hg and mean of 44 mm Hg.

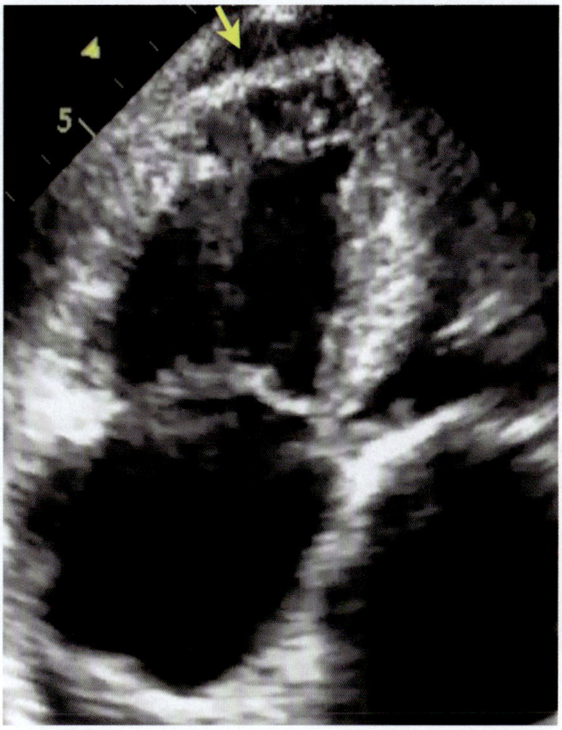

FIGURE 7.24 Right ventricle and right atrium in addition to the McConnell sign suggest that pulmonary embolus should be considered as part of the differential diagnosis (*yellow arrow*). A4C view.[19,20]

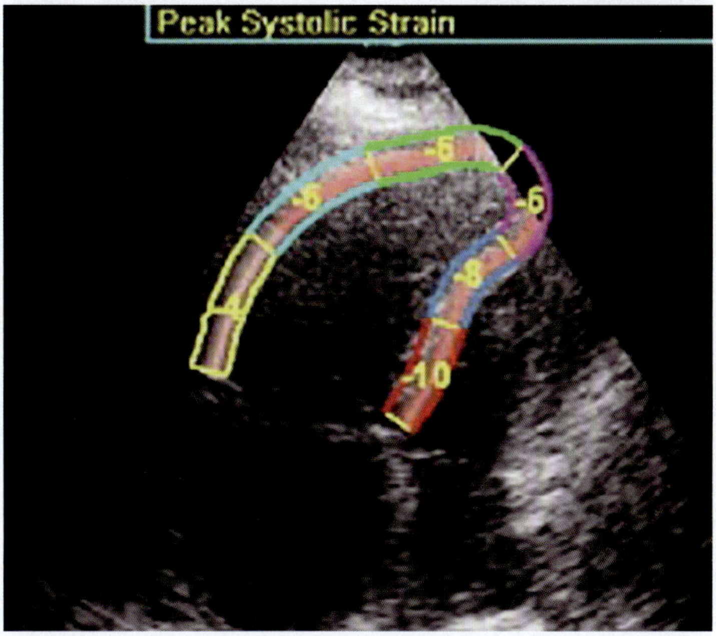

FIGURE 7.25 Global strain in the above individual shows markedly reduced strain numbers in the free wall of the RV and the septum (GS = −8.2%).[20]

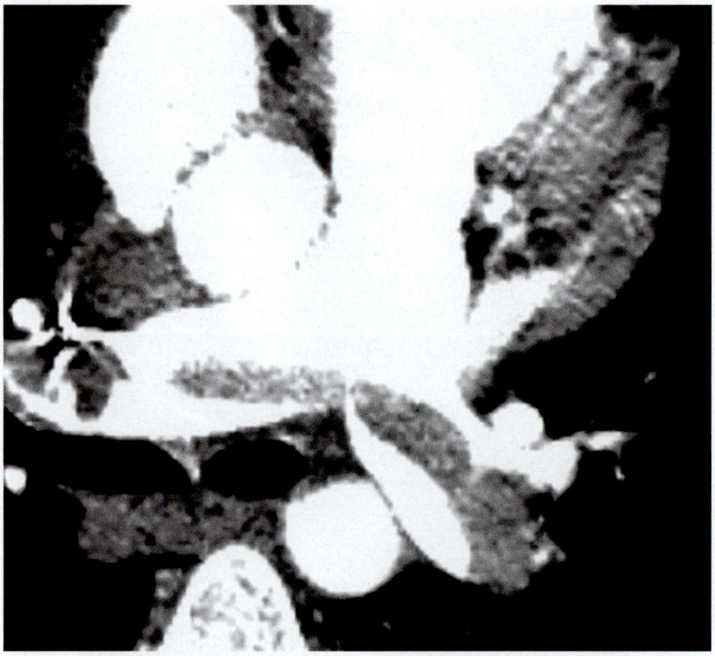

FIGURE 7.26 CT scan showing "saddle embolus" in addition to more distal emboli.

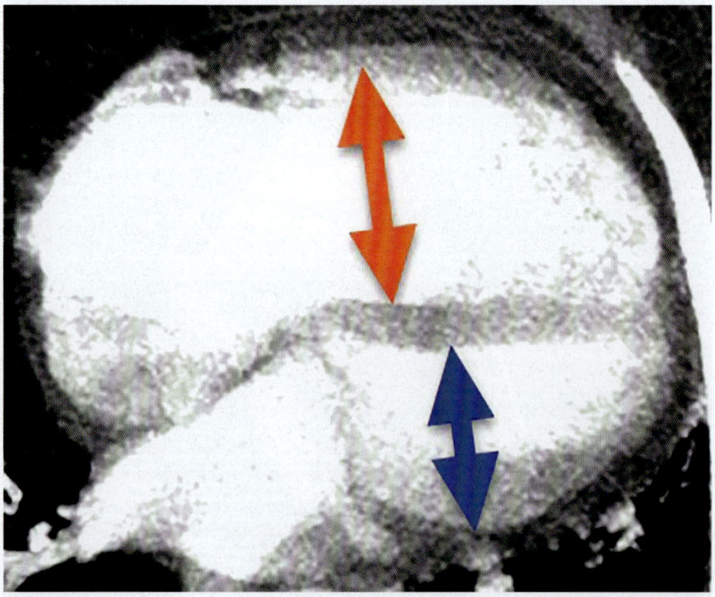

FIGURE 7.27 Very dilated right ventricle with a ratio of RVD 4-CH/LVD 4-CH > 1 suggests increased morbidity and mortality.[21,22]

SECTION 7

RIGHT VENTRICULAR MYOCARDIAL INFARCTION

Acute right ventricular infarction due to atherosclerotic coronary artery occlusion is usually associated with a proximal occlusion of the right coronary artery. The artery may be small and the acute marginal branches may be the largest branches of the artery and a posterior descending may or may not be present. On the other hand, the artery may be large and have many distal branches including a posterior descending and the occlusion is so high that the conus branch and the acute marginal branches are involved. With this situation, there is not only involvement with the inferior wall of the left ventricle but also involvement of the right ventricle. Cardiac output can be severely compromised in this situation with difficulty getting blood to the left side and high central venous pressures and hypotension. This syndrome presents difficulty in treatment in that sometimes large volumes of fluid must be used to prime the right ventricle in order to maintain adequate systemic cardiac output.

The echocardiogram can be helpful in demonstrating wall motion abnormalities of the free wall of the right ventricle. In addition it offers information about right ventricular and central venous pressures and the degree of tricuspid regurgitation.[23] Once the syndrome of right ventricular infarction is identified, usually volumes of fluid are needed to maintain blood pressure and cardiac output. The intra-aortic balloon pump is usually not helpful.

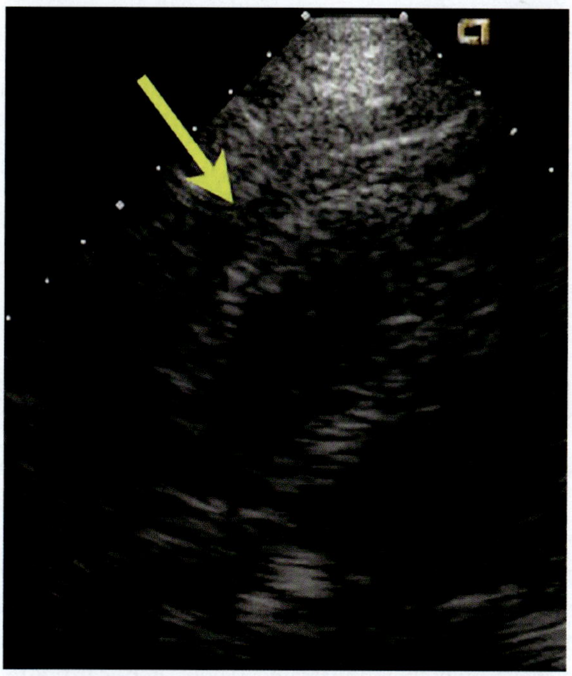

FIGURE 7.28 The echo showing wall motion abnormality (*yellow arrow*) in the free wall of the right ventricle. Modified 4C view.

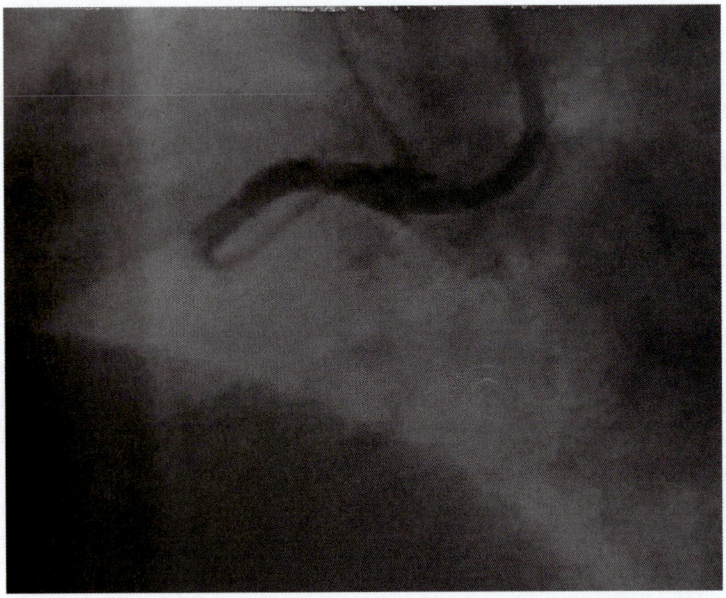

FIGURE 7.29 Coronary arteriogram demonstrating acute occlusion of the small right coronary artery after a conus branch. LAO view.

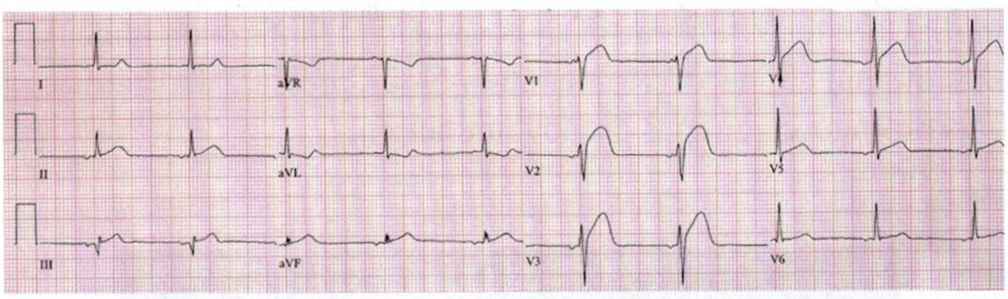

FIGURE 7.30 The EKG showing an ST vector pointing straight at leads V2 and V3 and thus toward the right ventricle. This initially was mistaken to be an anterior myocardial infarction due to occlusion of the left anterior descending but in fact was occlusion of a small right coronary artery. This EKG represents acute right ventricular infarction due to occlusion of a small codominant right coronary artery. In addition, there are changes in the inferior leads and a "low atrial" rhythm present.

SECTION 8

ARRHYTHMOGENIC RIGHT VENTRICULAR CARDIOMYOPATHY

This is a rare disorder in which there is fibrofatty replacement of the myocardium, usually the right ventricle but rarely the left. It is a genetic disease that is familial with autosomal dominant inheritance.

This characteristic abnormality is fibrofatty infiltration of the right ventricular myocardium. These areas have arrhythmia potential. Ventricular tachycardia is the usual arrhythmia. This entity has its own electrocardiographic wave called the "epsilon wave," which is illustrated below. Echocardiographic and cardiac magnetic resonance imagings are used to make the diagnosis along with the clinical situation and the electrocardiogram. Arrhythmogenic right ventricular cardiomyopathy (ARVC) is on the list of abnormalities that can result in sudden death in relatively young individuals.

Major efforts have been made to establish criteria that allow accurate diagnosis of this abnormality in all stages in hopes of finding adequate treatment modalities.[24-27]

CASE PRESENTATION

A 52-year-old woman who presented to the ER at age 37 years with right ventricular tachycardia (LBBB pattern) and subsequently has had multiple antiarrhythmic drugs plus a defibrillator and two ablations. The last one was both endocardial and epicardial. Earlier, she had an MRI that showed signs of fibrofatty infiltration of the right ventricle.

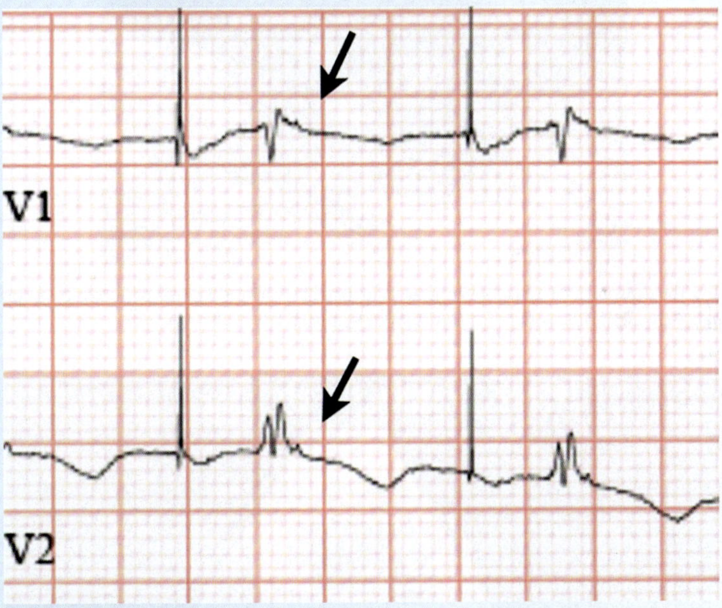

FIGURE 7.31 The right precordial leads showing atrial pacing and RBBB pattern and an after potential demonstrated by *arrows* and consistent with a seldom-seen "epsilon wave."

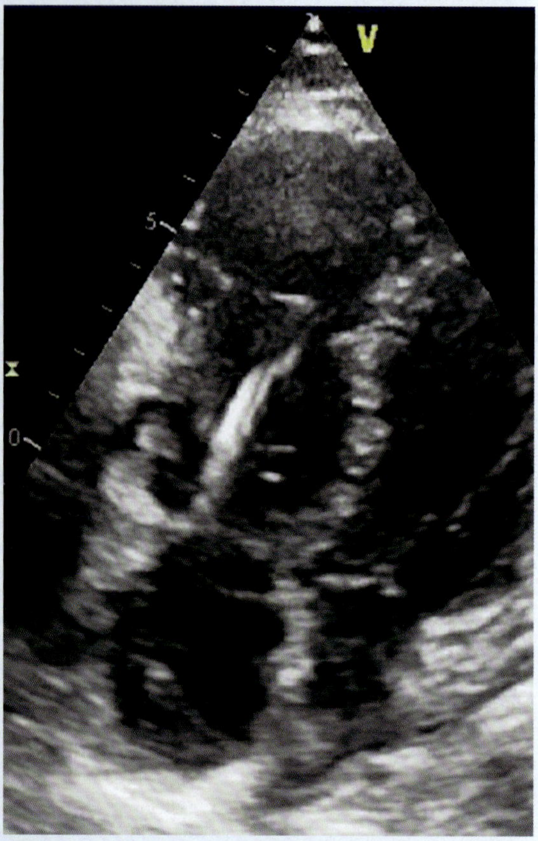

FIGURE 7.32 The unusual shaped right ventricle influenced by various degrees of fibrofatty dysplasia. No areas contract normally. The defibrillator wire is noted in the right ventricle. TTE, A4C view.

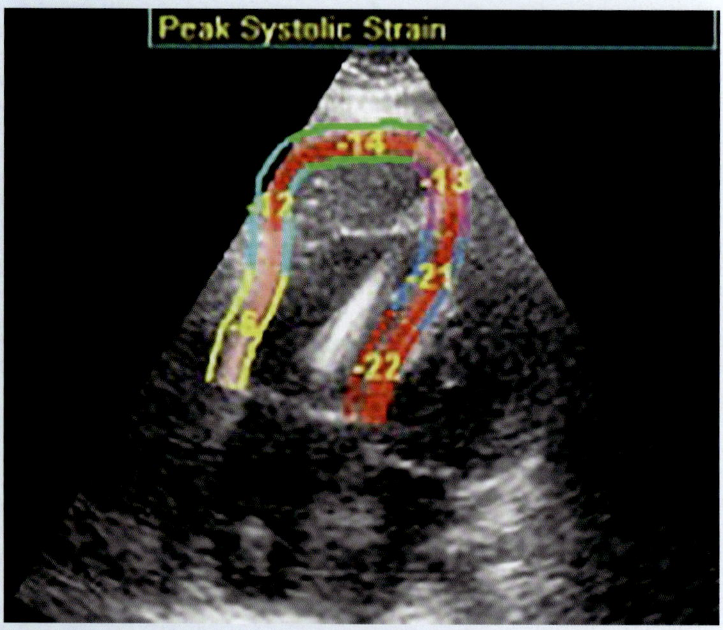

FIGURE 7.33 Global right ventricular strain very abnormal at—14.8%.

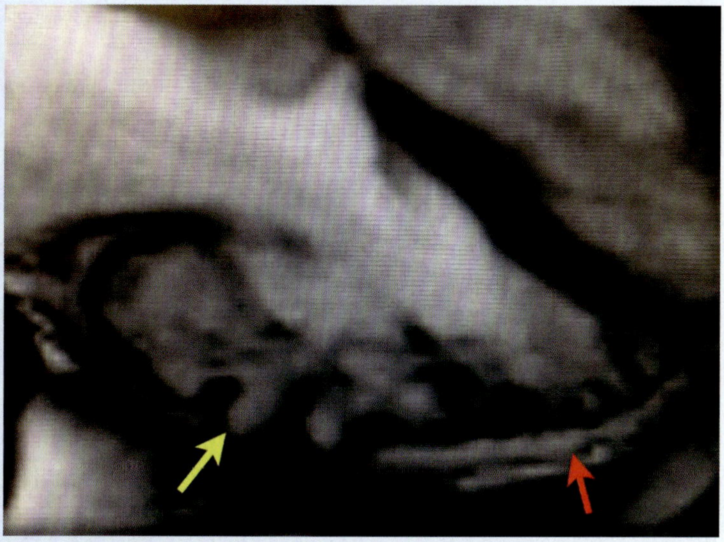

FIGURE 7.34 MRI (from the second patient in the digital version) demonstrating "fibrofatty" infiltration (*red arrow*) and aneurysmal areas at the more basal segments (*yellow arrow*).

REFERENCES

1. Ho SY, Nihoyannopoulos P. Anatomy, echocardiography and normal right ventricular dimensions. *Heart.* 2006;92(suppl 1):i2-i13.
2. Lang RM, Badano LP, Mor-Avi V, et al. Recommendations for chamber quantification by echocardiography in adults: an update from the American Society of Echocardiography and the European Association of Cardiovascular Imaging. *J Am Soc Echocardiogr.* 2015;28:1-39.
3. Rudski LG, Lai WW, Afilalo J, et al. Guidelines for the echocardiographic assessment of the right heart in adults: a report from the American Society of Echocardiography. *J Am Soc Echocardiogr.* 2010;23:685-713.
4. Lang RM, Goldstein SA, Kronzon I, Khandheria BK, Mor-Avi V. *ASE's Comprehensive Echocardiography*. 2nd ed. Philadelphia, PA: Elsevier (Saunders); 2016:157.
5. Hooper MM, Bogaard HJ, Condliffe R, et al. Definitions and diagnosis of pulmonary hypertension. *J Am Coll Cardiol.* 2013;62:D42-D50.
6. Bossone E, D'Andrea A, D'Alto M, et al. Echocardiography in pulmonary arterial hypertension: from diagnosis to prognosis. *J Am Soc Echocardiogr.* 2013;26:1-14
7. Rock PG, Popp RL. Noninvasive estimation of right ventricular systolic pressure by Doppler ultrasound in patients with tricuspid regurgitation. *Circulation* 1984;70:657-662.
8. Simonneau G, Gatoulis MA, Adatia I, et al. Updated clinical classification of pulmonary hypertension. *J Am Coll Cardiol.* 2013;62:D34-D41.
9. Galie N, Humbert M, Vachiery J, et al. 2015 ESC/ERS Guidelines for the diagnosis and treatment of pulmonary hypertension-web addenda. *Eur Heart J.* 2016;37(1):67-119.
10. Nanda NC, Gramiak R, Robinson TL, et al. Echocardiographic evaluation of pulmonary hypertension. *Circulation.* 1974;50:575-581.
11. Wood P. Pulmonary hypertension with special reference to the vasoconstrictive factor. *Br Heart J.* 1958;20(4):557-570.

12. Eisenmenger V. Die angeborenen Defekte der Kammerscheidewände des Herzens. The condition was first mentioned by Hippocrates, the Greek physician. *Zeitschr Klin Med.* 1897;32(suppl):1-28.
13. McGinn S, White PD. Acute for pulmonale resulting from pulmonary embolism: its clinical recognition. *JAMA.* 1935;104:1473-1480.
14. Ferrari E, Imbert A, Chevalier T, Mihoubi A, Morand P, Baudouy M. The ECG in pulmonary embolism, predictive value of negative T waves in the precordial leads—80 case reports. *Chest.* 1997;11:537-543.
15. Felner JM, Churchwell AL, Murphy DA. Right atrial thromboemboli: clinical, echocardiographic and pathophysiologic manifestations. *J Am Coll Cardiol.* 1984;4(5):1041-1051.
16. Miller G, Sutton G, Kerr I, et al. Comparison of streptokinase and heparin in treatment of isolated acute massive pulmonary embolism. *BMJ.* 1971;2:681-684.
17. Goldhaber SZ, Visani L, DeRosa M. Acute pulmonary embolism: clinical outcomes in the International Cooperative Pulmonary Embolism Registry (ICOPER). *Lancet.* 2012;353:1386-1389.
18. Torbicki A, Perrier A, Konstantinides S, et al. The task force for the diagnosis and management of acute pulmonary embolism of the European Society of Cardiology (ESC). Guidelines on the diagnosis and management of acute pulmonary embolism. *Eur Heart J.* 2008;29(18):2276-2315.
19. McConnell MV, Solomon SD, Rayan ME, et al. Regional right ventricular dysfunction detected by echocardiography in acute pulmonary embolism. *Am J Cardiol.* 1996;78:469-473.
20. Sosland RP, Gupta K. Images in cardiovascular medicine: McConnell's sign. *Circulation.* 2008;118:e517-e518.
21. Dang DK, Thilo C, Schoepf J, et al. CT signs of right ventricular dysfunction. Prognostic role in acute pulmonary embolism. *JACC Cardiovasc Imaging.* 2011;4(8):841-849.
22. Platz E, Hassanein AH, Shah A, Goldhaber SZ, Solomon SD. Regional right ventricular strain pattern in patients with acute pulmonary embolism. *Echocardiography.* 2012;29(4):464-470.
23. Goldberger JJ, Himelman RB, Wolfe CL, Schiller NB. Right ventricular infarction: recognition and assessment of its hemodynamic significance by two-dimensional echocardiography. *J Am Soc Echocardiogr.* 1991;4:140-146.
24. McKenna WJ, Thiene G, Nava A, et al. Diagnosis of arrhythmogenic right ventricular dysplasia cardiomyopathy. Task Force of the working group myocardial and pericardial disease of the European Society of Cardiology and of the Scientific Council on Cardiomyopathies of the International Society and Federation of Cardiology. *Br Heart J.* 1994;71:215-218.
25. Yoerger DM, Marcus F, Sherrill D, et al. Echocardiographic findings in patients meeting task force criteria for arrhythmogenic right ventricular dysplasia: new insights from the multi center study of right ventricular dysplasia. *J Am Coll Cardiol.* 2005;45:860-865.
26. Marcus FI, McKenna WJ, Sherrill D, et al. Diagnosis arrhythmogenic right ventricular cardiomyopathy/dysplasia. *Eur Heart J.* 2010;31(7):806-814.
27. Fontaine G, Giraumon G, Frank R, et al. Stimulation studies and epicardial mapping in ventricular tachycardia: study of mechanisms and selection for surgery. In: Kulbertus HE, ed. *Re-entrant Arrhythmias: Mechanisms and Treatment.* Baltimore, MD: University Park Press; 1977:334-350.

8

The Pericardium

SECTION 1

THE PERICARDIUM

The pericardium is a fibroelastic sac that contains the heart and the proximal segments of the aorta and pulmonary artery and a portion of the pulmonary veins and the venae cavae that are close to the heart. Embryologically, the heart invaginates into a spherical area that results in two layers, a visceral layer that is adherent to the heart and a parietal layer that surrounds the heart. The pericardium has two major sinuses that are created by pericardial reflections, the transverse sinus and the oblique sinus. The transverse sinus lies anterior to the superior vena cava and posterior to the aorta and pulmonary trunk. One can place a finger in the transverse sinus by starting at the left atrial appendage area and moving posterior to the great vessels. The transverse sinus continues posteriorly until it comes anteriorly between the superior vena cava and the ascending aorta. The oblique pericardial sinus lies posterior to the heart and can be visualized by lifting the heart and exploring the space between the pulmonary veins. The boundaries of the oblique pericardial sinus on the right are the inferior vena cava and the right pulmonary veins and on the left by the left pulmonary veins. Cardiac surgeons expose these sinuses as they lift the heart to inspect the posterior wall of the heart. The pericardial reflection onto the pulmonary veins limits the degree to which apex of the heart can be elevated. This anatomic feature becomes important during coronary bypass operations when bypass to posterior coronary vessels is needed. The transverse sinus will allow fluid to accumulate adjacent to the aorta and the pulmonary artery and surround the left atrial appendage. This can cause confusion on echocardiogram when a small amount of pericardial fluid lies adjacent to the ascending aorta. It gives the appearance of a double line that can raise the question of aortic dissection. Fluid in the transverse sinus that surrounds the left atrial appendage exposes the tip of the appendage and in "en face" views gives the appearance of a small mobile mass.

The intrapericardial portions of the above-mentioned vascular structures can become problematic. For example, in the setting of type A aortic dissection, the ascending aorta can "weep" serous fluid or even bleed into the pericardium if the aorta is disrupted. It is noteworthy that the pulmonary veins and a portion of the left atrium are extrapericardial and are not subjected to intrapericardial pressure. In the presence of tamponade or constriction, the extrapericardial relationship between the pleural space and the pericardial space results in only minor changes of flow into the left atrium during inspiration.[1]

The pericardial space contains a small amount of fluid, <50 mL, which acts as a lubricant minimizing friction during systole or diastole. This plasmalike, low-protein ultrafiltrate is likely expressed from the visceral pericardium and is drained by the adjacent lymphatic channels. When inflammation is present between the two layers of the pericardium, one can hear a "friction rub" during the systolic, diastolic, and atrial contraction phases of the cardiac cycle.[2]

These findings will be illustrated in Section 2: Pericardial Effusion.

SECTION 2

PERICARDIAL EFFUSION

The fibroelastic pericardial sac has elastic limits and can cause difficulty when pericardial fluid accumulates. Increased pericardial pressure is manifest by collapse of chambers that have the lowest pressure such as the right atrium and right ventricle. This collapse occurs during the phase of the cardiac cycle when the chamber pressures reach a nadir. For the right atrium, this occurs during late diastole and for the right ventricle during early diastole. With increasing pericardial pressure, the right and left ventricles compete for space resulting in the right ventricle filling at the expense of the left. During inspiration, the left ventricle has decreased available stroke volume because of decreased flow from extrapericardial veins and a left shifting of the interventricular septum. This results in compromise of stroke volume during inspiration and pulsus paradoxus in the peripheral circulation.

Cardiac compression from accumulation of pericardial fluid is a situation of many variables. One factor is the distensibility of the pericardial sac itself. Sometimes, accumulation of only a small amount of fluid or blood can result in cardiac tamponade. This situation can occur in cath lab or electrophysiology lab during procedures. Hemodynamic monitoring of systemic pressure may reveal inspiratory drop in blood pressure and indicate the presence of pericardial fluid. Echocardiography may show pericardial fluid and indicate the need for pericardiocentesis.

Interestingly, one of the functions of the pericardium is to contain the heart. When the heart dilates, the pericardium tends to limit diastolic expansion. This phenomenon is manifest when the pericardium is removed and diastolic volumes of the cardiac chambers increase. Sudden expansion of either ventricle in certain clinical situations can be harmful. For example, this becomes operative in the setting of pulmonary hypertension and pericardial effusion. Sudden removal of pericardial fluid can result in an even more dilated, thin-walled right ventricle, and hemodynamic deterioration can occur.

Doppler signs include exaggerated reciprocal changes in mitral and tricuspid Doppler inflow velocities. An inspiratory change in Doppler tricuspid inflow velocity of 60% is significant, whereas a reciprocal change in mitral Doppler inflow velocity of 30% is significant and indicates tamponade. In the presence of other conditions such as chronic obstructive lung disease, exaggerated inspiratory and expiratory velocities occur. Other abnormal ventricular filling patterns such as seen in atrial septal defect, aortic regurgitation, and pulmonary hypertension may alter these dynamics and make the diagnosis of cardiac compression challenging.[3-10]

Large amounts of pericardial fluid may cause the heart to swing from beat to beat, or this swinging may occur over several cardiac cycles. This causes the dramatic changes on the electrocardiogram that is called "electrical alternans." This can occur on every other beat or with groups of beats depending on the amount of fluid that is present and the heart rate.

MODERATE PERICARDIAL EFFUSION

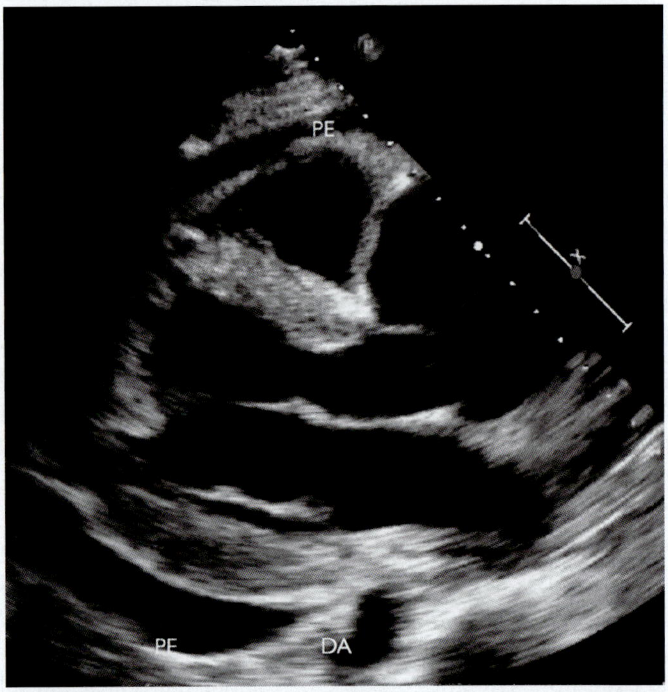

FIGURE 8.1 Pericardial effusion noted anterior to the right ventricular outflow tract and posterior to the left ventricle. The pericardial effusion (*PE*) does not extend posterior to the descending aorta (*DA*) as does a pleural effusion. The parasternal long-axis view offers the best opportunity to view the RV in the outflow area, and timing of the motion in late diastole reveals collapse at this vulnerable period of low pressure and indicates high pericardial pressure and a degree of tamponade. TTE, PLX view.

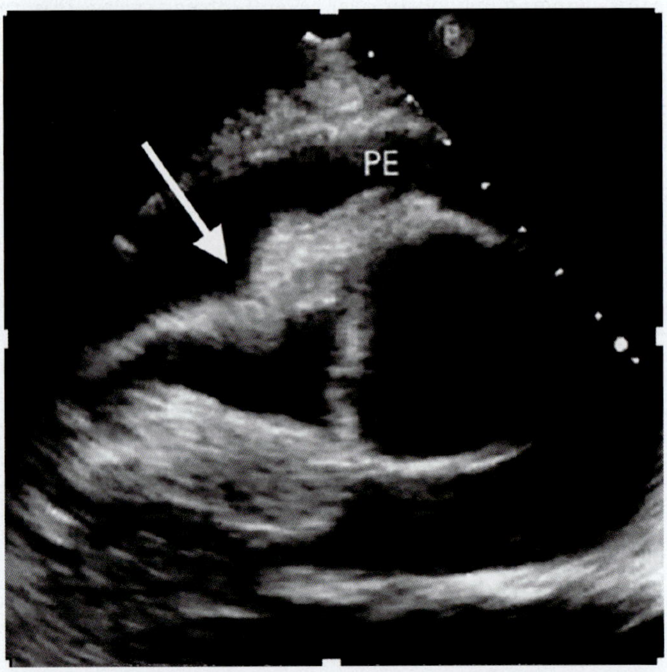

FIGURE 8.2 An early diastolic stop frame of the image on the left shows the RV collapsing (*white arrow*) under the influence of pericardial pressure, a sign of cardiac tamponade. PE, pericardial fluid.

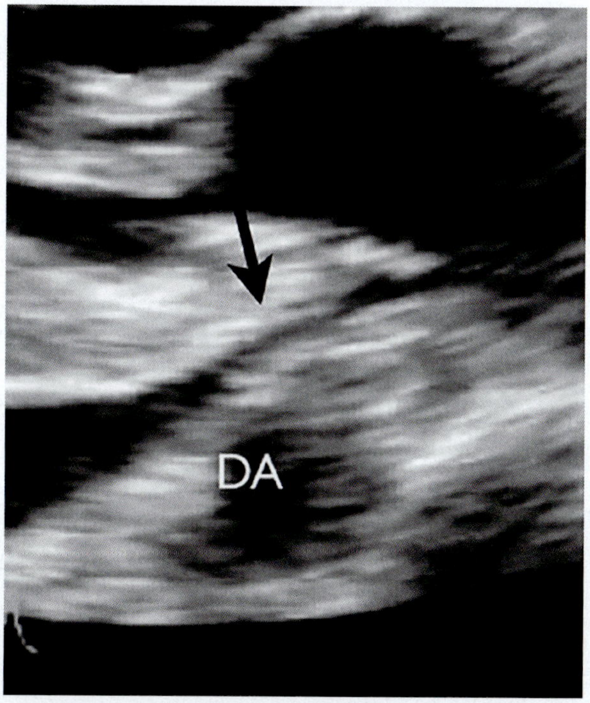

FIGURE 8.3 The pericardial effusion extends posterior to the mitral valve annulus (*black arrow*) and reflects upon the pulmonary veins leaving a space anterior to the descending aorta (*DA*).

LARGE PERICARDIAL EFFUSION

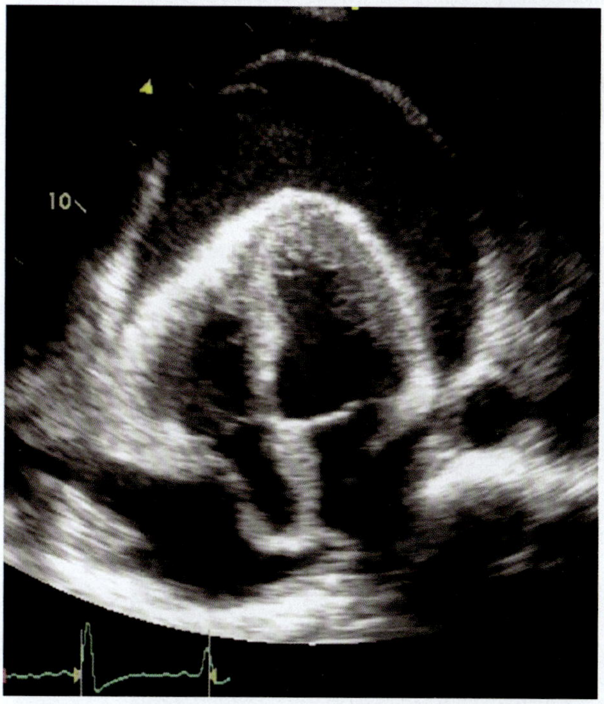

FIGURE 8.4 Large pericardial effusion with a "swinging heart."[11] This finding is usually seen with a very large effusion such as this one. The heart oscillates in a pendulum-like fashion. This occurs when the right amount of fluid is coupled with the right heart rate. Usually, there is one heartbeat with the heart located close to the chest wall and the next in a more posterior location. Note the competition between the pressure in the right atrium and the pericardial pressure resulting in the right atrium collapsing toward the tricuspid valve. The right atrium is collapsed the most in late diastole and early systole. TTE, A4C view.

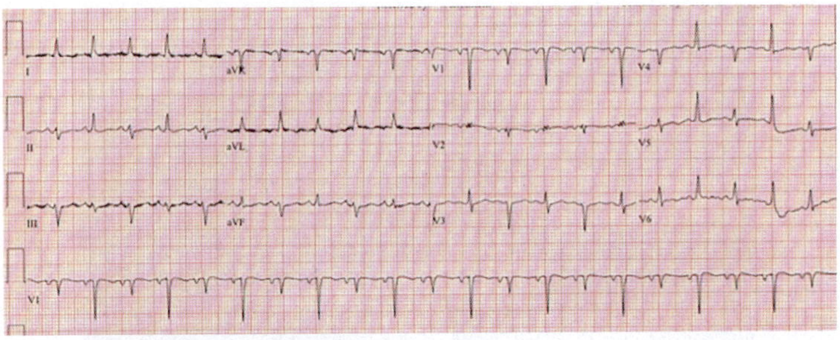

FIGURE 8.5 The EKG in such a patient with "electrical alternans"—this is especially notable in the leads that look at the heart in a profile that is near and far from the electrodes. These leads are V1 and V3-6 and leads II and aVF in this particular patient.

MITRAL AND TRICUSPID INFLOW VELOCITIES IN LARGE PERICARDIAL EFFUSION AND TAMPONADE

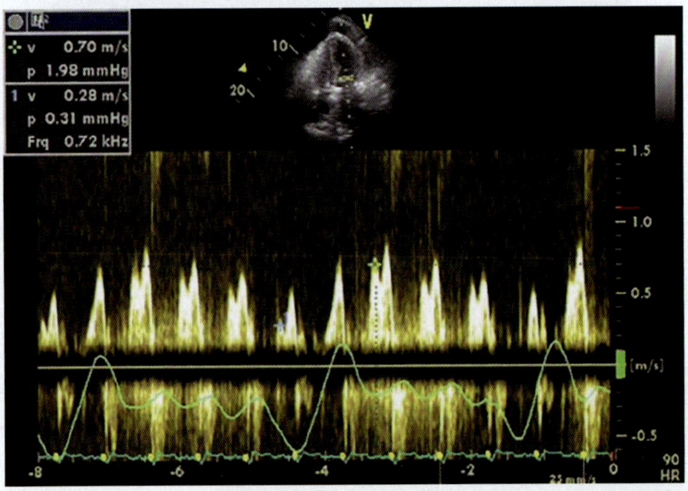

FIGURE 8.6 In this individual with large pericardial effusion and cardiac tamponade, the mitral inflow velocities vary from 0.70 to 0.28 m/s, a 60% change. Velocities above 30% are consistent with tamponade physiology. The respirometer may be slightly out of phase.[12-14]

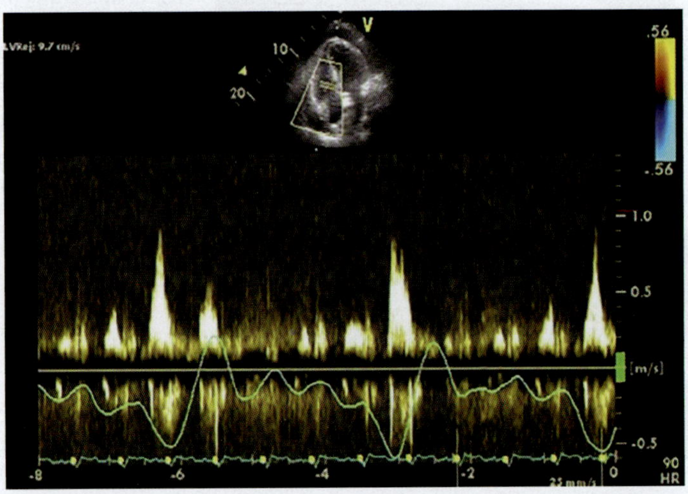

FIGURE 8.7 In this individual with large pericardial effusion and cardiac tamponade, the tricuspid inflow velocities vary from almost no inflow to 0.70 m/s, a very large change. Velocities >60% are consistent with tamponade physiology. The respirometer may be slightly out of phase.

Pulsus paradoxus and these types of respiratory-related changes in inflow velocities and integrals are not entirely specific for tamponade. As the respiratory efforts increase from any cause, one can understand how these flows might increase. Such conditions as severe dyspnea, pulmonary embolism, and COPD all can on occasions have exaggerated inflow velocities and some degree of paradoxical pulse.[14]

SECTION 3

CHRONIC PERICARDIAL EFFUSION

The "water bottle heart" on chest x-ray brings into play the differential of a large silhouette on chest x-ray especially with clear lung fields. Along with this finding is low voltage on electrocardiogram and on echo a large pericardial effusion and maybe a "swinging heart." On x-ray the diagnosis may not be clear, but the echocardiogram quickly establishes the diagnosis. Then, the etiology must be considered and ranges from causes unknown to malignancy.

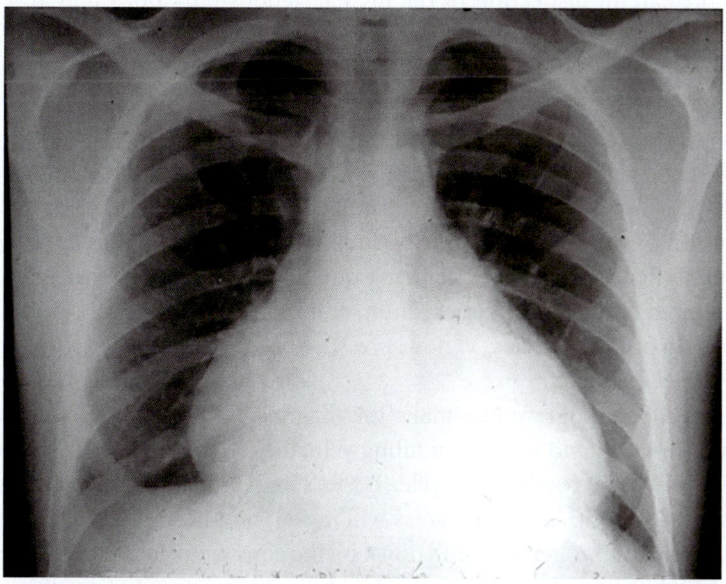

FIGURE 8.8 Large pericardial effusion on chest x-ray. Note the "water bottle" appearance, the large silhouette, and the clear lung fields. The area of the great vessels, left atrium, and ascending aorta is relatively narrow. If pericardial fluid accumulates slowly, individuals with large effusions may not have tamponade physiology. Rapid accumulation of fluid or blood will result in tamponade with smaller amounts of fluid or usually blood. The elastic limit of the pericardium in this situation is reached rapidly, and the pressure-volume relationship results in rapid rise in pressure and cardiac tamponade. This individual whose chest x-ray is illustrated on the left did not have tamponade physiology.

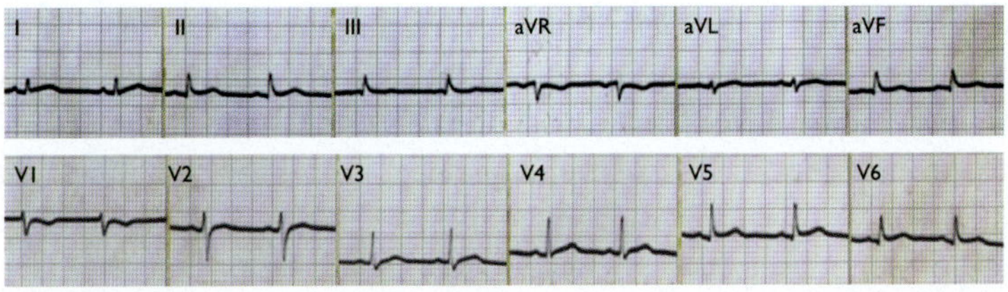

FIGURE 8.9 The EKG in the individual above showing a large pericardial effusion. He was relatively asymptomatic and has generally low voltage in every lead.

SECTION 4

CONSTRICTIVE PERICARDITIS

Constrictive pericarditis is often an elusive clinical diagnosis. Individuals with this problem present with edema and shortness of breath and jugular venous distention. What may be thought to be a third heart sound can be a pericardial knock. The ascites and peripheral edema are the same that are seen with dilated or restrictive cardiomyopathy. Heart failure with preserved ejection fraction is also a possibility in the differential diagnosis.[15]

More careful inspection of the jugular venous pulsations may reveal a rapid negative wave or "rapid Y descent," the bedside clue to the presence of constriction. Couple this with a pericardial knock, and clinical suspicion leads to more testing.

Intrapericardial space becomes limited when the pericardium becomes scarred and tightens around the ventricles. The right ventricle fills more prominently during inspiration as the intrathoracic pressure falls. The extrapericardial pulmonary veins fill the left-sided structures less, resulting in a septal shift toward the underfilled left ventricle. During quiet respiration, both ventricles are compromised by the scarred pericardium, and high and equal diastolic pressures are present in both ventricles. Venous pressure becomes high, and peripheral edema and ascites can occur.

The echocardiogram can make the diagnosis by revealing a shifting septum with inspiration and reciprocal filling velocities of the right and left ventricles as they relate to the respiratory cycle. Tissue Doppler diastolic velocities of the septal and lateral mitral annular areas will reveal "annulus reversus" consistent with the lateral annulus being bound down by the constrictive process. Rather than the usual higher lateral annular velocity when constrictive pericarditis is present, the septal annular velocity is the highest. In restrictive cardiomyopathy, the tissue Doppler numbers are very low but still maintain the usual septal/lateral velocity relationship.[15] When estimating filling pressures by using the E/e′ ratio, ordinarily, the higher this number, the higher the LV filling pressures. In the case of constrictive pericarditis, the opposite is true. E velocities are preserved because of high left atrial pressures and the e′ septal is preserved or increased and the ratio E/e′ is low despite high filling pressures. This is the opposite of what one expects, and this phenomenon is referred to as "annulus paradoxus."[16,17]

In the cardiac catheterization laboratory, the "square root" sign can be searched out and usually separates out constrictive pericarditis from restrictive cardiomyopathy. Equalization of diastolic pressures in the right and left ventricles at the end of diastole is characteristic of constrictive pericarditis. Monitoring of pressures simultaneously in the RV and LV reveals discordant changes in pressure in constrictive pericarditis. On inspiration, the left ventricular systolic pressure decreases whereas the right ventricular systolic pressure increases. Concordant changes occur with restrictive cardiomyopathy in that on inspiration, systolic pressure in both the right and left ventricles decreases.[17]

E velocities are preserved because of high left atrial pressures and the e′ septal is preserved or increased and the ratio E/e′ is low despite high filling pressures. This is the opposite of what one ordinarily expects with increasing filling pressures, and this phenomenon is referred to as "annulus paradoxus."[16,17]

In constrictive pericarditis, on inspiration, the left ventricular systolic pressure decreases whereas the right ventricular systolic pressure increases. Concordant changes occur with restrictive cardiomyopathy in that on inspiration, systolic pressure in both the right and left ventricles decreases.[18]

These points are illustrated in the following pages.

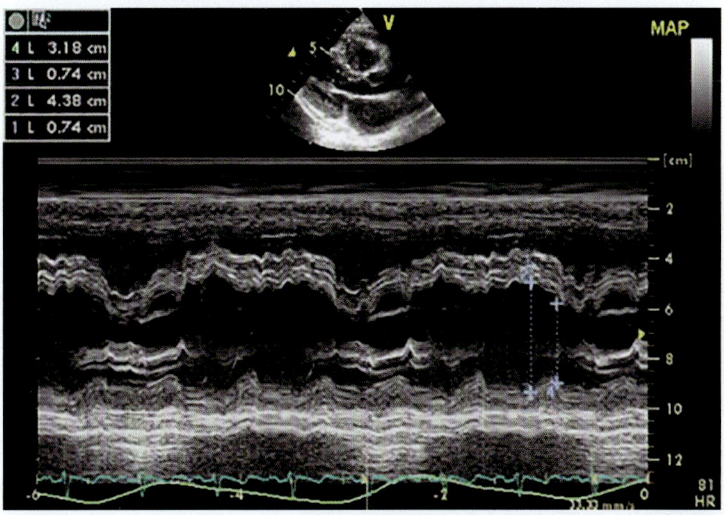

FIGURE 8.10 M-mode tracing through the mid-portion of the ventricles that demonstrates "septal shift" from right to left during inspiration.

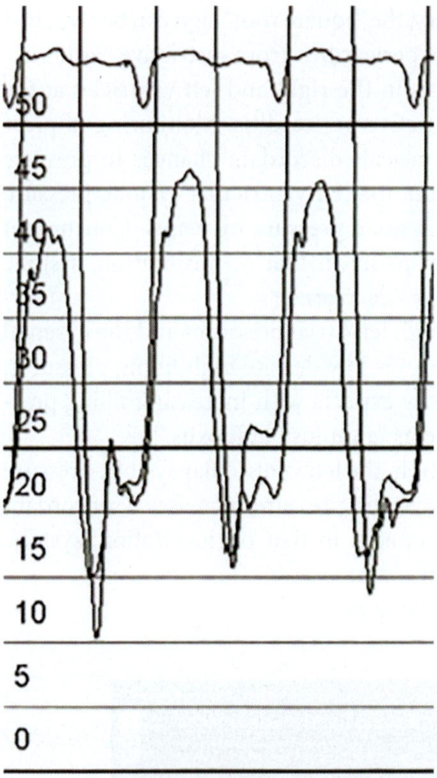

FIGURE 8.11 The simultaneous RV and LV tracings from the cath lab in the patient on the far left. Diastolic pressures tend to abruptly equalize in expiration creating a "square root sign." Systolic pressures tend to be discordant on inspiration.[18]

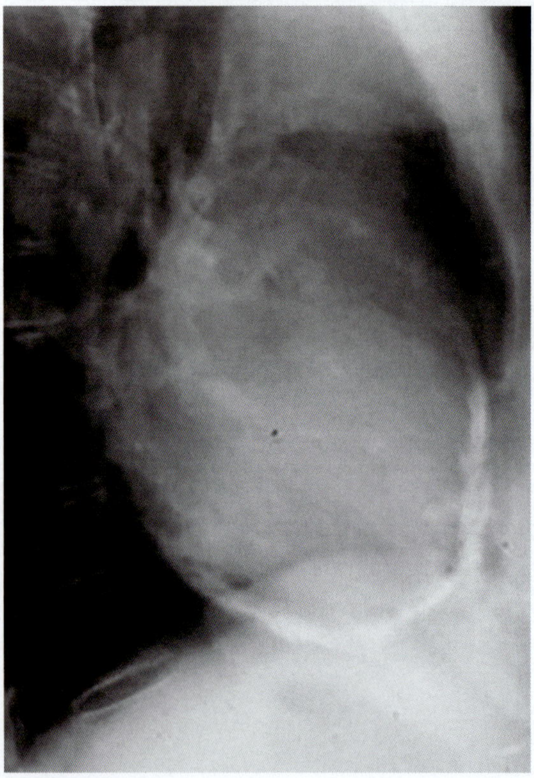

FIGURE 8.12 Calcified pericardium in another individual. In the past, this has been due to tuberculosis, but currently, this is rarely seen with the advent of anti-TB programs. This patient did not have tuberculosis. Lateral chest x-ray.

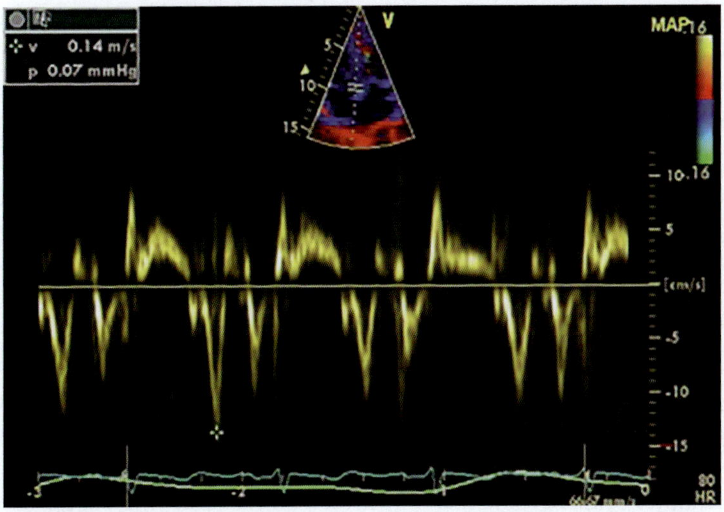

FIGURE 8.13 The tissue Doppler recorded from the septal side of the mitral annulus in the individual above that shows a velocity of 0.14 m/s, higher than the lateral e′ of 0.12 m/s. This is called "annulus reversus" or "annulus paradoxus."

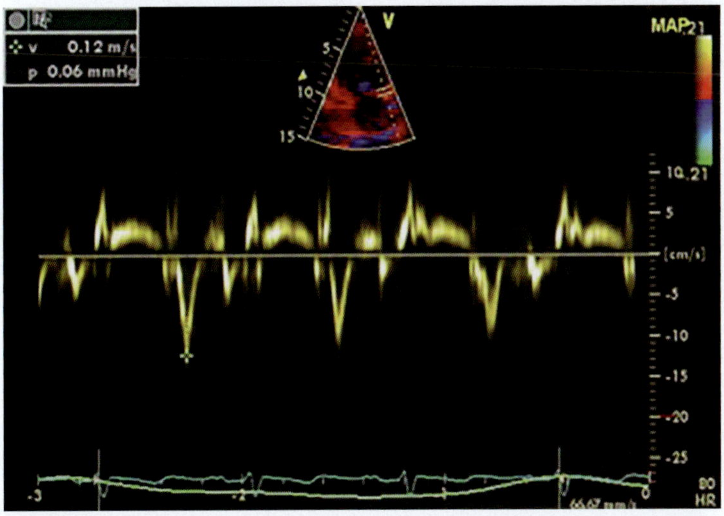

FIGURE 8.14 The lateral e′ reveals a velocity of 0.12 m/s, which is lower than the septal e′. These velocities also vary with respiration.

SECTION 5

ACUTE PERICARDITIS

When chest pain occurs especially in a young individual of college student age and the pain is aggravated by supine position and deep breathing, then pericarditis is on top of the clinical diagnosis list. Add to this a pattern of relief that is obtained by sitting up and leaning forward, and the possibility of acute pericarditis is even more likely. Auscultation for a three-component friction rub is indicated along with a careful look for PR segment depression and ST-segment elevation with a ST vector pointing to the apex. If the cardiac enzymes are elevated (troponin I), then the setting is suspicious for not only pericarditis with some element of myocardial involvement or myopericarditis. This can be further confirmed by CMRI that can show various degrees of subepicardial injury. The etiology of these syndromes is usually viral to include enteroviruses, group B coxsackievirus, and echoviruses. Other etiologies should be considered such as collagen vascular diseases and even malignancy. Treatment and follow-up will usually separate these different etiologies.

In these circumstances, the echocardiogram may be normal and there may be a variable amount of pericardial fluid. The CMRI can add to the diagnosis by imaging the pericardium, the extent of the fluid, and the presence or absence of myocardial involvement.

Examples of this problem are illustrated on the following pages.

CASE PRESENTATION

Pericarditis in a College Student

An 18-year-old freshman college student who presented to the ER with nausea, vomiting, and upper respiratory congestion of 1-day duration. Cough developed associated with chest pain with coughing. In the hospital, the troponin I peaked at 12.57 ng/mL. The history and this EKG are the first findings at hand for the emergency room physician from which to move to the correct diagnosis. The echocardiogram and the MRI have to come a bit later.

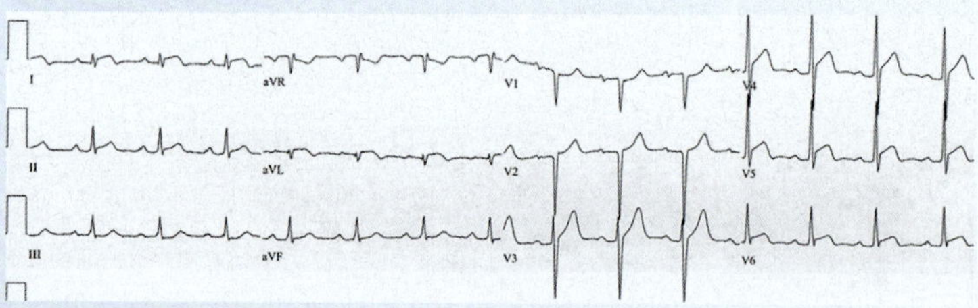

FIGURE 8.15 This EKG shows sinus rhythm with a borderline PR interval and a normal PR segment, a normal QRS complex, and abnormal ST segments. The ST vector points to the left and horizontal, and the T vector is abnormal also pointing toward lead III. The R waves are not prominent in lead V1-2. All of this is consistent with epicardial injury and needs to be put in context with the clinical situation.

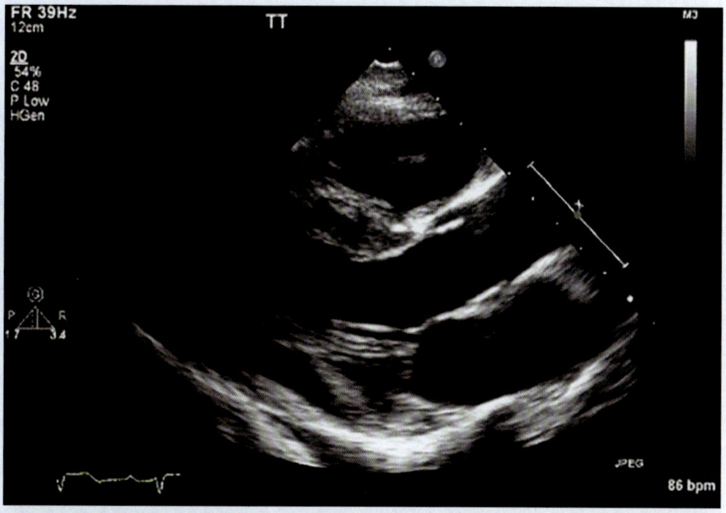

FIGURE 8.16 The left ventricle looks good, the relative chamber sizes look normal, and there are no regional wall motion abnormalities. There is no significant pericardial fluid noted.

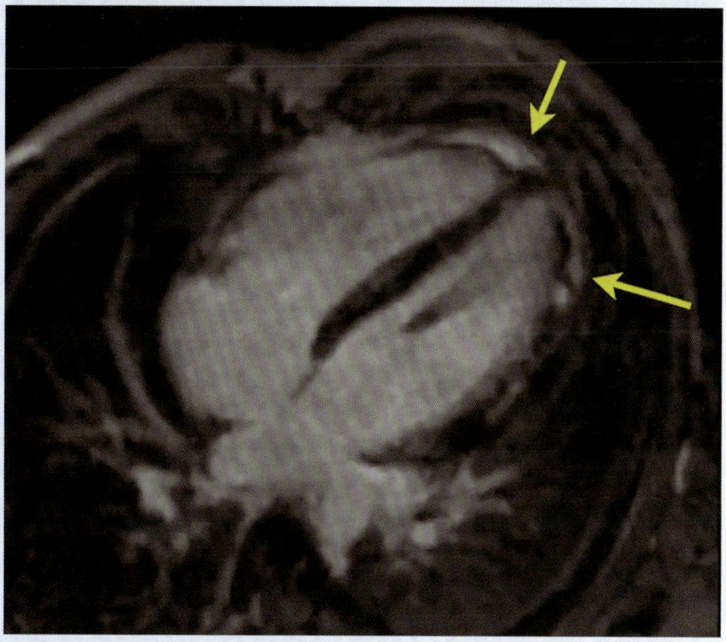

FIGURE 8.17 Four-chamber view of the MRI showing the pericardial inflammation and the subepicardial location of the myocardial edema (*yellow arrows*) consistent with myopericarditis.

SECTION 6

PLEURAL EFFUSIONS

Initial views from the parasternal views can uncover left pleural effusions. When such is visualized, it sometimes is appropriate to move to the posterior chest both left and right to assess for pleural effusion. This can be clinically helpful and is easy to perform if the patient can sit upright.

Correctly separating out pericardial effusion from pleural effusion is important. Remembering that the pericardium reflects onto the pulmonary veins anterior to the aorta identifies fluid in the pericardial space. Fluid that extends posterior to the aorta is likely pleural fluid. This is an important distinction and can be separated out by the echocardiogram.

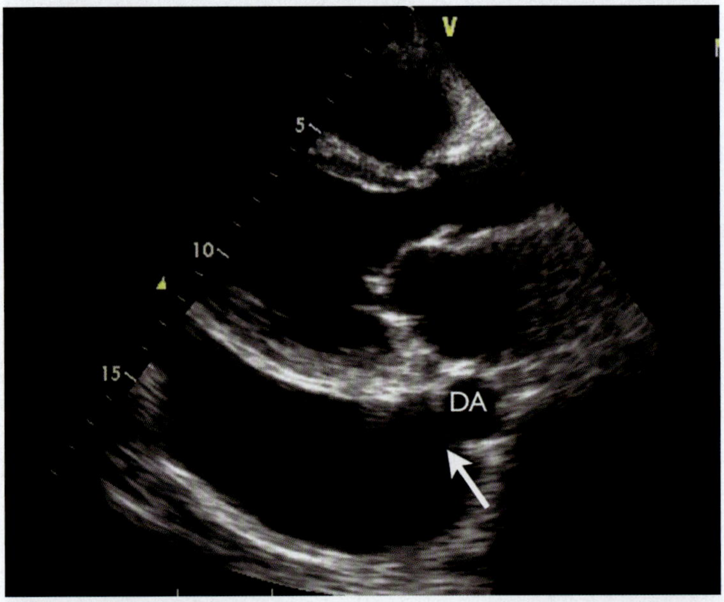

FIGURE 8.18 Posterior to the heart, there is a large accumulation of fluid. It is behind the left ventricle and extends posterior to the descending aorta (*DA*). Pleural effusions extend posterior to the descending aorta (*white arrow*) and pericardial effusions do not. TTE, PLX view.

SECTION 7

ADJACENT STRUCTURES

When examining the heart with ultrasound, the sonographer carefully interrogates the heart from all of the standard views. We look carefully at the sectors that are obtainable and analyze the images in those views. On occasion, there are structures that are visible outside of the usual views that are obtained. We usually extend the depth in the first parasternal views to evaluate for pleural effusion and then reduce the depth to include the posterior wall and pericardium. In other windows of examination such as the subcostal views, the liver is in clear view, and abnormalities such as cysts or solid metastasis are visible. Other areas adjacent to the cardiac chambers are visible such as solid tumors in the chest or mediastinum or solid tumors compressing the atria. When signals to such abnormalities are present, then the transducer can be manipulated in that direction to further define the abnormality.

Placing the transducer in other windows is also possible such as in the left posterior chest. This gives an assessment of a pleural effusion if present and even allows visualization of the heart when the effusion is large. So sometimes it is indicated to "view outside the box" so to speak and interrogate questionable structures around the heart. Although a definitive answer may not be available from ultrasound alone, clues to the need for additional imaging with CT or CMRI can be obtained.

An example of such imaging and the associated MRI images are illustrated on the following pages.

MEDIASTINAL TUMORS—HODGKIN LYMPHOMA

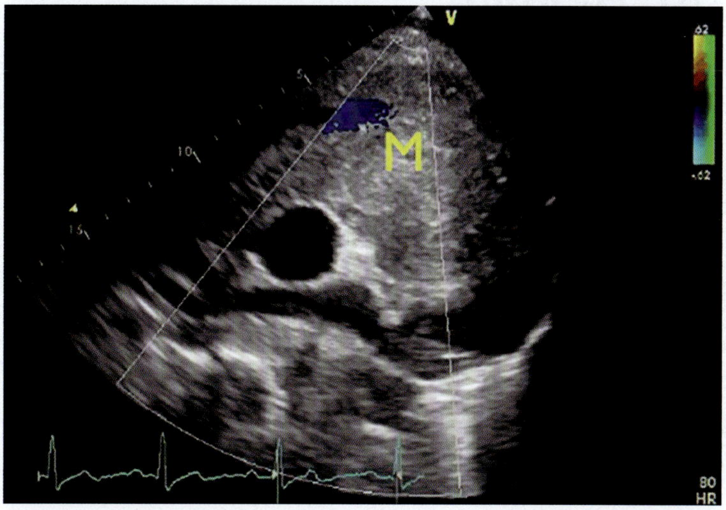

FIGURE 8.19 An even higher cross-sectional view at the level of the bifurcation of the pulmonary artery; the large mass (*M*) is seen to compress these structures. TTE, high cross-sectional view.

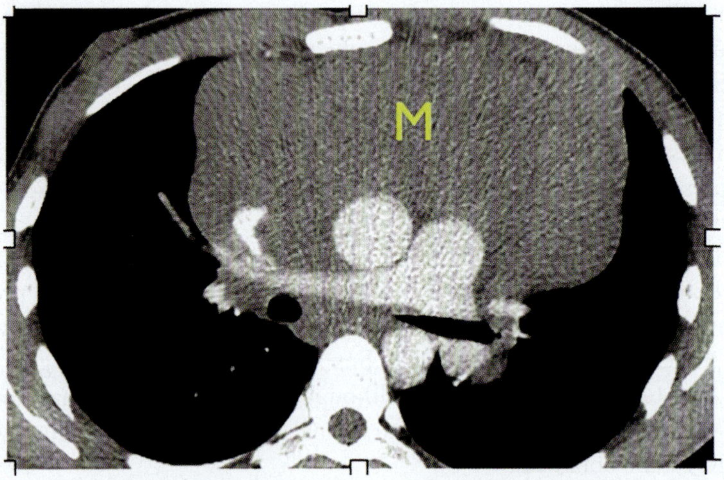

FIGURE 8.20 CT from a similar view as noted above on echo shows the solid consistency of this tumor (*M*) in the anterior mediastinum (Hodgkin lymphoma).

SECTION 8

HIATAL HERNIA

Ordinarily, one would not think of diagnosing a hiatal hernia by echocardiography. The esophagus is posterior to the left atrium and sometimes the right atrium. This can be a portion of the stomach with the esophageal-gastric region above the diaphragm (sliding hiatal hernia) or a portion of the stomach herniated alongside the esophagus above the diaphragm (paraesophageal hernia).

These structures may or may not be visible with ultrasound. If the structure is fluid filled, then it may have a masslike appearance, and if there is some air in this area, it can have a mixed appearance. By waiting a short period for peristalsis to take place, the structure may change—a clue to this area being part of the gastrointestinal tract.

A careful look at this area posterior to the heart can allow for correct identification of the structure and avoid alarm. An example of a hiatal hernia is in the following pages as it was viewed on echocardiography and then CMRI.

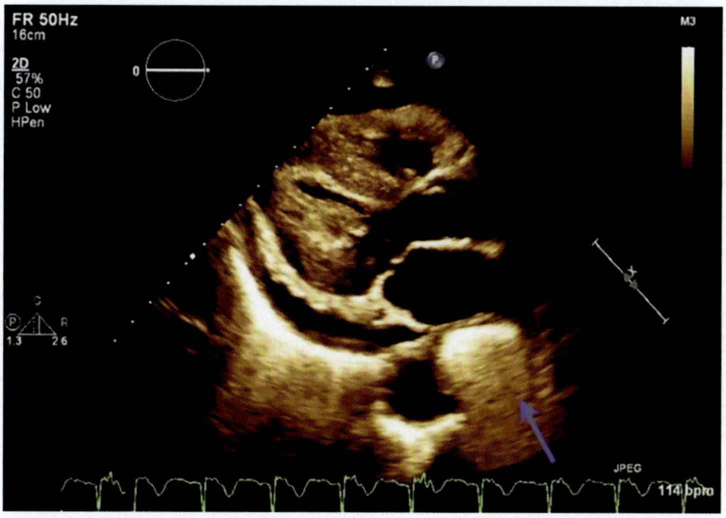

FIGURE 8.21 The images being prepared for the sip of carbonated beverage. The mass is posterior to and indenting the left atrium (*blue arrow*). It is just adjacent to the descending aorta. This image was done as a sip of ginger ale was given resulting in the "mass" lighting up with echogenic microbubbles. TEE, PLX view.

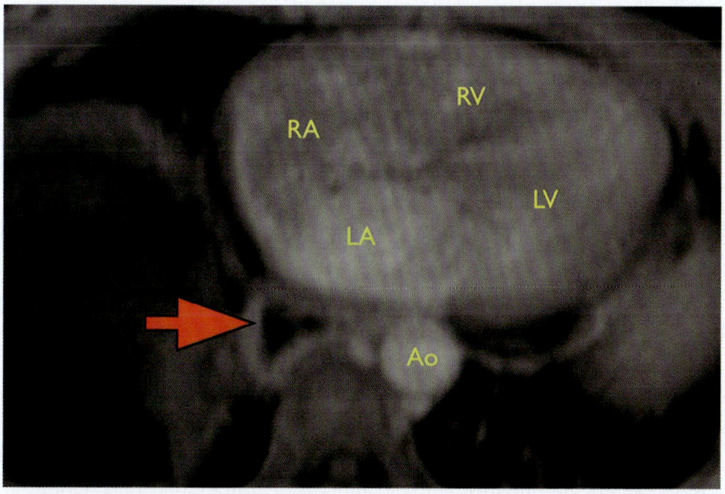

FIGURE 8.22 The MRI done for evaluation of the liver and portal circulation shows the cardiac silhouette and the air-filled esophagus posterior to the left atrium. Historically, the indentation of the left atrium on a barium-filled esophagus was used for assessment of left atrial size. In this situation, when there is a sliding hiatal hernia and the esophagus or herniated stomach is filled with solid or liquid, it can mimic a mass posterior to the heart. A small sip of carbonated drink can result in echogenic microbubbles that cause the contents of the esophagus to "light up" and differentiates the hiatal hernia from a solid and possibly malignant mass. LA, left atrium; LV, left ventricle; RA, right atrium; RV, right ventricle and Ao represents descending aorta. *Red arrow* points to herniated stomach.

REFERENCES

1. Lang RM, Goldstein SA, Kronzon I, Khandheria BK, Mor-Avi V. *ASE's Comprehensive Echocardiography*. 2nd ed. Philadelphia, PA: Elsevier (Saunders); 2016:593-613.
2. Spodick DH. *The Pericardium: A Comprehensive Textbook*. New York, NY: Marcel Dekker; 1997.
3. Horowitz MS, Schultz CS, Stinson EB, Harrison DC, Popp RL. Sensitivity and specificity of echocardiographic diagnosis of pericardial effusion. *Circulation*. 1974;50:239-247.
4. Singh S, Wann LS, Suchard GH, et al. Right ventricular and right atrial collapse in patients with cardiac tamponade—a combined echocardiographic and hemodynamic study. *Circulation*. 1984;70:966-971.
5. Gillam LD, Guyer DE, Gibson TC, King ME, Marchall JE, Weyman AE. Hydrodynamic compression of the right atrium: a new echocardiographic sign of cardiac tamponade. *Circulation*. 1983;68:294-301.
6. Munt BI, Moss RR, Erewal J. Pericardial disease. In: Otto CM, ed. *The Precise of Clinical Echocardiography*. 4th ed. Philadelphia, PA: Elsevier (Saunders); 2011:565-578.
7. Spodick DH. Acute cardiac tamponade. *N Engl J Med*. 2003;349:684-690.
8. Ariyaraja V, Spodick DH. Cardiac tamponade revisited: a postmortem look at a cautionary case. *Tex Heart Inst J*. 2007;34:347-351.
9. Kronzon I, Cohen ML, Winer HE. Cardiac tamponade by loculated pericardial hematoma: limitations of M-mode echocardiography. *J Am Coll Cardiol*. 1983;1:913-915.
10. Lang RM, Goldstein SA, Kronzon I, Khandheria BK, Mor-Avi V. *ASE's Comprehensive Echocardiography*. 2nd ed. Philadelphia, PA: Elsevier (Saunders); 2016:602.
11. Krueger SK, Zucker RP, Dzidzio BS, Forker AD. Swinging heart syndrome with predominant anterior pericardial effusion. *J Clin Ultrasound*. 1976;4:113.
12. Lang RM, Goldstein SA, Kronzon I, Khandheria BK, Mor-Avi V. *ASE's Comprehensive Echocardiography*. 2nd ed. Philadelphia, PA: Elsevier (Saunders); 2016:602-607.
13. Leeman DE, Levine MJ, Come PC. Doppler echocardiography in cardiac tamponade: exaggerated respiratory variation in transvalvular blood flow velocity integrals. *J Am Coll Cardiol*. 1988;11:572-578.
14. Hoit BD, Shaw D. The paradoxical pulse in tamponade: mechanisms and echocardiographic correlates. *Echocardiography*. 1994;11:477-487.
15. Lang RM, Goldstein SA, Kronzon I, Khandheria BK, Mor-Avi V. *ASE's Comprehensive Echocardiography*. 2nd ed. Philadelphia, PA: Elsevier (Saunders); 2016:607-613.
16. Ha, JW, Oh JK, Ling LH, Nishimura RA, Seward JB, Tajik J. Annulus Paradoxus. Transmittal flow velocity to mitral annular velocity ratio is inversely proportional to pulmonary capillary wedge pressure in patients with constrictive pericarditis. *Circulation*. 2001;104:976-978.
17. Asher CR, Klein AL. Diastolic heart failure: restrictive cardiomyopathy, constrictive pericarditis, and cardiac tamponade: clinical and echocardiographic evaluation. *Cardiol Rev*. 2002;10:218-229.
18. Talreja DR, Nishimura RA, Oh JK, Holmes DR. Constrictive pericarditis in the modern era: novel criteria for the diagnosis in the cardiac catheterization laboratory. *J Am Coll Cardiol*. 2008;51:314-319.

9

Neoplasms and the Heart

SECTION 1

CLASSIFICATION OF NEOPLASMS OF THE HEART

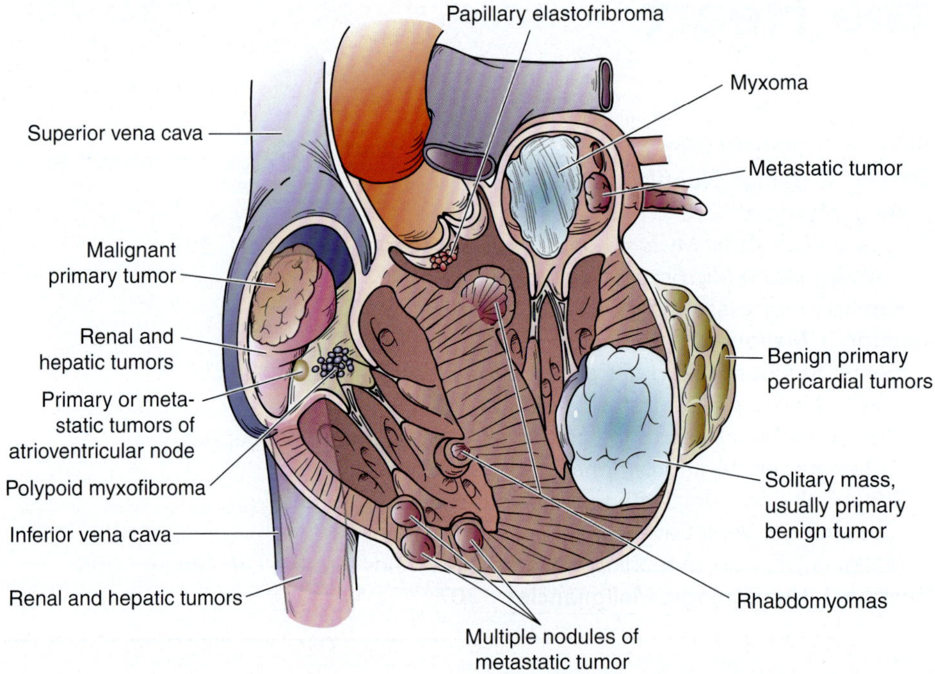

FIGURE 9.1 Patterns of involvement of the heart and pericardium by primary and secondary tumors. (Adapted from Buja LM. Cardiac tumors. In: Willerson JT, Sanders CA, eds. *Clinical Cardiology (The Science and Practice of Clinical Medicine)*. New York, NY: Grune & Stratton; 1977:400-404.)

- Primary benign neoplasms of the heart
  - Atrial myxomas
  - Papillary fibroelastomas
- Primary malignant neoplasms of the heart
  - Angiosarcoma
  - Rhabdomyosarcoma
  - Fibrosarcoma
  - Leiomyosarcoma
- Metastatic neoplasms of the heart
  - Carcinoma
  - Sarcoma
  - Hematologic malignancies
    - Leukemia
    - Lymphoma
    - Myeloma

SECTION 2

BENIGN NEOPLASMS

Numerous types of benign neoplasms can have their origin in the heart. Myxomas and papillary fibroelastomas account for the majority of these abnormalities. Additionally and less commonly, there are lipomas, fibromas, hemangiomas, and rhabdomyomas. The incidence of these neoplasms varies from children to adults with children more commonly having rhabdomyomas and fibromas. In contrast to those in adults, these neoplasms often occur in the myocardium and either have a mass effect or are arrhythmogenic.

This section illustrates myxomas and papillary fibroelastomas. Some of these images have been used in other sections but also fit well in this section of neoplasms of the heart.

ATRIAL MYXOMA

Atrial myxoma is a benign tumor of the heart and is one of the most discussed abnormalities in cardiology. Myxomas are common topics on teaching rounds, medical conferences, textbooks, and board examinations. They have a wide variety of clinical manifestations, physical findings, and appearances on various imaging techniques. The clinical manifestations vary from fever anemia and high sedimentation rate to diastolic rumbles and "tumor plops." The common ones are embolization and symptoms due to valve obstruction. A diastolic rumble and symptoms of exercise-induced shortness of breath as seen in mitral stenosis can be mimicked by large atrial myxomas. A diastolic rumble can be present with valve obstruction as seen in rheumatic valve stenosis, but in the case of a myxoma, a "tumor plop" is substituted for an opening snap especially when it is a left-sided tumor. Today, hearing such a sound is a rare occurrence since these tumors are often discovered earlier in the course of their natural history. "Tumor plops" are generally of a lower pitch than opening snaps.

Imaging techniques have moved the discovery of atrial myxomas earlier in their natural history. Echocardiography has played a major role in early discovery of myxoma, thus leading to resection before the dreaded embolic consequences have occurred. Computerized tomography (CT) and cardiac magnetic resonance imaging (CMRI) have also played a role in the early diagnosis of myxoma. CT scans with contrast for abnormalities such as pulmonary embolus can uncover left atrial myxomas as will be illustrated later. CMRI also has the same potential to discover these masses early in their course. Even coronary arteriography has the potential to discover an unusual coronary artery leading to a "tumor blush" with motion suggesting that is a myxoma.

Atrial myxomas have some unusual characteristics under the microscope. They contain lots of myxoid tissue and few cells. Myxomas have an endocardial lining and underneath have scarce myxoma cells that have a propensity to congregate around vascular tissue within the tumor. They have venous lake–like areas that empty into the surrounding chamber. This phenomenon can be seen in one of the following illustrations.

Large Left Atrial Myxoma on 2D and 3D Echocardiography

Determining the site of origin of the tumor is important for the surgeon. The use of 2D and 3D imaging can reveal the origin especially if the myxoma has a pedicle. Surgeons are very familiar with these sites of origin. Identification of the site of origin by imaging techniques gives the surgeon the best opportunity for complete removal.

In this example on 3D, one can see the pedicle of the myxoma tugging on the atrial septum in the region near the aorta.

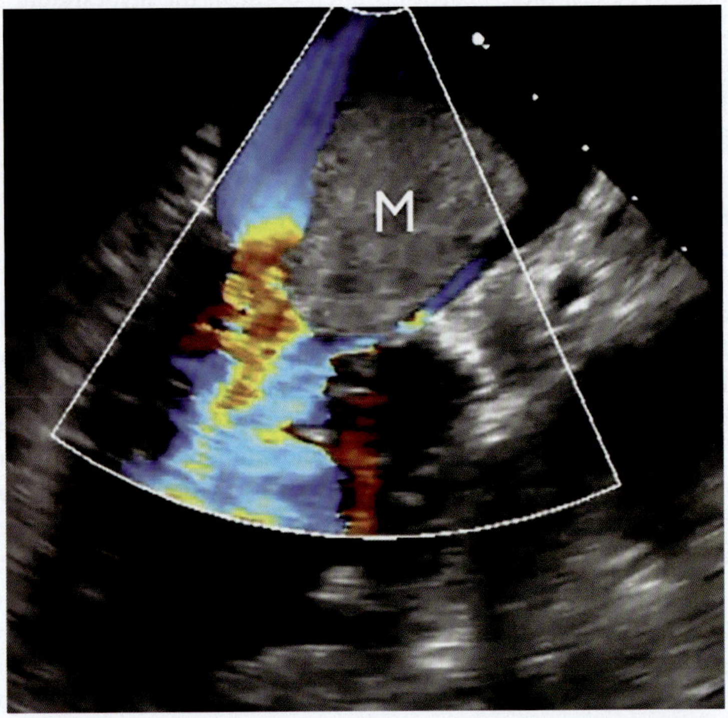

FIGURE 9.2 LA myxoma demonstrated as it partially obstructs the MV orifice in diastole. Repeated pounding of the tumor on the mitral valve can cause damage—this has been called "wrecking ball effect." M, myxoma. TEE, 114° view with color Doppler.

Myxomas on Microscopic View

Under the microscope, myxomas have a characteristic appearance. The dominant feature is the myxoid tissue that has interspersed a scant number of spindlelike myxoma cells. Additionally, there are large venous sinusoidlike vessels that exit to the chamber of origin. Around these vascular structures, the myxoma cells congregate in a halolike fashion in the perivascular region. The junction of the tumor itself and usually the adjacent atrial wall is well defined microscopically with no invasion of that adjacent tissue. The principles of removal of myxoma is to remove the origin of the base of the tumor—that is remove the wall of the atrium from which it arose. The other principle is to carefully remove the tumor intact, thus avoiding fragmentation and subsequent embolization of myxoma tissue.

The microscopic appearance of these tumors is shown in Figure 9.3.

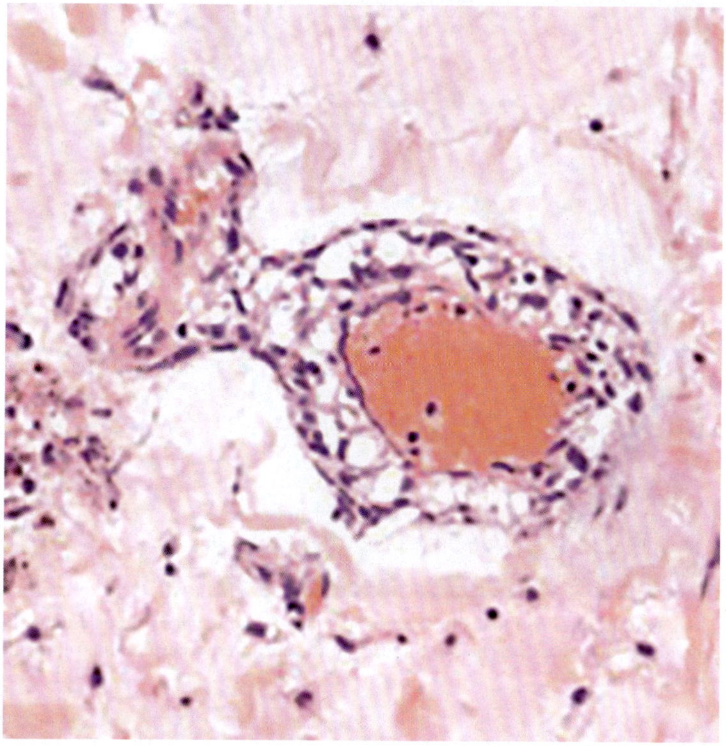

FIGURE 9.3 A halo of myxoma cells surrounding a vessel.

PAPILLARY FIBROELASTOMA

These benign tumors are small and usually attached to the aortic valve most commonly but sometimes attached to the mitral valve and rarely in other areas of the heart. They usually have a stalk and therefore have some mobility. Most commonly, they are single; however, as in the following example, they may be multiple. Under the microscope, they have a characteristic appearance described as a "sea anemone" in that they have hyaline material lined with endothelium. These do have embolic potential that comes to mind when these small tumors are visualized on echocardiography and have been removed surgically when this has occurred.

The following illustrations demonstrate one of these tumors at postmortem examination and one that was discovered as part of an evaluation for hypertrophic cardiomyopathy. The example of the mitral valve had embolized to the retina and was subsequently removed.[1]

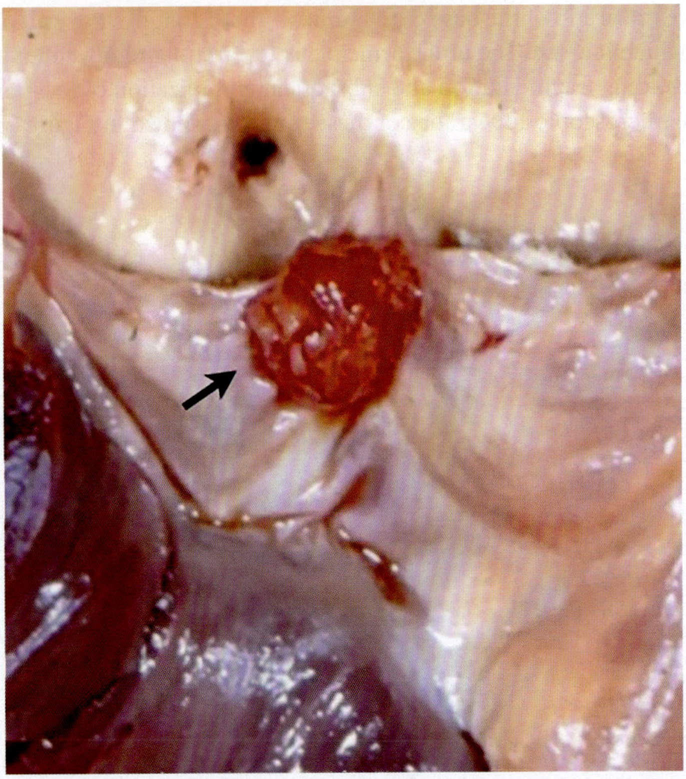

FIGURE 9.4 An autopsy specimen that shows an incidentally found papillary fibroelastoma. It appears as a small rounded multilobulated mass attached to the edge of the aortic valve cusp on the ventricular side of the valve (*black arrow*).

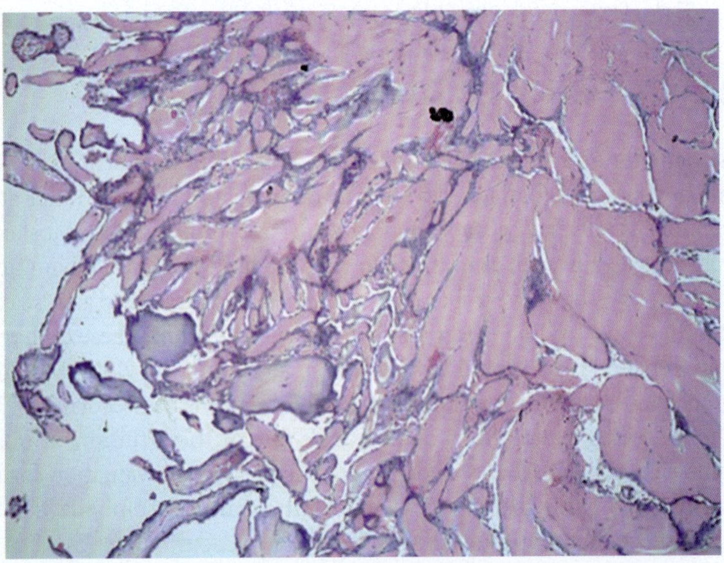

FIGURE 9.5 Microscopic view of the above papillary fibroelastoma demonstrating mucopolysaccharide-rich material covered with endothelium. Sea anemone–like appearance.

SECTION 3

MALIGNANT NEOPLASMS

Early diagnosis and more effective treatment have resulted in more unusual late manifestations of the disease. Cardiac involvement with neoplasms seems more common. Treatment modalities such as chemotherapy and radiation in themselves have their own set of adverse effects. Fortunately, the most common primary neoplasms of the heart are benign (myxoma). Primary malignant neoplasms of the heart are rare with sarcoma being at the top of the list. These neoplasms are aggressive and difficult to treat.

Secondary or metastatic neoplasms spread to the heart in four different pathways: through the blood or the hematogenous route, lymphatic spread, transvenous extension, and direct extension. Hematogenous spread results in myocardial or endocardial metastasis as seen with melanoma, lymphoma, and sarcoma. Lymphatic spread occurs as seen with tumors nearby in the lung or breast and results in pericardial and epicardial involvement. Renal and hepatic tumors metastasize by transvenous extension up to the vena cava into the right atrium or in the case of lung cancer through the pulmonary veins. Mesothelioma of the pleura, mediastinum, and pericardium undergo direct extension into the pericardial sac. Hematologic malignancies, leukemia, and lymphoma can appear in the heart. Large numbers of leukemic cells can become stagnant and create masslike areas in the heart. Lymphomas can shed tumor fragments that become lodged in various areas of the heart.

Cancer tends to metastasize to certain anatomic areas more than to others. The pericardium is the most common site for metastasis followed by the epicardium and the endocardium. Melanoma as a tumor has the strongest propensity to metastasize to the heart. Lung and breast tumors are more common in the population and are most often found involving the heart at postmortem examination.[2,3]

Neoplasms involving the heart are often discovered by echocardiography. Other modalities such as computerized tomography (CT) and cardiac magnetic imaging (CMRI) are used for surveillance, often uncovering cardiac metastasis from malignant tumors. Once discovered, these cardiac metastases are often limiting factors and are difficult to treat.

In addition, cancer treatments themselves to include radiation and chemotherapy can result in damage to various parts of the heart. Echocardiography offers monitoring opportunities of the effects of adriamycin, herceptin, and other agents. Serial ejection fraction measurements and, more recently, strain measurements have been studied in attempts to identify adverse effects early in the disease course. The effects of herceptin in particular can be reversible if identified early. Not only can systole be monitored but diastole also has been under investigation as a marker of early myocardial dysfunction in those undergoing treatment for cancer. The long-term effects of radiation on valves and the atherosclerotic process in coronary arteries can be assessed by echocardiography.

In the following panels, some of these findings are presented to illustrate the interaction of cancer and the heart.

HEMATOGENOUS SPREAD OF CANCER TO THE HEART: THE LEFT VENTRICLE WITH MYOCARDIAL METASTASIS

Each of these examples illustrates the tendency of malignancies to spread to the heart by way of the coronary circulation. Diffuse widespread nodular metastasis is found throughout the myocardium.

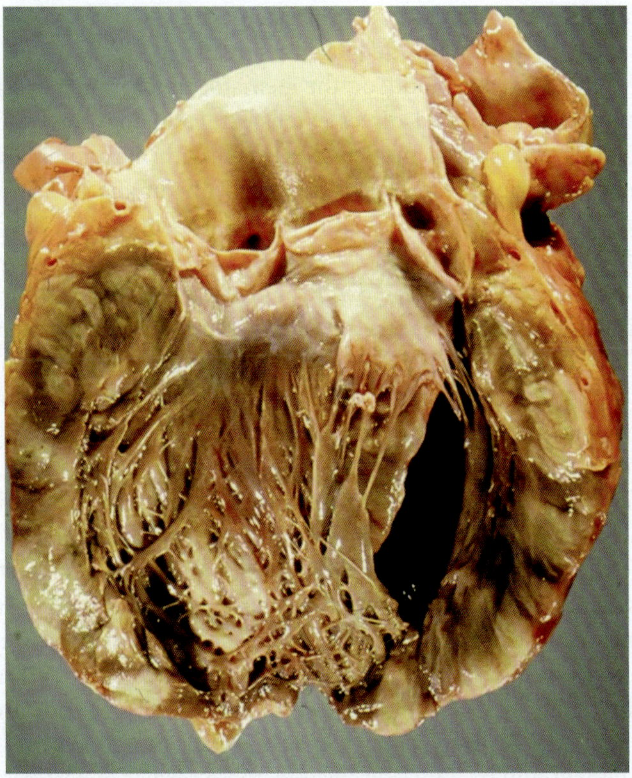

FIGURE 9.6 Histiocytoma metastatic to the left ventricle.

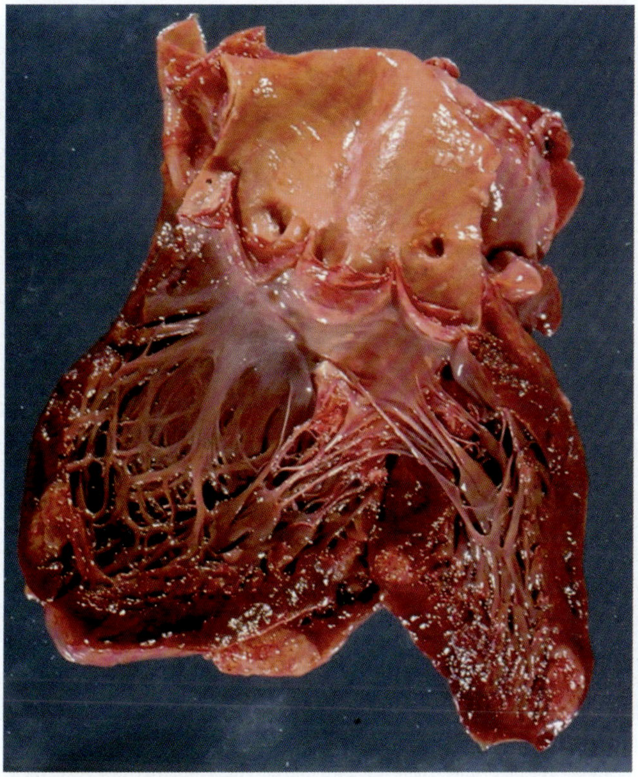

FIGURE 9.7 Lung cancer metastatic to the left ventricle.

CASE PRESENTATION

Metastatic Sarcoma to the Left Ventricular Endocardium and Almost Obstructing the Left Ventricular Outflow Tract, Hematogenous Spread Endocardial Metastasis

This gentleman, ~40 years old, had a known sarcoma and despite treatment developed this endocardial metastasis. He did receive radiation but experienced sudden cardiac death shortly after these images.

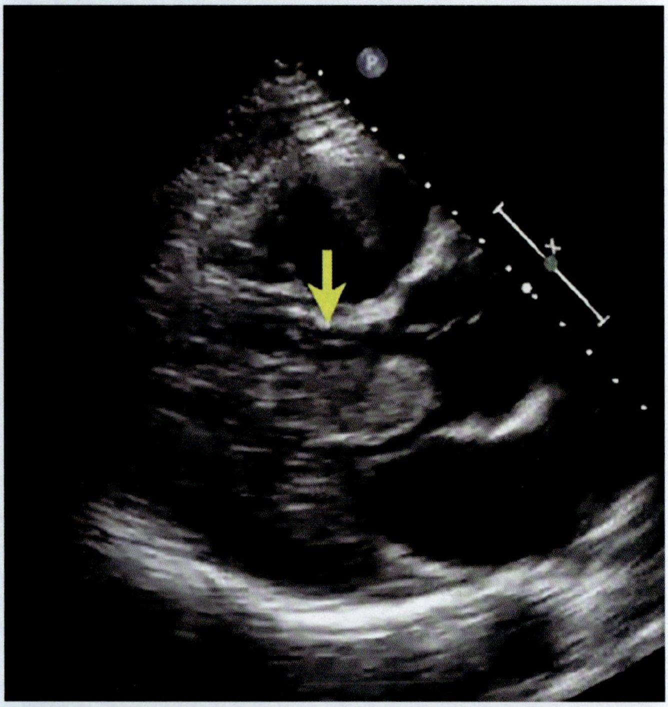

FIGURE 9.8 Metastatic sarcoma noted in the left ventricle and arising from the endocardium, approaching and nearly obstructing the LVOT (*yellow arrow*). There was a 40–mm Hg gradient across the LVOT. Micro of the above tumor shows nuclei of multiple types and shapes and chromatin variability. From Okene E, Parikh A, Clay M, Williams R III, Clements SD. Metastatic sarcoma: a rare case of left ventricular outflow tract obstruction. *J Heart Cardiol.* 2015;1(1):1-2.

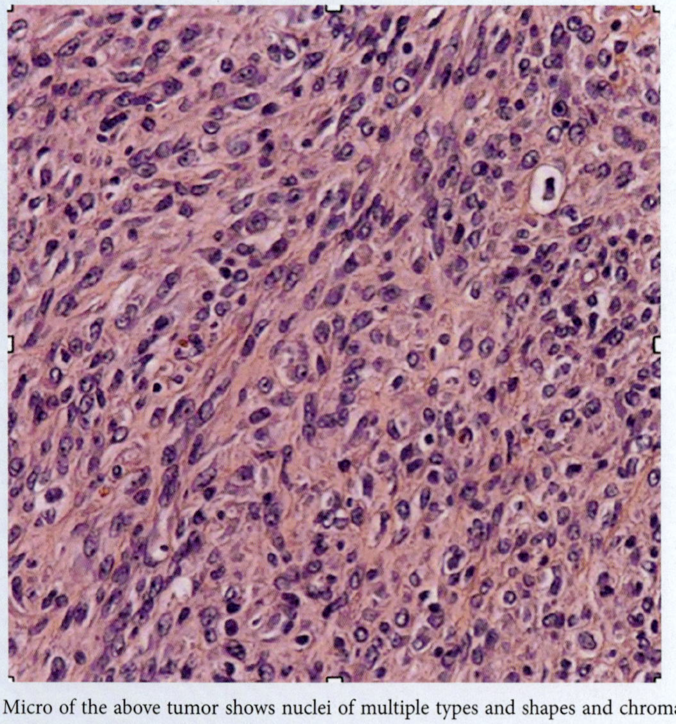

FIGURE 9.9 Micro of the above tumor shows nuclei of multiple types and shapes and chromatin variability. From Okene E, Parikh A, Clay M, Williams R III, Clements SD. Metastatic sarcoma: a rare case of left ventricular outflow tract obstruction. *J Heart Cardiol.* 2015;1(1):1-2.

MELANOMA METASTATIC TO THE LEFT ATRIAL WALL AND INTERATRIAL SEPTUM, HEMATOGENOUS AND LYMPHATIC SPREAD

Melanoma is a tumor that knows no boundaries. Additionally, the primary tumor may be in the skin or other places and be many times smaller than the metastasis. It is the tumor that has the strongest propensity to metastasize to the heart. It may choose the pericardium, endocardium, or myocardium in that order. Treatment is difficult, but some progress has been made in recent years.

The following illustration is that of an individual who has pericardial effusion implying metastasis there and also within the wall of the atria producing a masslike effect. This tumor involves the interatrial septum and the wall of the left atrium.

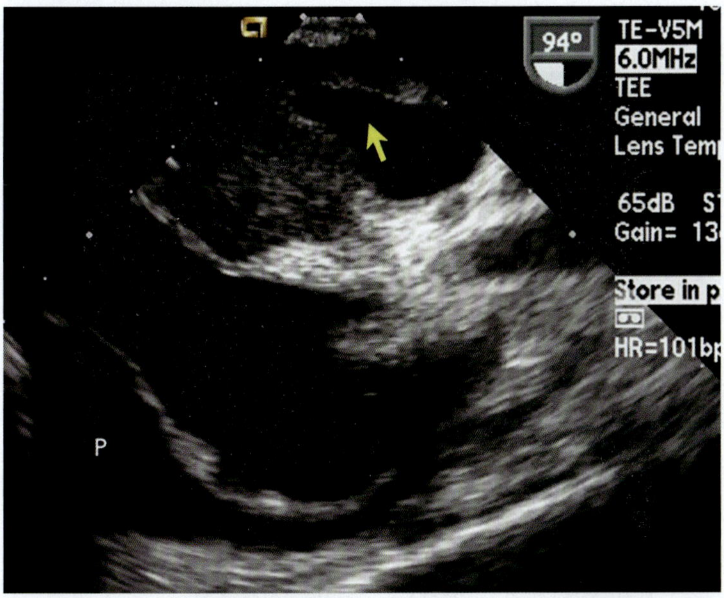

FIGURE 9.10 Additional TEE views show the tumor involving the interatrial septum and wrapping around (*yellow arrow*) the posterior wall of the left atrium. In addition, there is a pericardial effusion anterior to the right atrial appendage. PE, pericardial effusion. TEE, 94° view.

Melanoma can metastasize anywhere, and of all tumors that metastasize to the heart, melanoma does this most commonly. Breast and lung metastasis are the most commonly found cancers in the heart because of their overall higher frequency in the general population. However, melanoma, while less common, has the greatest tendency to metastasize to the heart.

RENAL CELL CARCINOMA WITH EXTENSION TO THE RIGHT ATRIUM FROM THE INFERIOR VENA CAVA

Renal cell carcinoma is the most common tumor to have metastasis to the heart by way of invading and growing up the inferior vena cava. When these tumors are visualized by echocardiography, the first diagnosis on the differential list is benign right atrial myxoma. Once a stalk is searched for unsuccessfully and the inferior vena cava is investigated, the answer becomes more obvious. A right atrial mass and an inferior vena cava filled with tumor put renal cell carcinoma with vena cava and right atrial extension on top of the list. Other tumors can do this including hepatic cell carcinomas and rarely pelvic tumors. Once the diagnosis is established, the surgical approach is needed, and urologic surgeons elicit the help of the cardiac surgeons for a combined approach.

Examples of these large tumors that spread by invasion of large veins and extent to the heart follow.

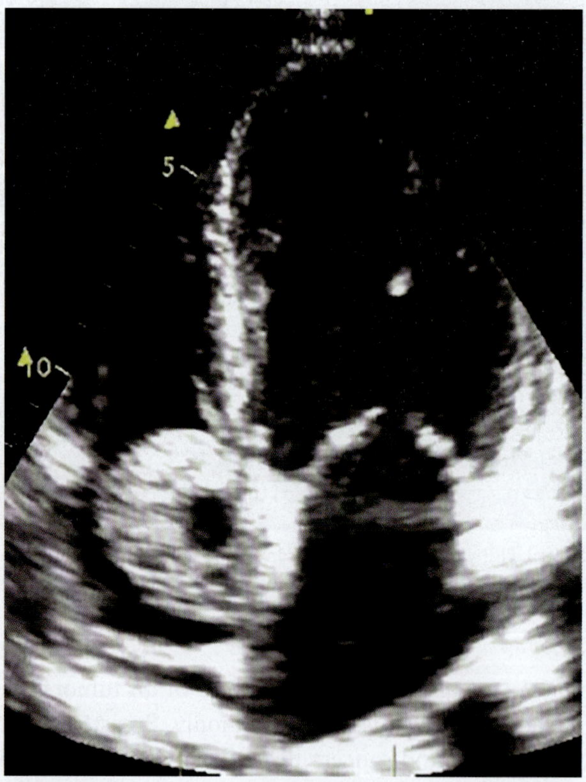

FIGURE 9.11 Right atrium filled with a rounded mass without a well-defined attachment. The central hypoechoic area could be vascularity or a large area of necrosis. A4C view.

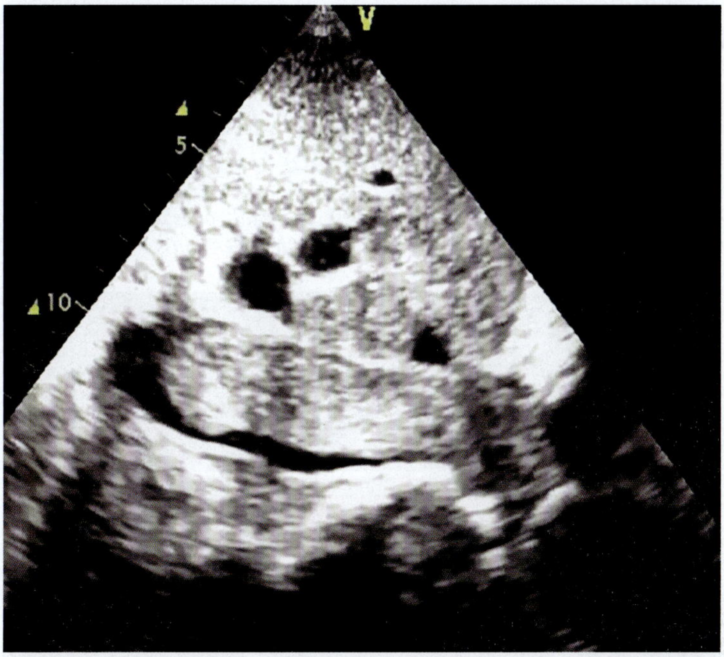

FIGURE 9.12 An important part of evaluation of a right atrial mass is to view the inferior vena cava as shown here in this patient. The cava is filled with tumor coming from below and extending into the right atrium. This information now suggests that this is a tumor extending from below. If originating from the renal vein, it is most often renal cell carcinoma. TTE, subcostal view.

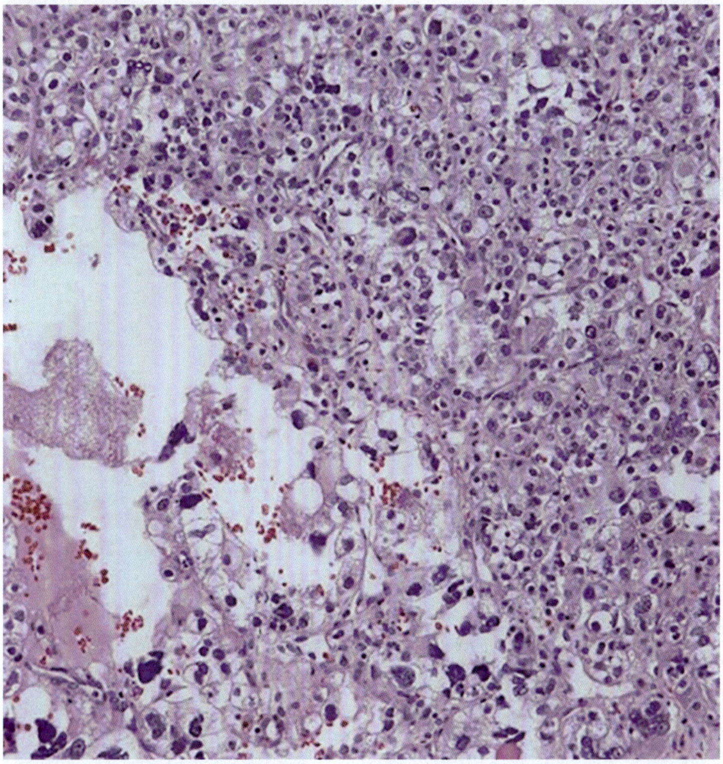

FIGURE 9.13 Microscopic view of this tumor showing clear cells and Fuhrman nuclear grade 4 changes. This vascular invasion led to the tumor progressing up the vena cava to the right atrium.

CASE PRESENTATION

Renal Cell Carcinoma Metastatic to the Right atrium With Near-Total Obstruction of the Inferior Vena Cava (CMRI Images)

A 67-year-old lady presented with shortness of breath on exertion, edema of the lower extremities, and fatigue. She was found to have a large RA mass.

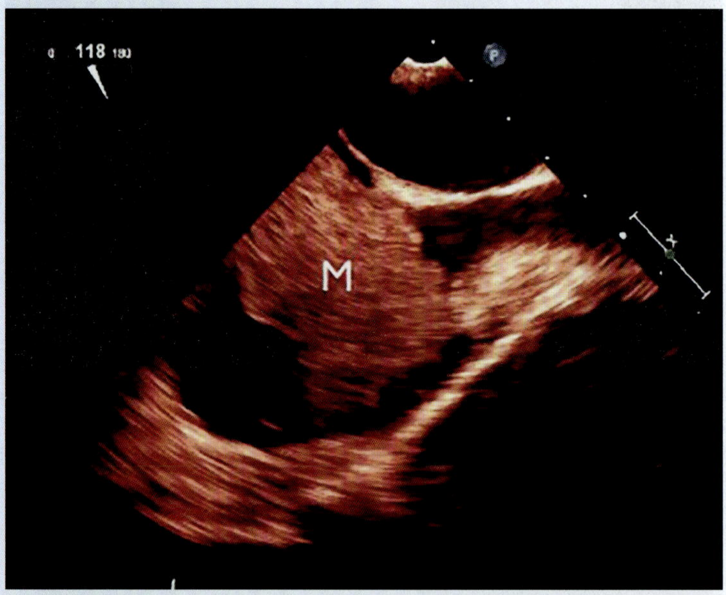

FIGURE 9.14 The large mass from the SVC-IVC view showing that it comes from the IVC. M, mass. TTE, 118° view.

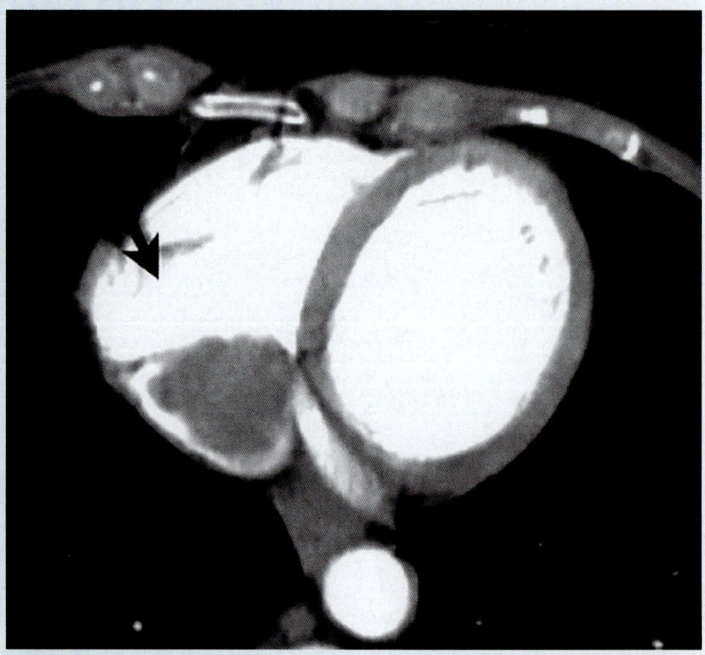

FIGURE 9.15 CT scan with dense contrast opacification of all chambers showing the tumor in the right atrium (*black arrow*).

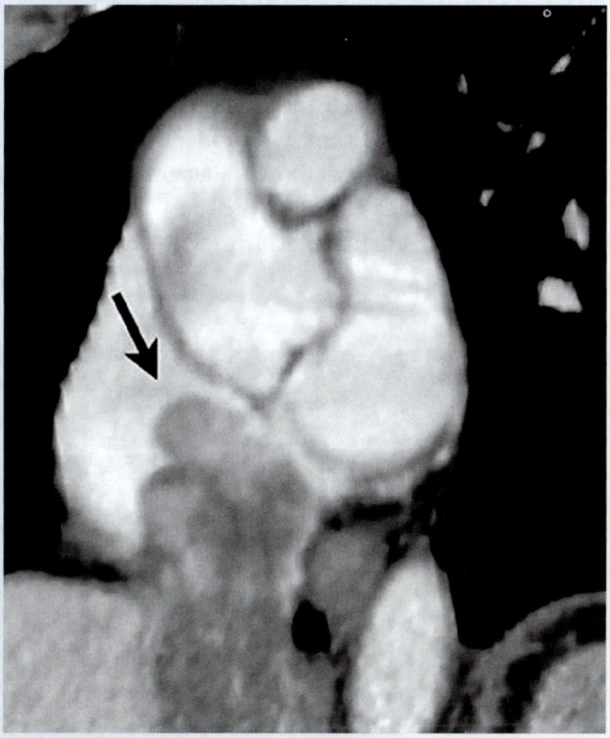

FIGURE 9.16 A lateral view of the heart on CT showing the multilobulated tumor extending up into the right atrium from the IVC (*black arrow*).

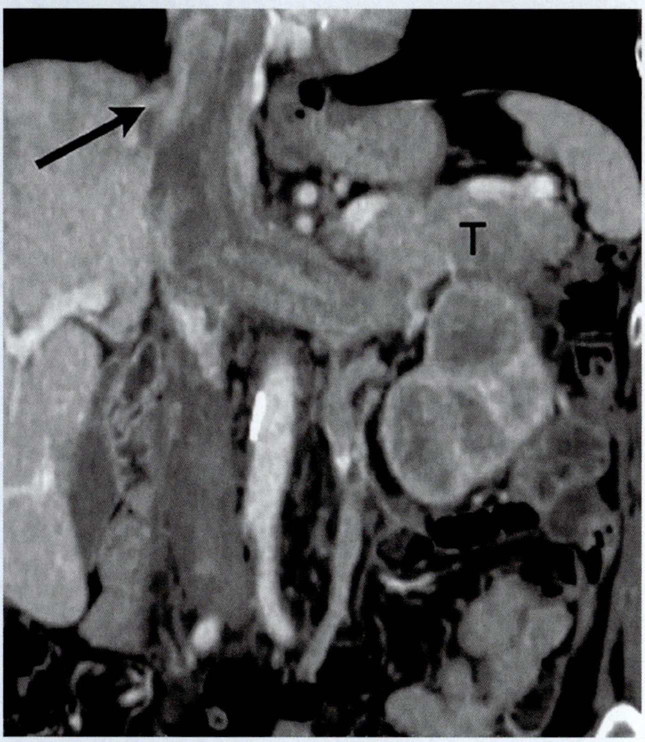

FIGURE 9.17 Frontal view of the CT showing the renal tumor (*T*) as it extends up the IVC to the right atrium (*black arrow*).

MALIGNANT TUMORS EXTENDING VIA PULMONARY VEINS INTO THE LEFT ATRIUM

Malignant tumors in the lung can extend via the pulmonary into the left atrium. The most common tumors are primary tumors of the adjacent lungs. Lung and breast cancer are on top of the list as tumors that are found involving the heart in one manner or another because they are the most common tumors. The tumor that has the greatest propensity to metastasize to the heart is melanoma with sarcoma being a close second.[4]

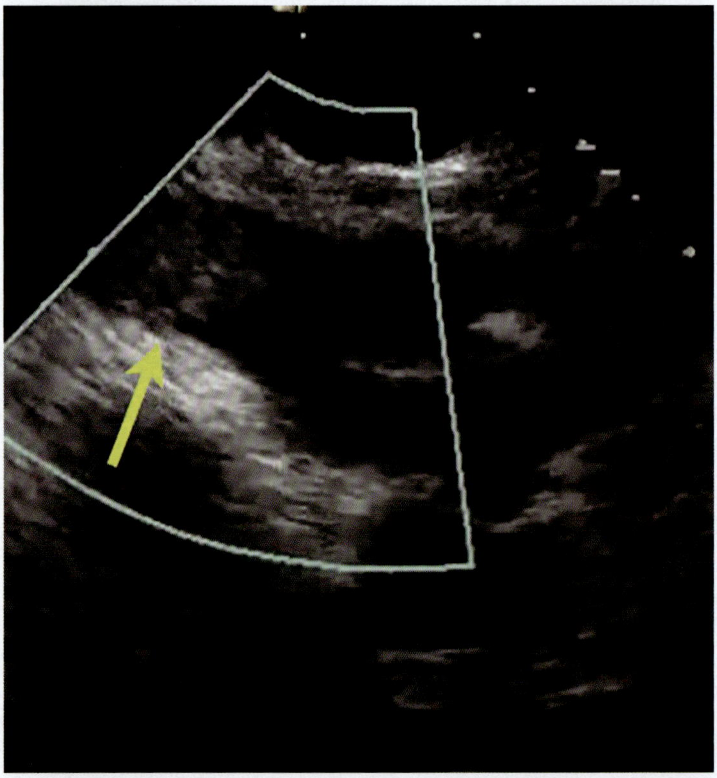

FIGURE 9.18 TEE demonstrates a pulmonary vein with a tumor mass (*yellow arrow*) extending to the left atrium. TEE, 27° view.

SECTION 4

HEMATOLOGIC MALIGNANCIES

CASE PRESENTATION

Plasmacytoma of the Heart[5]

A 78-year-old gentleman presented with a cardiac mass that was subsequently on myocardial biopsy and was determined to be a plasmacytoma. Chemotherapy and radiation therapy later were successful in treating this area, and it essentially disappeared. The patient had a history of a similar mass in the axillary area about 20 years before, which also had been successfully treated.

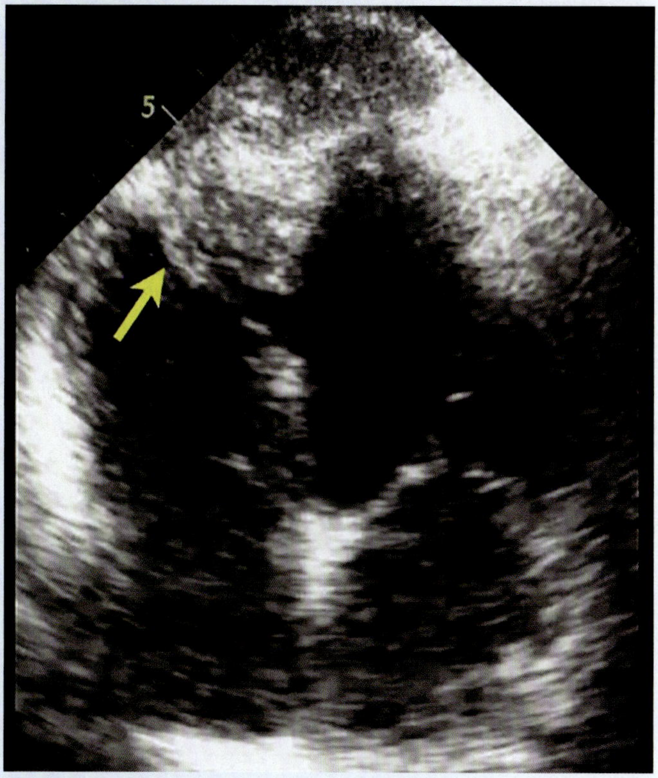

FIGURE 9.19 A rare plasmacytoma is shown above that involves the apex of both ventricles (*yellow arrow*) and the interventricular septum. TTE, A4C view.

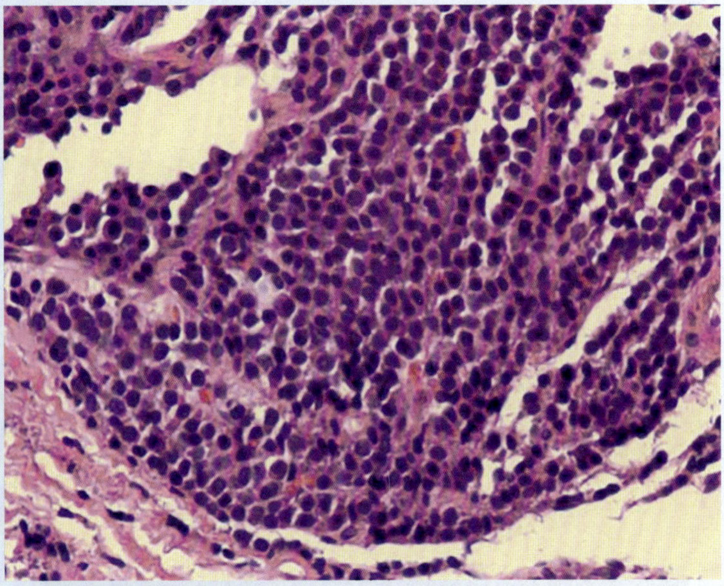

FIGURE 9.20 Microscopic view of right ventricular septal biopsy that shows clusters of plasma cells.

REFERENCES

1. Kalarich KW, Wnriquez-Sarano M, Gura GM, et al. Papillary fibroelastoma: echocardiographic characteristics for diagnosis and pathologic correlation. *J Am Coll Cardiol.* 1997;30:784-790.
2. Goldberg AD, Blankstein R, Padera RF. Tumors metastatic to the heart. *Circulation.* 2013;128:1790-1794.
3. Bussani R, De-Giorgio F, Abbate A, Silvestri F. Cardiac metastasis. *J Clin Pathol.* 2007;60(1):27-34.
4. Buja LM. The multifaceted manifestations of cardiac tumors. *Tex Heart Inst J.* 2012;39(1):84-85.
5. Vrettou AR, Heffner LT, Rossi PJ, Clements SD Jr. Cardiac plasmacytoma: a rare clinical entity. *Tex Heart Inst J.* 2014;41(5):554-557.

10

Congenital Heart Disease

SECTION 1

ECHOCARDIOGRAPHY AND CONGENITAL HEART DISEASE

Progress has been made in the diagnosis of congenital heart diseases. In the past, careful physical examination along with the electrocardiogram and the chest x-ray was the mainstay of making a preliminary diagnosis. Once this assessment was made, cardiac catheterization, hemodynamics, angiography, and analysis of complex catheter courses laid the groundwork for the cardiac surgeon.

Currently, echocardiographic techniques allow for the precise diagnosis of congenital heart diseases. This includes the location of shunts, great vessel arrangements, atrioventricular valve orientations, and many other abnormalities, all of which can be displayed on the echo screen in both two and three dimensions. Doppler assessments allow for pressure and flow calculations and shunt quantifications. Echocardiography along with CMRI have revealed so much anatomic and physiologic information that cardiac catheterization with angiography have become focused on gathering information that is missing from the diagnostic equation.

Structural heart interventions with devices for shunt closure and valve replacement have filled in the time slots in the diagnostic cardiac catheterization laboratories and have altered the procedures done by cardiac surgeons.

The specialty of adult congenital cardiology has been born from the excellent work done by pediatric cardiologists, pediatric cardiac surgeons, and adult cardiologists interested in this area, and they have allowed our patients to reach adulthood and lead normal lives.

This chapter deals with the diagnosis of congenital heart disease focusing on common, relative simple abnormalities and not dealing with very complex congenital cardiac abnormalities. For the emergency room physician, the primary care physician, and the internist to the cardiologist, the diagnosis of congenital heart disease in the adult patient is challenging. There are certain basic clues in the general examination, the electrocardiogram, and the echocardiogram that should allow the correct diagnosis to be made.

Bicuspid aortic valve is the most common congenital abnormality of the heart, and it is presented in more detail in the section on the aortic valve and aorta.

Examples of common congenital abnormalities in the young person and adult are discussed in the following pages.

SECTION 2

PATENT FORAMEN OVALE

Although bicuspid aortic valve is the most common congenital abnormality of the heart if we label patent foramen oval (PFO) as a congenital abnormality, it might be the most common. Actually, we consider PFO to be a part of our development that is incomplete and not a frank defect. In ordinary circumstances, it poses no problem, but in special situations, it can cause difficulty. In the setting of high right-sided pressures with pulmonary embolus or pulmonary hypertension from another etiology, high right atrial pressures will result in a PFO opening up and allowing right-to-left shunting. In the setting of a PFO with a relative short tunnel, simple maneuvers such as deep breathing, coughing, sneezing, and Valsalva maneuver can open the PFO and cause right-to-left shunting. This physiology comes into play in the setting of SCUBA diving when decompression difficulties occur.[1]

PFO at times can be a major factor in cryptogenic stroke. Small thrombi from the legs can migrate up the vena cava to the right atrium and in the right clinical setting can cross to the arterial circulation. The extreme of this situation is the pulmonary embolus in transit that crosses to the left circulation and causes a stroke. An additional relationship exists with PFO and migraine headaches. The incidence of migraine headaches in those who have a PFO is higher than in the general population. One explanation is that vasoactive substances bypass the lungs by crossing through the PFO producing migraine headaches by altering the vasculature of the brain.[2-4]

LARGE PATENT FORAMEN OVALE

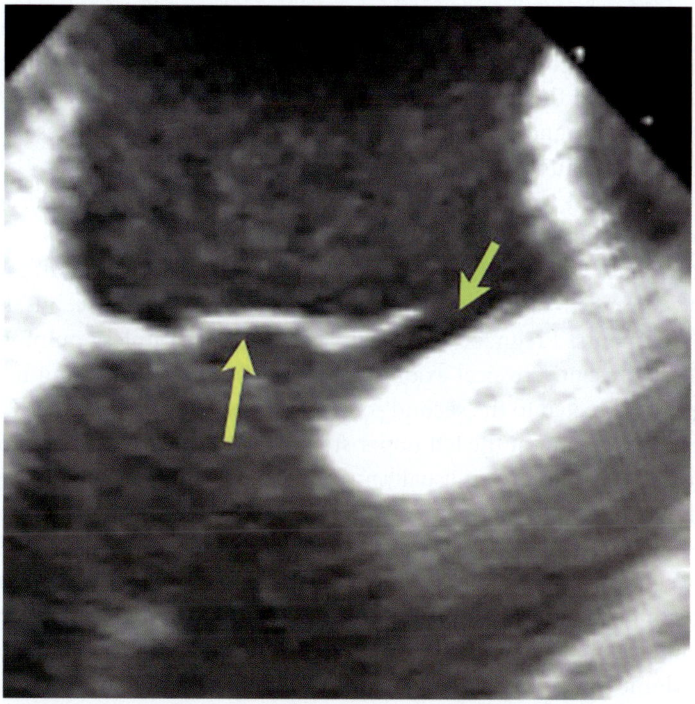

FIGURE 10.1 A freeze frame from the image above that shows the thin portion of the interatrial septum on inspiration as it shifts to the left side (*yellow arrow*) opening up the tunnel of the PFO (*green arrow*).

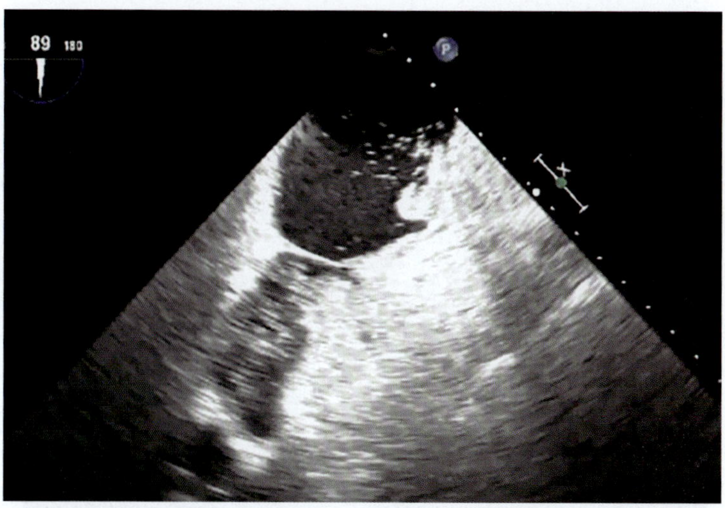

FIGURE 10.2 "Bubble study" showing a negative stream coming from the left side and then with inspiration a puff of contrast crosses from right to left. TEE, 89° view.

SECTION 3

ATRIAL SEPTAL DEFECT

OSTIUM SECUNDUM ATRIAL SEPTAL DEFECT

Ostium secundum atrial septal defects (ASDs) are the most common type of ASD. Embryologically, this defect occurs when the septum secundum does not completely cover the fenestration in the septum primum. ASDs can be of various sizes and shapes and can be multiple or can be like "Swiss cheese." They result in left-to-right shunting because of the low resistance pathway to the compliant right atrium and ventricle, and this will remain so unless the complication of pulmonary hypertension develops.

Individuals with this defect may go unrecognized until adulthood. Careful history taking will often reveal intolerance to vigorous exercise, but they are usually participants. Pregnancy is usually tolerated well unless pulmonary hypertension is present. Physical examination may not be so revealing unless careful attention is directed to the second sound uncovering fixed splitting. There may be an ejection murmur at the left upper sternal border from excessive flow.

The electrocardiogram is usually not normal and shows incomplete right bundle-branch block. In older individuals with larger ASDs, the chronic volume overload of the right atrium and ventricle results in dilated chambers and atrial fibrillation.

The echocardiogram plays a major role in making this diagnosis and defining the anatomy and physiology. The location of the defect and its relationship to the aorta and the superior and inferior vena cava and the direction and quantification of the shunt can be determined. Current therapies of these defects with closure devices all require exact definition of the size of the defect, the anatomy of the remaining interatrial septum, and the relationship to the adjacent aorta. The definition of the aortic rim is important to anchor the edges of the implanted device.[5]

Examples of secundum atrial septal defects are noted in Figures 10.3 and 10.4.

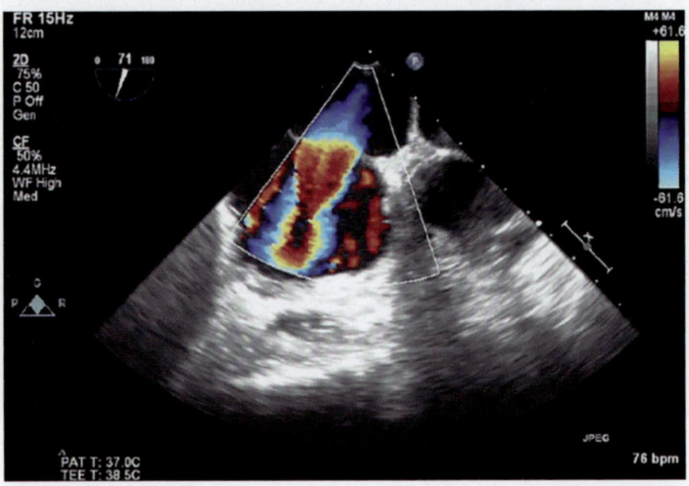

FIGURE 10.3 Flow through the secundum ASD (blue on color Doppler with aliasing in the middle of the jet).

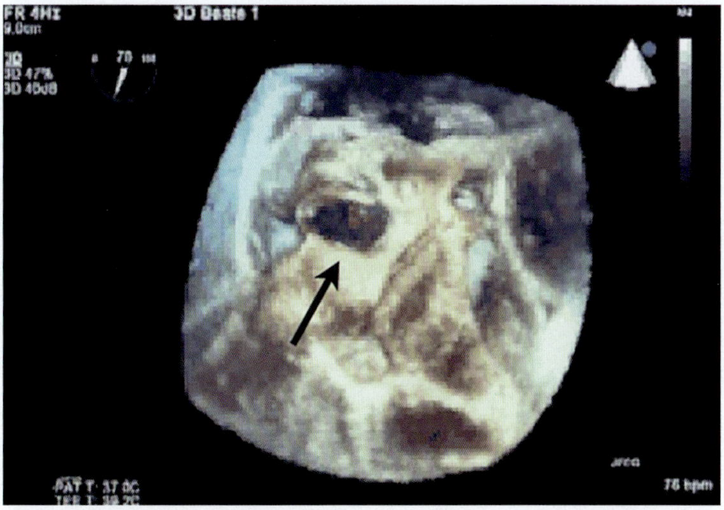

FIGURE 10.4 3D view of the defect from the left side (*black arrow*).

TEE-GUIDED CLOSURE OF A SECUNDUM ASD WITH AN AMPLATZER DEVICE

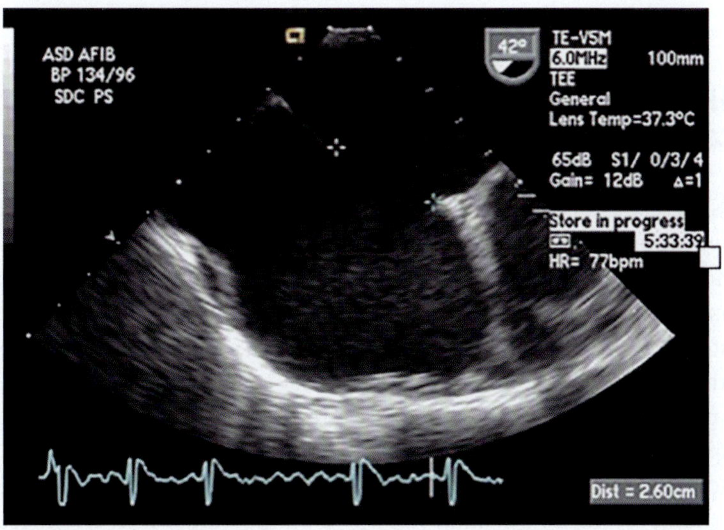

FIGURE 10.5 TEE 42° view showing the defect in the atrial septum and the aortic rim—which should be at least 5 mm in order to minimize complications.

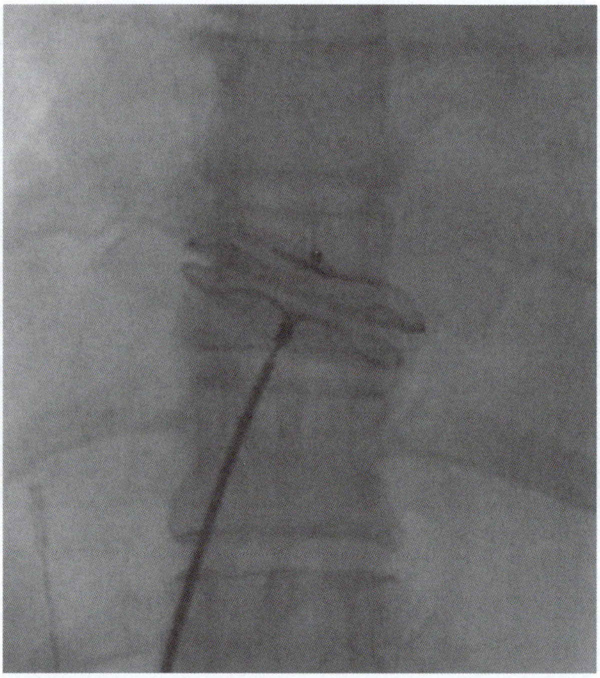

FIGURE 10.6 Once both disks are out from the guiding catheter, they assume their original shape and close on the defect.

COMPLICATIONS OF SECUNDUM ATRIAL SEPTAL DEFECT

If ASD escapes detection in childhood, in later life it may surface because of a complication. The most dreaded complication of these defects is the development of increased pulmonary vascular resistance and pulmonary hypertension. This complication can be progressive to the point of shunt reversal and the development of cyanosis. ASD, ventricular septal defect, and patent ductus arteriosus are the three congenital abnormalities that most commonly result in shunt reversal. The presence of one of these defects, a reversed shunt and cyanosis, forms the components of Eisenmenger syndrome.

Actually, Eisenmenger in 1897 first described the syndrome of the presence of a shunt, reversed flow, and cyanosis in an individual with a ventricular septal defect. Currently, this terminology is used for any shunt that results in increased pulmonary vascular resistance and shunt reversal with cyanosis.[6,7]

In addition to pulmonary hypertension, chronic volume overload of the right atrium and ventricle can lead to dilated dysfunctional chambers, right heart failure, ascites, and atrial fibrillation. In this setting, the presence of right heart failure,ascites and incomplete right bundle-branch block are clues to the diagnosis. Echocardiography will usually solve the problem.

SECTION 4

VENTRICULAR SEPTAL DEFECT

Congenital ventricular septal defect comes in many forms including muscular defects, inflow defects, and outflow defects both infracristal and supracristal. Defects in the inflow area of the right ventricle are very close to the tricuspid valve and the perimembranous area of the ventricles. The septal leaflet of the tricuspid valve often has its origin in the middle of the membranous portion of the interventricular septum and poses options for shunting to take place. Below the tricuspid valve, the shunt is to the right ventricle, and above the septal leaflet, it is directed to the right atrium (Gerbode defect). Muscular defects can be of various locations and can be multiple often orienting around the moderator band.

Other defects in the direction of the right and left ventricular outflow tracts may be infracristal or supracristal. The infracristal defects are identified as their jets relate to the aortic valve and are located at the 9 o'clock region or more toward the body of the right ventricle. The supracristal defects are high up in the interventricular septum and have a 12 o'clock orientation as related to the aorta in cross section and lie under the right cusp of the aortic valve. These defects are notorious for resulting in poor support of the right coronary cusp of the aortic valve and can cause aortic regurgitation of various degrees. Repair of this defect often requires intervention of one type or another on the aortic valve. The resulting aortic regurgitation may change in an abrupt fashion, and for this reason, long-term follow-up is needed. These types of defects do not lend themselves to percutaneous interventions.[8,9]

In summary, congenital ventricular septal defects can be in several locations including the muscular portion of the septum, the perimembranous area (inflow area of the right ventricle), and the supracristal area (the outflow area). When located in the right ventricular outflow area, they can interfere with the support of the right cusp of the aortic valve. The outflow tract ventricular septal defects can be problematic and be associated with prolapse of the right cusp and aortic regurgitation. These latter types of defects often require follow-up looking for evidence of aortic regurgitation.

Some of these defects are shown in Figures 10.7 and 10.8.

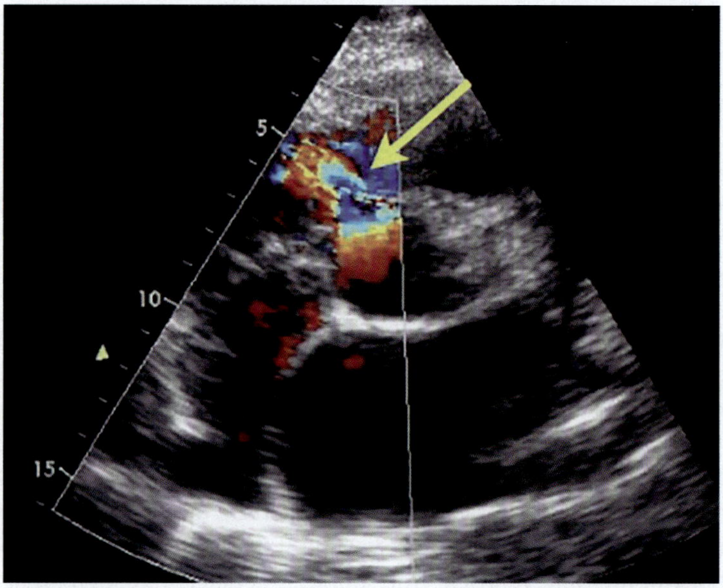

FIGURE 10.7 In the high cross-sectional view with the left ventricular outflow tract in the middle of the picture, the jet across the VSD is located at the 10 o'clock position. This location is characteristic of an "inflow VSD."

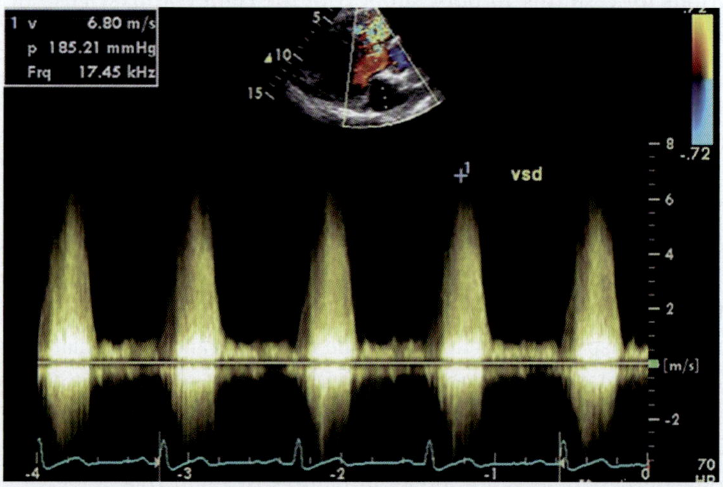

FIGURE 10.8 The vigorous jet is sampled with continuous wave Doppler and the jet has a velocity in the 6.8 m/s range. This calculated number can be subtracted from the systemic blood pressure, and an estimate of right ventricular systolic pressure can be obtained—in this situation probably very low.

Figure 10.9 is a diagram of ventricular septal defects and their location relative to a cross section of the aortic valve.

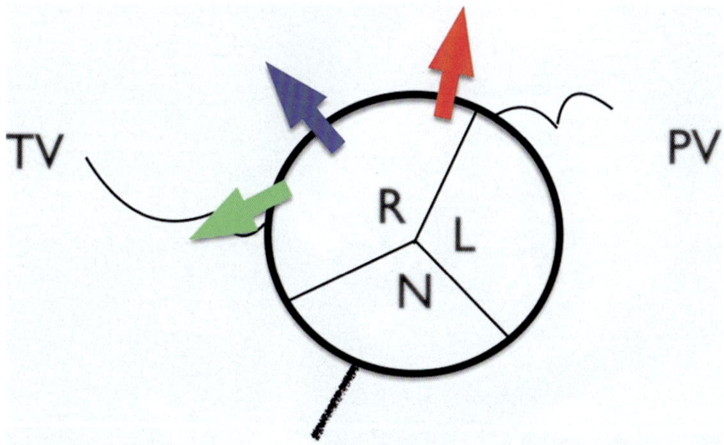

FIGURE 10.9 *Blue arrow*, perimembranous ventricular septal defects; *Red arrow*, supracristal ventricular septal defects; *Green arrow*, perimembranous defects and Gerbode-type defects; TV, tricuspid valve; PV, pulmonic valve.

SECTION 5

TETRALOGY OF FALLOT

Tetralogy of Fallot was first described in 1673 by Steno of Denmark, and Fallot coined the term tetralogy in 1888. The four famous abnormalities to include right ventricular hypertrophy, overriding aorta, ventricular septal defect, and right ventricular infundibular stenosis constitute the tetralogy.

The clinical syndrome of a cyanotic child that has learned to squat down for relief of cyanotic spells is well known to clinicians. The process of squatting increases systemic resistance and causes preferential shunting into the pulmonary circulation through the stenotic infundibulum of the right ventricle.

Surgery for this defect started with the Blalock-Taussig anastomosis in 1944 at John Hopkins Hospital. In the 1970s, a total repair of the defect was performed, and from there, infants have grown to adulthood. In present-day times, adult congenital clinics have these survivors returning for follow-up. Individuals with these repairs have their onset of issues. These individuals then have prosthetic valves and all the issues that they bring. Additionally, the right ventriculotomy is arrhythmogenic in itself.[10] Follow-up of these individuals with repaired tetralogy of Fallot is so important that guidelines have been set as recently at 2014.[11]

Occasionally, an adult will appear in our clinics that has uncorrected tetralogy of Fallot. An example of this is shown in Figures 10.10 and 10.11.

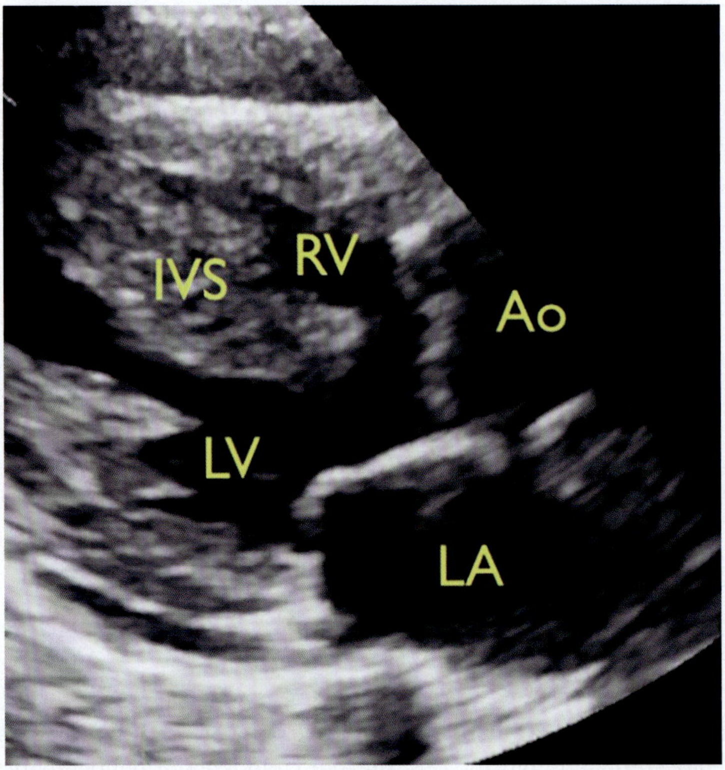

FIGURE 10.10 Still frame of the LV during late diastole showing the aorta overriding the interventricular septum. Ao, aorta; RV, right ventricle; LV, left ventricle; IVS, interventricular septum; LA, left atrium.

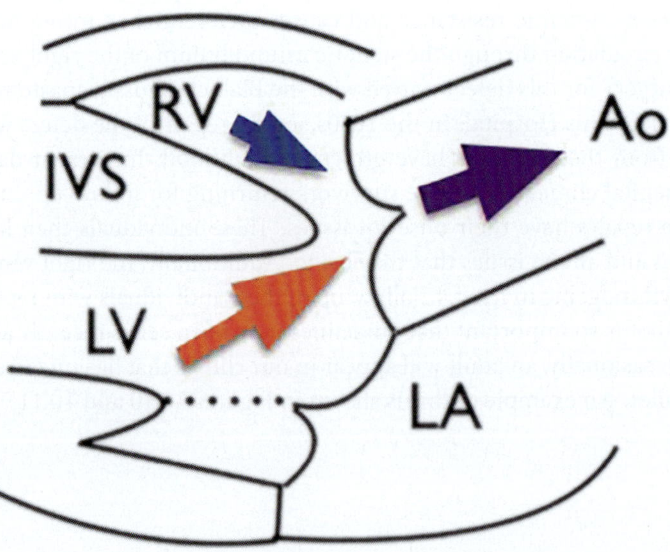

FIGURE 10.11 Diagram of the IV septum overriding the ascending aorta offering opportunity for outflow opportunity for flow into the aorta or the pulmonary circulation (which has high resistance because of infundibular stenosis). *Blue arrow* indicates unsaturated blood and *red arrow* indicates oxygenated blood. Ao, aorta; RV, right ventricle; LV, left ventricle; IVS, interventricular septum; LA, left atrium.

SECTION 6

PATENT DUCTUS ARTERIOSUS

Patent ductus arteriosus is a common congenital abnormality in newborns and in this setting lends itself to multiple interventions. In the older person, it is a rare abnormality. It is feared as a diagnosis because of the complication of pulmonary hypertension. In the adult, if pulmonary hypertension develops, it causes the classic right-to-left shunt into the aorta and causes differential clubbing and cyanosis of the lower extremities and not of the upper.

If a loud continuous murmur is present, that implies that there is a gradient between the aorta and pulmonary artery and severe pulmonary hypertension is not present. When a shunt is present from the aorta to pulmonary artery, this puts an extra load on the left ventricle and it becomes dilated from volume overload.

Echocardiography in the adult requires searching for this abnormality in high cross-sectional views that identify the bifurcation of the pulmonary artery. Flow into the pulmonary artery comes anterior from the aorta in the region of the ligamentum arteriosum and creates reversed flow in the pulmonary artery in diastole. If gradients are sufficient, shunting will continue throughout the cardiac cycle. If significant pulmonary hypertension is present, there will be reversed shunting and Eisenmenger physiology will develop. Therefore, a loud murmur is a good sign and no murmur is not.[9,12,13]

An example of an individual with a patent ductus arteriosus is shown in Figures 10.12 and 10.13.

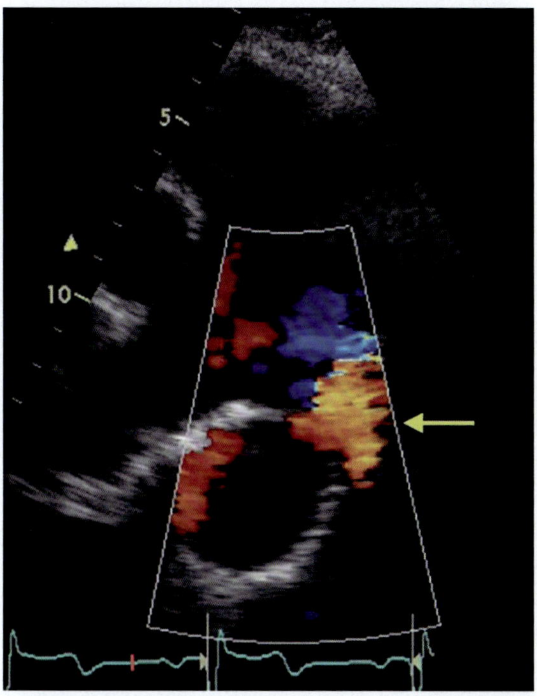

FIGURE 10.12 A very large pulmonary artery is demonstrated with flow in diastole into the pulmonary artery from the aorta (the red flow indicated by the *yellow arrow*), and in systole, the flow reverses and goes into the aorta and wraps around the aorta. This implies that the systolic pressures in the pulmonary artery exceeds that in the aorta and results in reversal of flow, whereas in diastole, the aortic pressure exceeds that in the pulmonary artery and the flow is reversed. Variations in the peripheral resistance in each of these circulations dictate the direction of flow. At the bedside, this patient had cyanotic toes and not so much fingers, and in addition, clubbing of the toes was present without the fingers being clubbed. This is a classic bedside finding in patent ductus with Eisenmenger physiology.

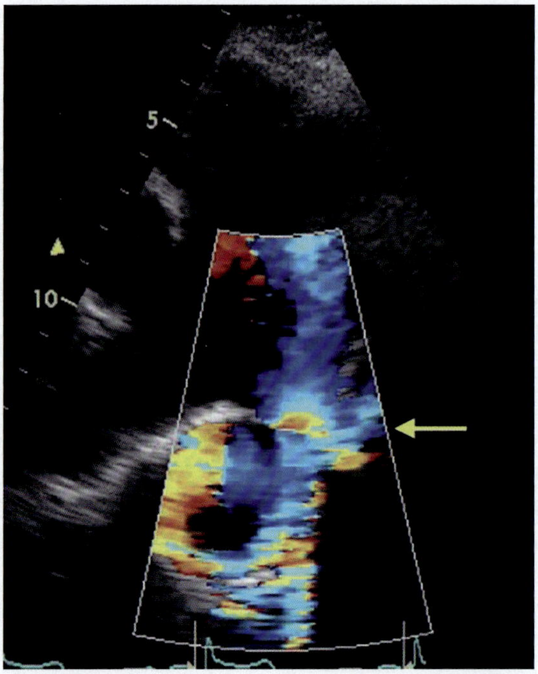

FIGURE 10.13 Systolic frame showing PISA forming in the pulmonary artery (*yellow arrow*) and the jet extending into the aorta at the ligamentum arteriosus causing some degree of cyanosis and resulting in differential cyanosis in the toes vs the fingers.

EISENMENGER PHYSIOLOGY AND RIGHT VENTRICULAR HYPERTROPHY ON ELECTROCARDIOGRAM

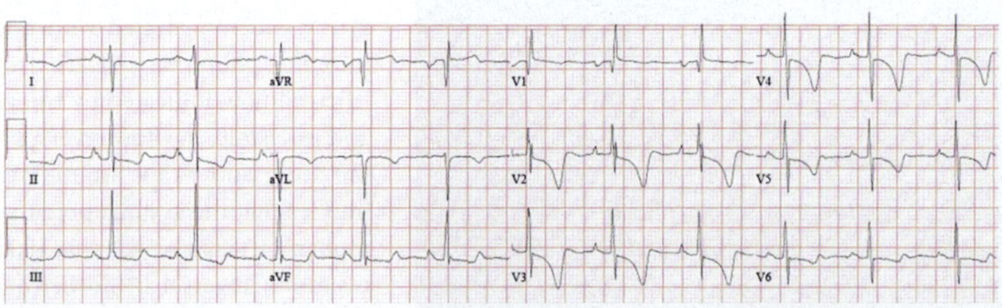

FIGURE 10.14

The initial EKG in the condition of patent ductus arteriosus shows left atrial enlargement and left ventricular enlargement. The physiolory is such that the left ventricle is doing systemic work in addition to supporting the circuit through the ductus and back through the pulmonary circulation. Once the pulmonary vascular resistance increases, the pulmonary artery pressure becomes higher or even systemic and the right ventricle becomes hypertrophied. At this point right ventricular hypertrophy makes itself manifest on the EKG as is noted in the above patient.

The electrocardiogram (Fig. 10.14) shows right atrial abnormality with a tall first portion of the P wave in lead II and a rightward axis of about 110° and a "qR" pattern in lead V1. Associated are the T-wave changes with a T vector pointing toward aVR. The T vector is pointed away from the right ventricle and suggests "right ventricular strain pattern" associated with the elevated right-sided pressures to systemic levels. Many times, this EKG was read as showing "ischemia" implying that the left ventricle is ischemic—it is the right ventricle that is responsible for these changes.

SECTION 7

EBSTEIN ANOMALY

Ebstein anomaly of the tricuspid valve is one of the most studied abnormalities in congenital heart disease. The classic presentation in a newborn with a large silhouette is difficulty breathing in the first few days of life that improves in a short time. Once the pulmonary vascular resistance decreases after the first 5 days or so the burden on the right ventricle is lessened and clinical improvement occurs. At this point the clinical situation may be tolerated for many years depending on the degree of abnormality.

In adults with this abnormality, there is not much to hear with the stethoscope; however, on occasion, a large mobile downwardly displaced anterior tricuspid leaflet may scrap against the anterior wall of the RV and cause a scratchy systolic sound, or it may "pop" like a sail upon close and cause an early systolic sound.

Couple the large cardiac silhouette with an electrocardiogram that has the largest P waves ever (save tricuspid atresia) and "splintered QRS" complexes and an "atypical" RBBB pattern, and the diagnosis is made. In a few individuals with this abnormality, ventricular preexcitation will be present.

The echocardiogram defines the abnormality showing the downwardly displaced tricuspid valve with the index as mentioned below making the diagnosis. The natural history depends on the degree of tricuspid valve regurgitation and any of the many associated abnormalities such as ASD.[14]

An example of Ebstein abnormality is shown in Figure 10.15.

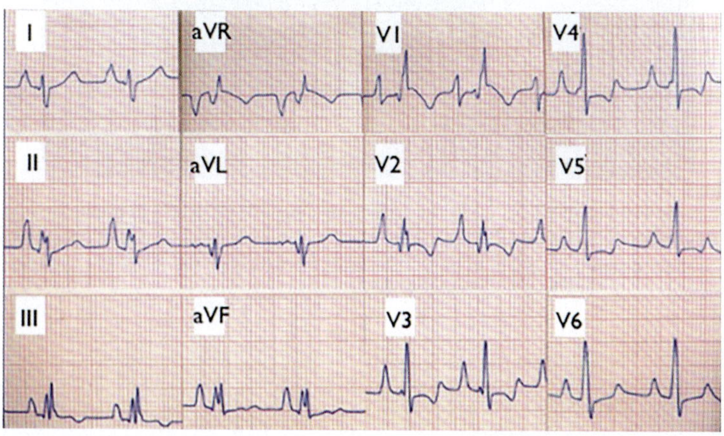

FIGURE 10.15 Large P waves especially in lead II and unusual right bundle-branch block exhibiting a bizarre "splintered" configuration in the precordial leads.

Ebstein anomaly of the tricuspid valve consists of a downward displacement and hypoplasia of the septal leaflet of the tricuspid valve, hypoplasia of the posterior leaflet, and a very large prominent fenestrated anterior leaflet that has various degrees of tethering. This large leaflet may be very mobile and flail open and closed. Sometimes, when it closes, it causes a loud sound that is called a "sail" sound. The degree of downward displacement, the fenestrations, and the degree of tethering of the large leaflet are related to its insufficiency and the degree of tricuspid regurgitation. Downward displacement into the right ventricle of the septal leaflet of the tricuspid valve relative to the mitral annulus of 8 mm/m^2 or greater defines this anomaly. A portion of the ventricle by virtue of the tricuspid valve being downwardly displaced becomes "atrialized." Often, the tricuspid regurgitation is severe and results in a very large right atrium and very large P waves on ECG.

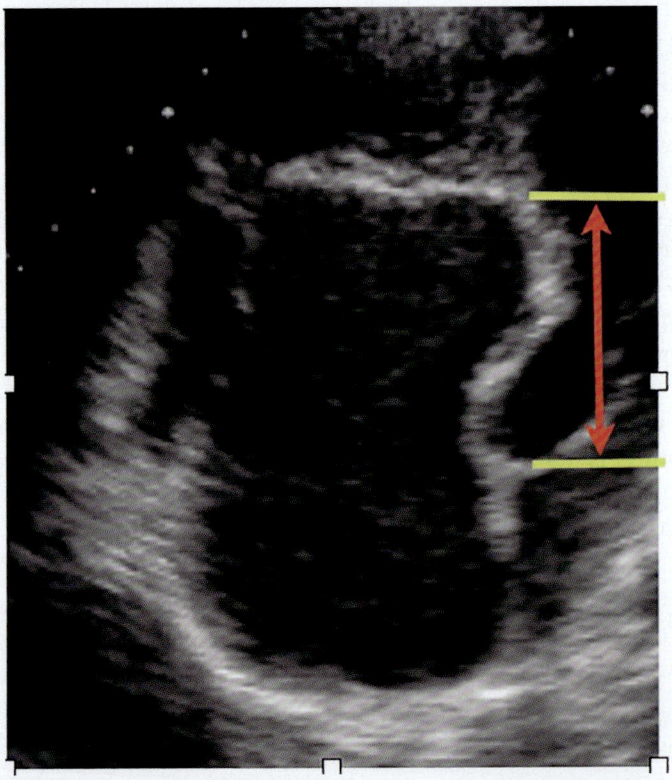

FIGURE 10.16 In Ebstein anomaly, one of the criteria for diagnosis especially in milder cases is that the distance from the mitral to the tricuspid valve insertions into the septum in the A4C view is 0.8 cm/m^2 or greater. In this example, the total distance is 4.8 cm, so those criteria are far exceeded. The *yellow lines* indicate the tricuspid leaflet insertion and the mitral leaflet insertion with the *red arrow* indicating the distance between.

SECTION 8

ANOMALOUS LEFT CORONARY ARTERY FROM THE PULMONARY ARTERY (ALCAPA)

Rarely, a newborn develops shortness of breath while feeding and the mother notes something is wrong. This can be a presenting symptom of anomalous left coronary arriving from the pulmonary artery. Left ventricular dysfunction due to ischemia or infarction of the left coronary territory results from steal of blood from this territory. The heart dilates, and pulmonary edema can result. This syndrome to include the heart failure symptoms and the EKG changes of anterior myocardial infarction was first described by Bland, White, and Garland and bears their name.[15]

Survival to adulthood can occur without major infarction or heart failure. Sometimes these individuals present later in life with dilated hearts and mitral regurgitation or even ventricular arrhythmias. When diagnosed early enough, surgical techniques allow connection of the left coronary artery to the aorta and reestablished flow in the appropriate direction down the left coronary.

Later in life, a well-developed fistulous connection develops and creates a left-to-right shunt and produces a continuous murmur over the precordium. The clinical situation, the electrocardiogram, the echocardiogram, the coronary arteriography, and the computerized tomographic angiography (CTA) each have diagnostic clues to the correct diagnosis.

Echocardiography plays a role in the diagnosis of anomalous coronary artery. Identification of the origin of each coronary is an important part of evaluation of the newborn in distress and the adult with a question of an anomaly. These can be established by echocardiography and lead to the correct diagnosis. In the case of ALCAPA, not only can the abnormally large right coronary be identified but the flow disturbance in the pulmonary artery can establish the presence of a fistulous connection.

In Figures 10.17 and 10.18, echocardiography, coronary arteriography, and CTA are illustrated.

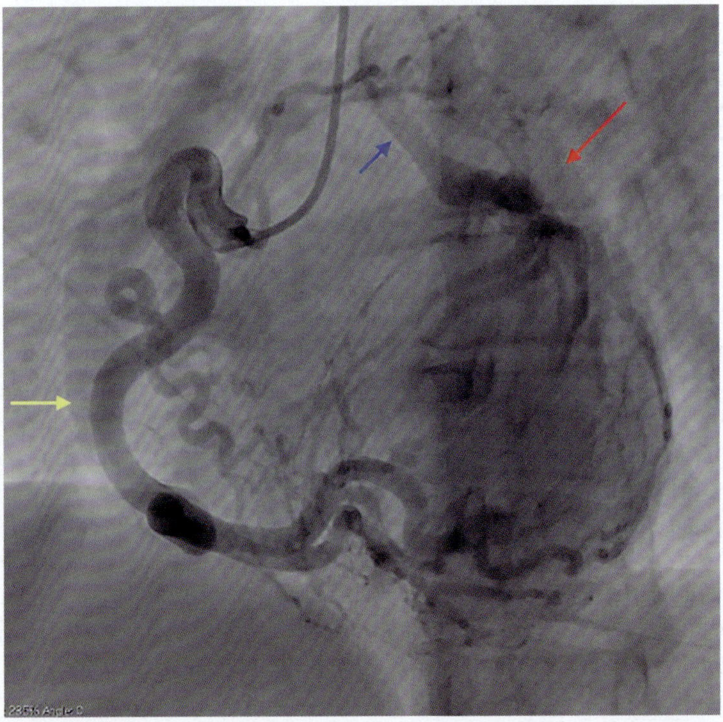

FIGURE 10.17 The multipurpose catheter has been rotated clockwise, and a very large right coronary (*yellow arrow*) has been engaged and contrast has been injected. Flow rushes down this large artery and courses through collaterals to the left system (*red arrow*), which in turn empties into the pulmonary artery (*blue arrow*). The native left artery never connects with the left coronary sinus but comes very close. This anatomy allows surgical correction by closing the fistulous connection with the pulmonary artery and connecting the left main to the aorta.

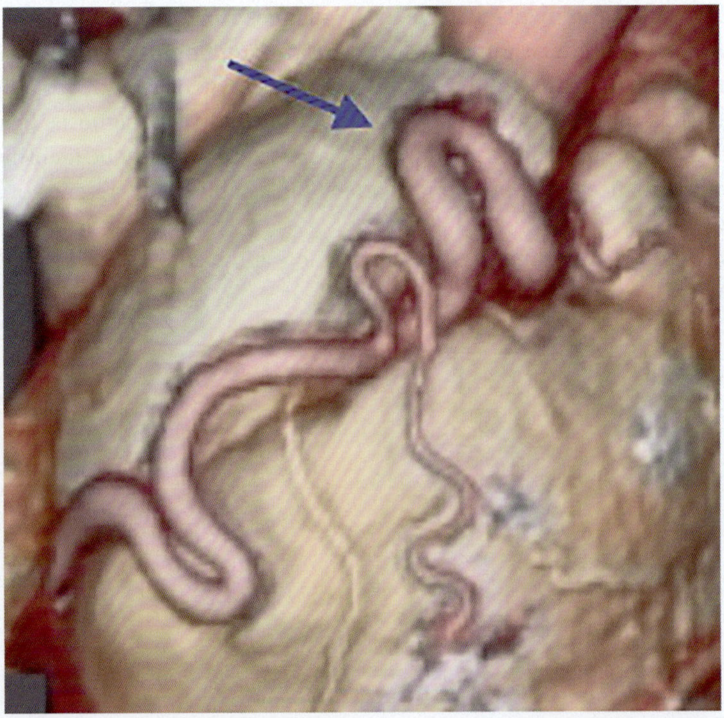

FIGURE 10.18 Close-up view of the large tortuous right coronary artery on the epicardial surface. It enlarges and becomes tortuous because of excessive flow (*blue arrow*).

REFERENCES

1. Schwerzmann CS. Recreational scuba diving, patent foramen oval and their associated risks. *Swiss Med Wkly.* 2001;131:365-374.
2. Messe SR, Silverman IE, Kizer JR, et al. Practice parameter: recurrent stroke with patent foramen oval and atrial septal aneurysm. *Neurology.* 2004;62:1042-1050.
3. Butera G, Giodi-Aoccai GGL, Carminati M, et al. Systemic review and meta-analysis of currently available clinical evidence on migraine and patent foramen oval percutaneous closure: much ado about nothing? *Catheter Cardiovasc Interv.* 2010;75:494-504.
4. Dowson A, Mullen MJ, Peatfield R, et al. Migraine intervention with STARFlex technology (MIST) trial: a prospective, multicenter, double-blind, sham-controlled trial to evaluate the effectiveness of patent foramen oval closure with STARFlex septal repair implant to resolve refractory migraine headache. *Circulation.* 2008;117:1397-1404.
5. Webb G, Gatzoulis MA. Atrial septal defects in the adult. Recent progress and overview. *Circulation.* 2006;114:1645-1653.
6. Eisenmenger V. Die angeboren defect der Kammer scheidewand des Herzenes. *Z Klin Med.* 1897;32(suppl):1.
7. Wood P. Pulmonary hypertension. *Br Med Bull.* 1952;8:348-353.
8. Ammash NM, Warnes CA. Ventricular septal defects in adults. *Ann Intern Med.* 2001;135:812-824.
9. Warnes CA, Williams RG, Bashore TM, et al. ACC/AHA 2008 guidelines for the management of adults with congenital heart disease: executive summary. *Circulation.* 2008;118:2395-2451.
10. Neill CA, Clark EB. Tetralogy of Fallot. The first 300 years. *Tex Heart Inst J.* 1994;21(4):272-279.
11. Valente AM, Cook A, Festa P, et al. Multimodality imaging guidelines for patients with repaired tetralogy of Fallot: a report from the American Society of echocardiography developed in collaboration with the Society for Cardiovascular Magnetic Resonance and the Society for Pediatric Radiology. *J Am Soc Echocardiogr.* 2014;27:111-141.
12. Schneider DJ, Moore JW. Patent ductus arteriosus. *Circulation.* 2006;114:1873-1882.
13. Wang JK, Liau CA, Huang JJ, et al. Transcatheter closure of patent ductus artists using Gianturco coils in adolescents and adults. *Catheter Cardiovasc Interv.* 2002;55:513-518.
14. Jost CHA, Connolly HM, Detrain JA, Edwards WD, Danielson GK. Ebstein's anomaly. *Circulation.* 2007;115:277-285.
15. Bland EF, White PD, Garland J. Congenital anomalies of the coronary arteries: a report of an unusual case associated with cardiac hypertrophy. *Am Heart J.* 1933;8:787-801.

11

Multimodality Imaging and Structural Heart Interventions

SECTION 1

ECHOCARDIOGRAPHY IN STRUCTURAL HEART DISEASE

Recent advances in technology have led to the development of new devices and procedures that have greatly improved our ability to effectively treat structural heart abnormalities. Implementation of these procedures has been effective alternative treatment to surgery for several congenital and acquired diseases. The advent of transcatheter valve implantation techniques constitutes one of the main breakthroughs of the last decade. Such development and implementation are mostly related to continuous progress in cardiac imaging including echocardiography. Indeed, multimodality cardiac imaging has become essential for providing accurate patient selection, monitoring interventional procedures, and optimizing the success rate and minimizing complications. In this chapter, we present examples that demonstrate the critical importance of the use of echocardiography and multimodality imaging for the initial planning, intraoperative monitoring, and assessing of the results acutely and at follow-up of patients undergoing common structural heart and valve therapeutic interventions.

SECTION 2

PARAVALVULAR LEAKS

Prosthetic valves of any type are subject to unintended blood flow around the perimeter of the valve at the valve-tissue interface termed paravalvular leak. This is more common when the valve has been replaced a second time. Paravalvular leaks can be difficult to identify clinically. They are often difficult to auscultate and may manifest as unexplained heart failure or hemolysis.

For echocardiographic interrogation of an aortic prosthesis, views from the apex and parasternal views offer an evaluation of the left ventricular outflow tract (LVOT) and identification of regurgitant paravalvular jets. Echocardiographic assessment of mitral valve paravalvular leak is often more difficult due to acoustic shadowing from the prosthesis. Indirect measures such as pulmonary vein reversal and pulse and continuous Doppler interrogation of the annular areas can be helpful. Transesophageal echocardiogram (TEE) is often needed to view the prosthesis from the atrial perspective to make the diagnosis. In the clinical setting of a mitral prosthetic valve, and hemolysis or unexplained heart failure, TEE is recommended to further evaluate the valve characteristics and surrounding areas.

Current structural heart techniques allow for mitral and aortic paravalvular leaks to be treated with vascular occlusion devices. Once the leak is identified and localized, echocardiographic guidance in the cardiac catheterization laboratory is needed to confirm wire placement through the defect and successful placement of the closure device. Assessing relationships between prosthetic valve leaflets and devices is also aided by two- and three-dimensional echocardiography.[1]

AORTIC PARAVALVULAR LEAKS

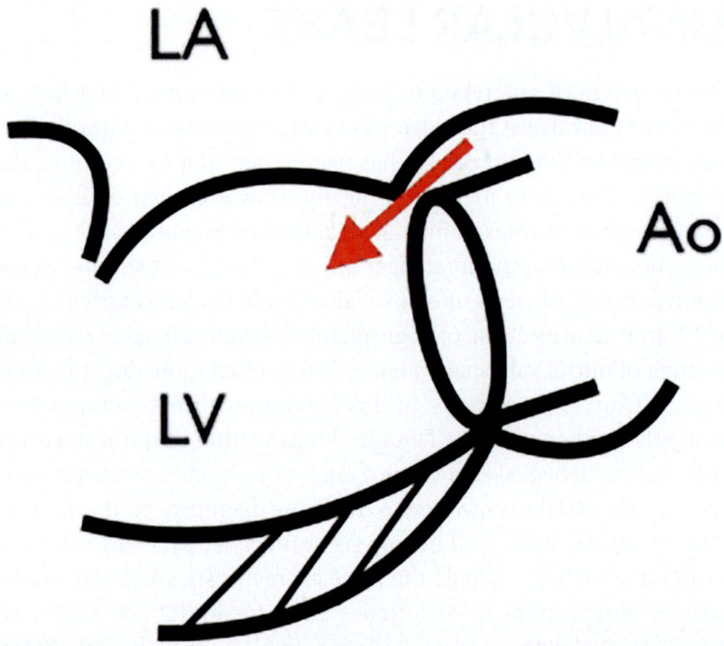

FIGURE 11.1 Aortic paravalvular leaks are easily identified by transthoracic echocardiography. The location can usually be identified by transthoracic echo; however, if this is not entirely clear, transesophageal echo can add more information. Fluoroscopic images can also localize the leak, but the combination of all of these modalities makes catheter and wire approaches much easier and quicker. The more information that is obtained in the planning stages, the easier and more efficient the procedure. Preprocedural preparation by the structural team and imaging team is important. Imaging allows for targets to be identified and quickly approached at the time of the procedure. Ao, aorta; LA, left atrium; LV, left ventricle.

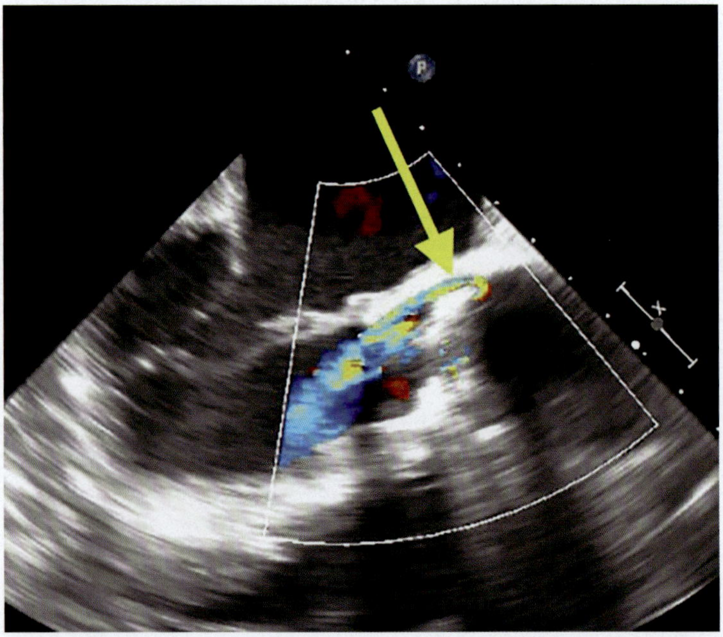

FIGURE 11.2 This image defines the aortic paravalvular leak to be on the posterior aspect of the valve and anterior to the anterior mitral valve leaflet. Color Doppler shows this jet (*yellow arrow*).

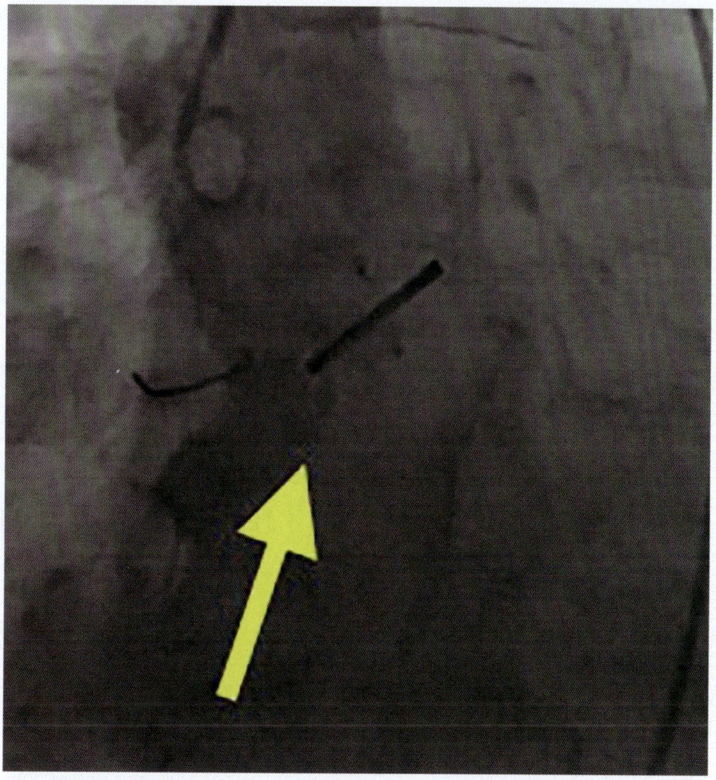

FIGURE 11.3 Angiogram demonstrates the leak from this ascending aortic infection using a pigtail catheter. The regurgitant jet is to the left of the valve ring in this frontal projection (*yellow arrow*).

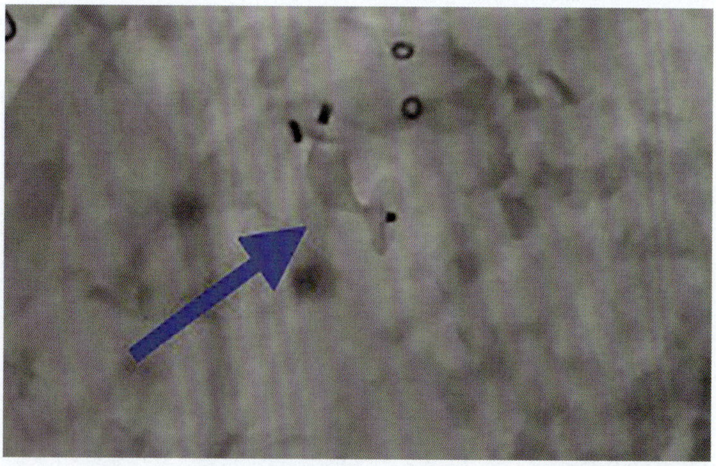

FIGURE 11.4 In another individual with a paravalvular leak, a small hourglass-shaped closure device (*blue arrow*) with its two end markers is seen across and closing a defect.

MITRAL PROSTHETIC VALVE PARAVALVULAR LEAK

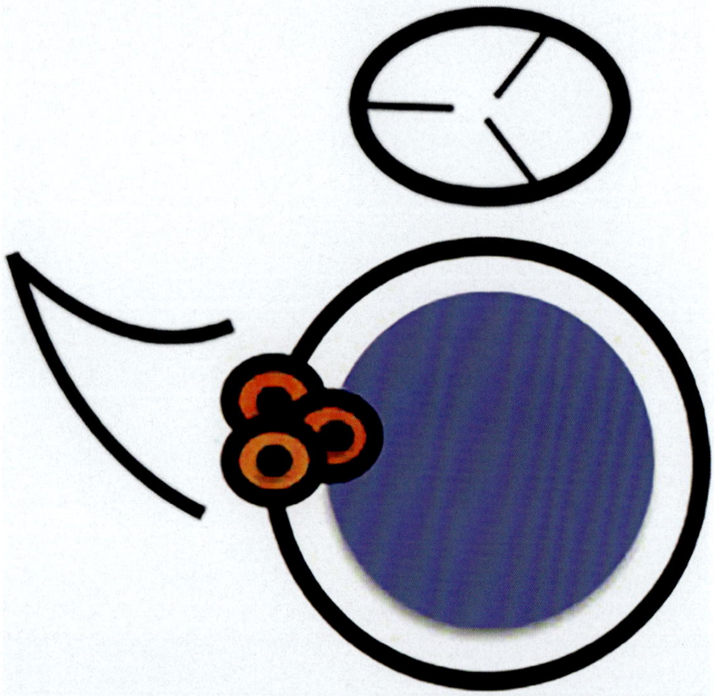

FIGURE 11.5 Mitral paravalvular leaks are more occult than aortic paravalvular leaks. They hide behind the acoustic shadows of the prosthetic valve. They may manifest themselves as hemolysis or heart failure. Transesophageal views from the atrium allow the mitral valve to be viewed clearly and makes leaks around valve easily identified. From this view acoustic shadowing is avoided. Usually they are located close to the left atrial appendage; however, the second most common location is medially close to the interatrial septum and aorta. This latter location requires special effort to cross the septum and loop around back toward the aortic valve and interatrial septum to wire the lesion and place vascular plugs. The illustration here is one located in the typical location near the LAA.

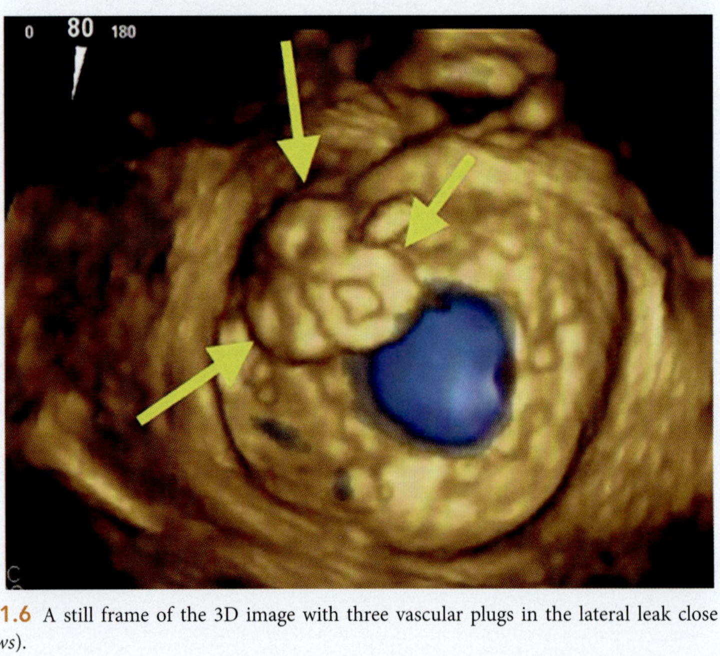

FIGURE 11.6 A still frame of the 3D image with three vascular plugs in the lateral leak close to the LAA (*yellow arrows*).

SECTION 3

TRANSCAVAL TRANSAORTIC VALVE REPLACEMENT

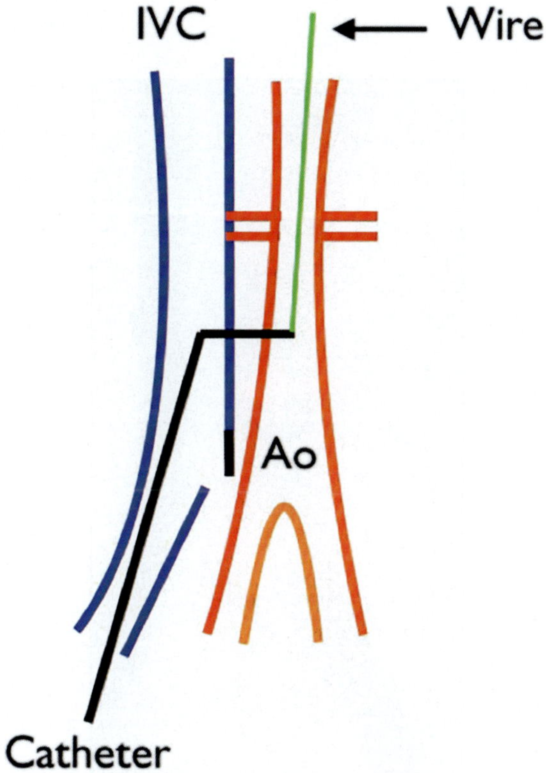

FIGURE 11.7 Stick diagram of a transcaval TAVR. Vena cava on the left side of the diagram (IVC) and aorta (Ao) on the right. A right angled catheter is advanced up the IVC and an activated wire (*green line*) is advanced through the wall of the IVC into the aorta. The wire is captured from the aorta by a snare catheter and pushed up the aorta. Larger catheters can follow and the TAVR can be deployed via this route. Closure is obtained by an Amplatzer closure device.

Vascular access for transaortic valve replacement (TAVR) remains challenging in individuals with peripheral arterial disease particularly in individuals with small, calcified, and tortuous iliofemoral vessels. Alternative approaches have included the transaortic approach through a small upper midsternotomy incision, transapical approach with access through a small left thoracotomy, and the transcarotid approach through the right carotid. Recently, there has been success with the transcaval approach. In this approach, a region approximately midway between the renal and the aortic bifurcation is identified for crossing. The aorta and inferior vena cava are relatively close together in this location. In choosing this location, one has to consider the position of the closure device making sure that it does not interfere with the adjacent vascular branches. Using an angled catheter and a Bovie wire, one can burn from the inferior vena cava to the aorta. The wire can be advanced into the aorta, snared, and advanced up to the descending thoracic aorta, and then a catheter can follow. Wire exchanges can be done for a stiffer wire, and the delivery catheter system can be advanced up the vena cava, across to the aorta, and up to the ascending aorta for deployment. Upon deployment and then withdrawal of the catheter, the connection between the aorta and vena cava can be closed with a vascular occlusion device. Location of the closure device such that the disks do not interfere with adjacent major arterial branches is important. Thus far, the bleeding risk has been low and the success rate has been high.[2]

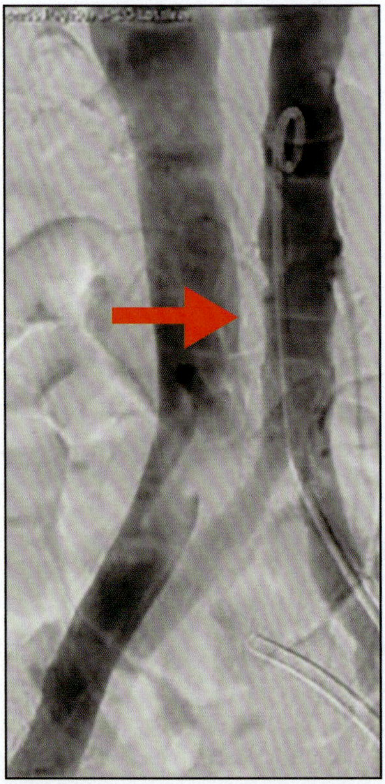

FIGURE 11.8 A stop frame of this image is analyzed for choosing the appropriate location for crossing from the vena cava to the aorta. This is usually midway between the renal and aortic bifurcation. The *red arrow* indicates the approximate location.

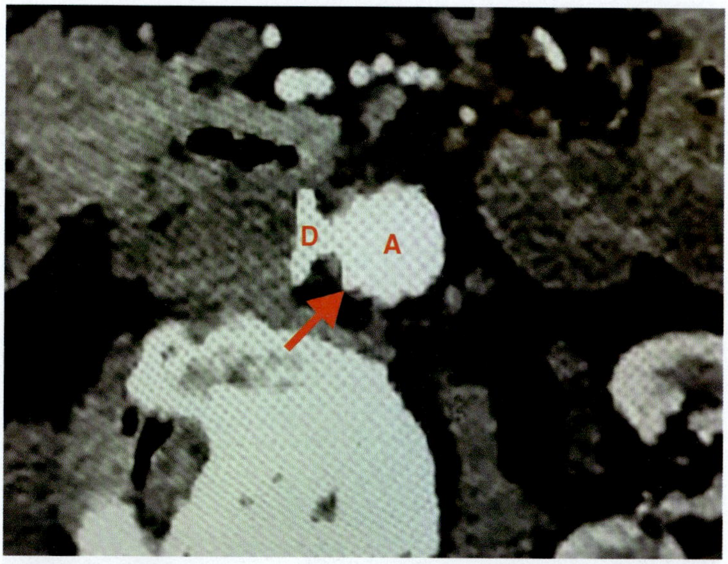

FIGURE 11.9 Upon completion of the valve deployment, an appropriately sized vascular occlusion device is placed across the defect from the aorta to the vena cava. In this example, contrast is present in the aorta and there is no leak to the vena cava. Red A, aorta; red D, vena cava side of the device. *Red arrow* indicates the aortic side of the closure device.

SECTION 4

ASSESSMENT OF THE SIZE OF THE LEFT VENTRICULAR OUTFLOW TRACT

The LVOT as viewed from the parasternal long axis view has a dimension that in some of our equations is assumed to be a circle in cross section. This assumption when factored into the equation for the area of a circle gives one a cross-sectional area that can be used for sizing of a TAVR. This turns out not to be entirely true. Early on in the experience with TAVR, special attention was paid to paravalvular leaks, and their significance and the valve sizing process was questioned. The use of three-dimensional echo and 3D reconstruction of CT revealed that the LVOT was actually elliptical in shape and the dimensions and the overall cross-sectional areas could impact the sizing process for TAVR.

In addition to sizing of the LVOT, it is important to know the relationships of the coronaries to the eventual position of the TAVR. The height of the coronaries from annulus is critical in prevention of interference of the valve with the coronary ostia. A dimension of 6 mm or less can compromise the ostia and alters the type and size of the valve to be chosen. These dimensions can be obtained by echocardiography and CT measurements.

At the present time, this process is used commonly for accurate sizing of TAVR procedures, and improvement of results and fewer paravalvular leaks occur. Examples of this measuring are noted in the sections that follow.

Cardiac Q Lab measurement of LVOT area and not ST junction + coronary height are shown in Figure 11-10.

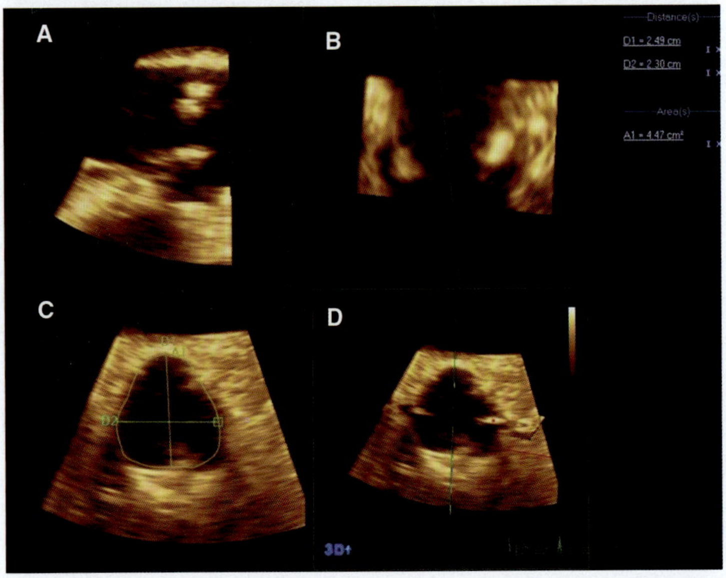

FIGURE 11.10 Multiplanar reconstruction (MPR) of the LVOT and aortic annulus is shown above. MPR allows for assessment of the full 3D volume in separate planes to obtain the most accurate measurement of the aortic annulus. **A** is the long axis plane of the left ventricular outflow tract. **B** is the orthogonal plane through the center of the LVOT. **C** is the short axis of the aortic annulus. Due to the irregular shape, the diameter is measured in at least two places (D1 and D2) and the annular area is traced. In the above example, an annular area of 4.47 cm^2 would correlate to a 26-mm Edwards SAPIEN 3 transcatheter heart valve. **D** is the full 3D volume set in which all planes are represented and is used as a reference.

SECTION 5

CMRI AND QUANTITATION OF MITRAL REGURGITATION

PRINCIPLES OF CARDIAC MAGNETIC RESONANCE FOR IMAGING AND QUANTIFICATION OF REGURGITANT LESIONS

Imaging

- CMR is the gold standard for ventricular volumetric quantification and ejection fraction measurements.
- CMR is not limited by acoustic windows or body habitus.
- The anatomy of the mitral valve apparatus can be investigated in any imaging plane, which offers a good opportunity for determination of etiology.

Quantification

- Regurgitant volume can be quantified without specific hemodynamic assumptions or consideration of regurgitant jet direction.
- Phase contrast imaging derives flow velocity from the entire orifice without assumptions of flat transorifice flow or specific geometric shape.
- CMR identifies myocardial fibrosis or scar that can aid in determination in the etiology of any associated myopathic process and provides important prognostic information.

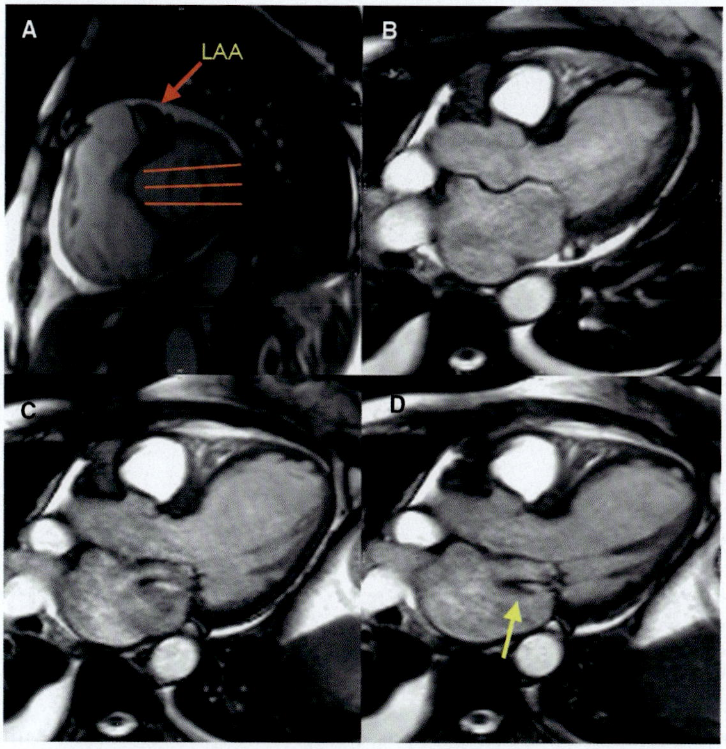

FIGURE 11.11 In the magnetic imaging above, specific cine imaging planes across the various scallops of the mitral valve have been selected. Using the short axis image **(A)**, planes are selected (*red lines*) from lateral to medial that interrogate the A1-P1 **(B)** and the A3-P3 coaptations **(C)**. The regurgitant jet is more prominent in the A3-P3 image **(D)** suggesting a more medial origin of the mitral regurgitation jet (*yellow arrow*).

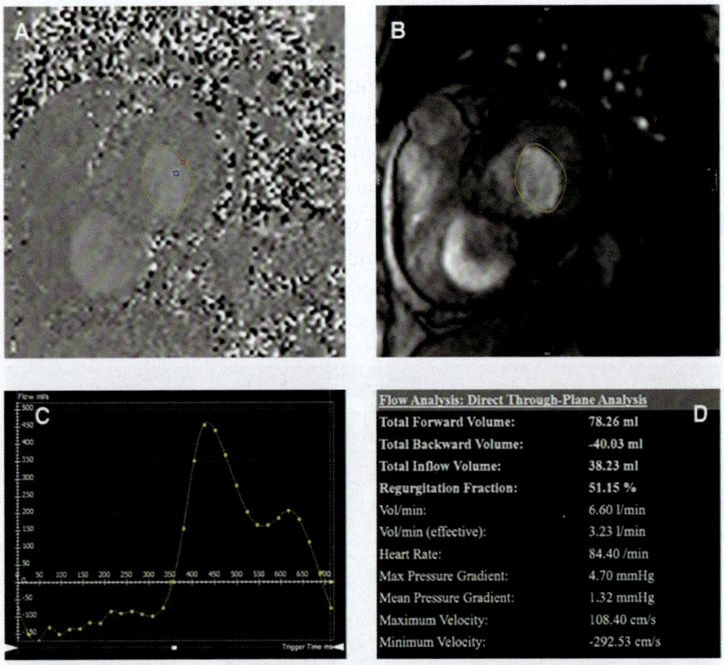

FIGURE 11.12 Direct method of assessing mitral regurgitation by through-plans phase contrast imaging of the mitral flow (**A**). Anatomical images of the mitral inflow scan (**B**). During the cardiac cycle, forward and backward flow can be directly measured. There is backward flow during systole and forward flow with a large E wave in diastole (**C**). Quantification of flow calculated a regurgitant volume of 40 mL and regurgitant fraction of 51% (**D**).

SECTION 6

COMPUTERIZED TOMOGRAPHY AND DIMENSIONAL ASSESSMENT FOR TAVR

Both CT and CMRI are useful in assessing candidates for TAVR. Annular measurements, sinotubular junctional measurements, and assessment of the annulus to the origin of the coronaries are all possible with these modalities. CT is used most commonly. Valve calcification and the calcium burden can easily be assessed.

These modalities along with echocardiography all are part of the planning process for TAVR and other structural heart procedures. These modalities are a moving target with advances that will continue to move this arena forward in the future.

CROSS-SECTIONAL AREA OF THE AORTIC ANNULUS ON CT AND LOCATION OF CORONARY ARTERIES

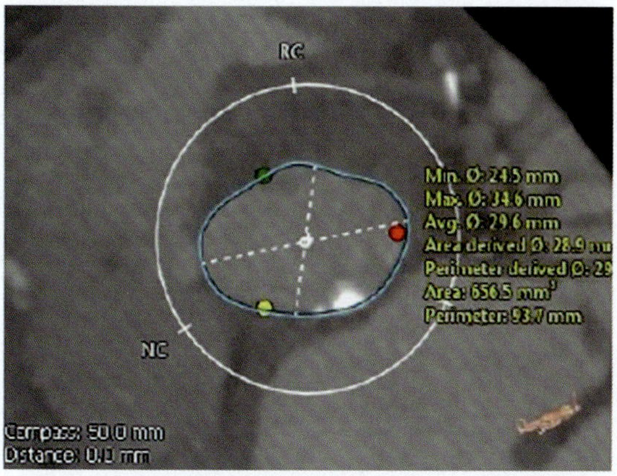

FIGURE 11.13 Measurement of the LVOT by CT allowing for a cross-sectional area and choosing of a valve size. An area of 656.5 mm^2 suggests that a 29-mm valve should be chosen. The three dots are markers for the three lowest points of the aortic valve cusps defining the annular plane.

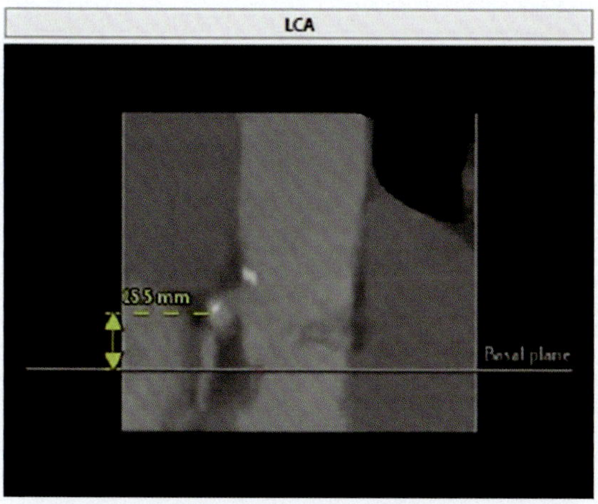

FIGURE 11.14 The lower edge of the left coronary artery in this view is 15.5 mm above the aortic annulus. This measurement allows avoiding a compromise of the coronary ostium by the upper portions of a percutaneous valve.

Multimodality Imaging and Structural Heart Interventions

REFERENCES

1. Ruiz CE, Jelin V, Kronzon I, et al. Clinical outcomes in patients undergoing percutaneous closure of periprosthetic paravalvular leaks. *J Am Coll Cardiol.* 2011;58:2210-2217.
2. Greenbaum AB, O'Neill WW, Paone G, et al. Cabal-Aortic access to allow transcatheter aortic valve replacement in otherwise ineligible patients: initial human experience. *J Am Coll Cardiol.* 2014;63:2795-2804.

INDEX

Note: Page numbers in *italics* denote figures, those followed by t indicate tables

N